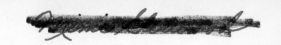

Proteins of the Nervous System

Editors

Diana Johnson Schneider

Neurosciences Research Program
Massachusetts Institute of Technology
Brookline, Mass.

Ruth Hogue Angeletti

Washington University School of Medicine
St. Louis, Missouri

Ralph A. Bradshaw

Washington University School of Medicine
St. Louis, Missouri

Alfonso Grasso

Laboratorio di Biologia Cellulare
Rome

Blake W. Moore

Washington University School of Medicine
St. Louis, Missouri

Raven Press • New York

Made in the United States of America

International Standard Book Number 0-911216-54-5
Library of Congress Catalog Card Number 73-79287

Preface

The field of neurochemistry has experienced considerable development in the last decade, primarily due to the development of new chemical and biological techniques and their application to the study of the nervous system. Notable among these are the newer separation methods for proteins, including cellulose ion-exchange chromatography and gel electrophoresis. Methods for the separation of membrane proteins on detergent gels and purification of receptor proteins by affinity chromatography have been particularly powerful tools for studying proteins of the nervous system. At the same time, there have been many recent developments in physical and chemical methods for studying protein structure and properties, thus allowing more sophisticated analyses of primary structure, three-dimensional conformation, and immunochemical properties.

One of the most exciting developments has been the availability of cloned tissue culture lines derived from various types of nervous system cells, such as gliomas, neuroblastomas and Schwannomas. These retain many of the characteristics of differentiated cells in the nervous system, including process formation, action potential propagation, transmitter synthesis, and the production of nervous system-specific proteins. There have also been developments in other methods of obtaining pure or enriched cell types for study, such as batch separation of neurons and glia and wet or dry dissection of single cells. Methods for subcellular fractionation to yield nerve-ending particles, synaptic vesicles, and, in particular, pure membranes such as myelin and synaptic membranes, have undergone major developments.

In view of the fact that the field of proteins in the nervous system has and continues to develop so rapidly, it was thought that it would be profitable to hold a conference on this subject and to publish the proceedings. The field was limited to work on proteins which, on the basis of current evidence, seem to have something to do with specific nervous system function but are not directly involved in enzymatic reactions, and was limited to those aspects where well-defined proteins are known or will undoubtedly be identified in the near future. Toward this end, the conference "Proteins of the Nervous System" was organized and convened at Cortona, Italy, from September 10 to 17, 1972. The chapters of this book are derived mainly from the lectures of the invited speakers with the comments of the participants interspersed where appropriate. It is hoped that the success of this conference will be passed on to the rest of the scientific community through the pages of this volume.

The organizing committee wishes to thank the Mayor of Cortona for his hospitality and friendly welcome. We would also like to thank Messrs. Favilli and Solfanelli of the Azienda Autonoma di Soggiorno e Turismo Cortona for their extensive assistance. The organizers gratefully acknowledge the use of Villa Passerini, which was provided through the courtesy of Professor Gilberto Bernardini of the Scuola Normale di Pisa, for the formal sessions of the conference. We would also like to thank the Scientific Affairs Division of the North Atlantic Treaty Organization who supplied the major economic support for the conference, and Eli Lilly-Italia s.p.a., Gruppo Lepetit s.p.a., Hoechst-Italia s.p.a. and Merck, Sharpe and Dohme-Italia s.p.a. for their generous donations.

Finally, we wish to recognize and acknowledge the enthusiasm and cooperativity of all the participants of the workshop, without which there would have been no exchange of ideas and thoughts which comprise the substance of this report.

D. Johnson Schneider
R. A. Hogue-Angeletti
R. A. Bradshaw
A. Grasso
B. W. Moore

Contents

Contributors

Pietro U. Angeletti, Laboratorio di Chimica Biologica, Istituto Superiore di Sanità, Rome, Italy.

Ruth Hogue Angeletti, Washington University School of Medicine, St. Louis, Missouri 63110, USA.

Samuel H. Barondes, University of California at San Diego, School of Medicine, La Jolla, California 92037, USA.

Ralph A. Bradshaw, Washington University School of Medicine, St. Louis, Missouri 63110, USA.

W. C. Breckenridge, Centre de Neurochimie du C.N.R.S. and Institut de Chimie Biologique, Faculté de Médecine, Université Louis Pasteur, Strasbourg, France.

Pietro Calissano, Laboratorio di Biologia Cellulare, via Romagnosi 18A, Rome, Italy 00196.

Edwin H. Eylar, Merck Institute for Therapeutic Research, Rahway, New Jersey 07065, USA.

Jordi Folch-Pi, Harvard Medical School, Boston, Massachusetts 02115, McLean Hospital, Belmont, Massachusetts 02178, USA.

William A. Frazier, Washington University School of Medicine, St. Louis, Missouri 63110, USA.

G. Gombos, Centre de Neurochimie du C.N.R.S. and Institut de Chimie Biologique, Faculté de Médecine, Université Louis Pasteur, Strasbourg, France.

Alfonso Grasso, Laboratorio di Biologia Cellulare, Rome, Italy.

Harvey R. Herschman, Department of Biological Chemistry and Laboratory of Nuclear Medicine, University of California at Los Angeles School of Medicine, California 90024, USA.

Bruce S. McEwen, Rockefeller University, New York, New York 10021, USA.

Blake W. Moore, Department of Psychiatry, Washington University School of Medicine, St. Louis, Missouri 63110, USA.

Walter J. Moore, Brain Research Group, Chemical Laboratory, Indiana University, Bloomington, Indiana 47401, USA.

Ian G. Morgan, Centre de Neurochimie, du C.N.R.S. and Institut de Chimie Biologique, Faculté de Médecine, Université Louis Pasteur, Strasbourg, France.

Diana Johnson Schneider, Neurosciences Research Program, Massachusetts Institute of Technology, Brookline, Massachusetts 02146, USA.

Michael L. Shelanski, Laboratory of Biochemical Genetics, National Heart and Lung Institute, National Institutes of Health, Bethesda, Maryland 20014, USA.

G. Vincendon, Centre de Neurochimie du C.N.R.S. and Institut de Chimie Biologique, Faculté de Médecine, Université Louis Pasteur, Strasbourg, France.

Victor P. Whittaker, Department of Biochemistry, University of Cambridge, Cambridge, England.

Proteins of the Nervous System
Raven Press, New York © 1973

Brain-Specific Proteins

Blake W. Moore

I. INTRODUCTION

The differentiation of any cell leads to the synthesis of certain proteins which are responsible for its specific functions. In the nervous system, this includes such functions as the conduction of action potentials, synaptic transmission, and the establishment of specific connections. Proteins similar in evolutionary history, structure, or other parameters may have different but related functions in different tissues. However, it is highly probable that the specific functions of the nervous system, and of neurons in particular, are to a large extent mediated by proteins which are unique to the nervous system, and are not found in other organs. The study of the biosynthetic control and developmental biology of such proteins is therefore of great importance when studying the relationship of proteins to functions in the nervous system.

There are several approaches that can be used to choose those proteins which are probably involved in specific nervous system functions. One approach is to select proteins which are obviously related to certain structures known to be important in the operation of the nervous system, such as the proteins of myelin, microtubules, synaptic membranes, or synaptic vesicles. Another is to study proteins involved in specific functions of the nervous system, such as metabolic pathways known to be of great importance for neural function, for example, neurotransmitter biosynthesis and degradation.

A third approach, one that has been taken by our laboratory, has been the systematic search for proteins which are both specific to the nervous system and found in the nervous systems of a wide range of species. This approach is based on the premise that a protein which has been conserved during evolution but is not required in any other tissue has an important function that is specific to the nervous system. Our laboratory has until recently concentrated on the soluble proteins of the nervous system, but we are now using this same approach to study neural membrane proteins.

1

II. METHODOLOGY

The first step in the detection of nervous system-specific, species-nonspecific proteins is the preparation of two-dimensional "protein maps" of the soluble proteins of the nervous system and other organs. These are prepared by first chromatographing the proteins on DEAE-cellulose, and then subjecting the fractions obtained by this procedure to gel electrophoresis (Moore and McGregor, 1965). The resulting protein patterns can be compared visually to determine if there are any proteins seen only in the nervous system. Those proteins which appear to be specific to the nervous system are then purified to homogeneity by means of standard purification procedures, using their position on the two-dimensional maps or on electrophoretic patterns alone as an assay.

Neither the two-dimensional map method nor polyacrylamide gel analyses are specific or sensitive enough to provide conclusive evidence that the purified protein is actually nervous system-specific. Our next step, therefore, was the development of a more sensitive and specific assay, namely the preparation and use of antiserum to the protein. Immunological methods such as complement fixation and radioimmunoassay are extremely sensitive and specific, and permit rigorous testing for specificity to the nervous system, as well as for cross-species testing for the presence and similarities of analogous proteins.

Once such a specific and sensitive assay method is available, it is possible to utilize many approaches that may eventually uncover the function of the protein, such as its localization to a specific cell type, its behavior during development, and its synthesis and regulation in tissue culture or cell-free protein synthetic systems.

This approach can best be illustrated with the S-100 and 14–3–2 proteins, which have been intensively studied by our laboratory and are undoubtedly both nervous system-specific and species-nonspecific. The most obvious difference between "protein maps" of brain and other tissues is the presence in brain of a large amount of material in the map region corresponding to small molecular weight acidic proteins. Both S-100 and 14–3–2 are such proteins and appear in this region. They were purified to homogeneity by a step-wise sequence of ammonium sulfate fractionation, DEAE-cellulose chromatography at pH 7, Sephadex G-150 chromatography, and DEAE-Sephadex chromatography at either pH 7 or pH 5 (Moore, 1965, 1972). This is a fairly general scheme of purification that can be used for almost any protein in the nervous system. The molecular weights of S-100 and

14–3–2 are approximately 24,000 and 50,000 daltons, respectively, and neither contains detectable amounts of carbohydrate, lipid, or nucleic acid.

III. DEMONSTRATION OF NERVOUS SYSTEM SPECIFICITY

That S-100 and 14–3–2 are specific to the nervous system was indicated by the standard agar diffusion (Oechterloney method) for the detection of antigen-antibody reactions (Moore and Perez, 1968; Fig. 1). Reaction of the antibody to each protein could be demonstrated only for brain tissue.

This is not a highly sensitive method for the determination of specificity, and we therefore turned to the more sensitive and specific method of complement fixation (Wasserman and Levine, 1961; Moore and Perez, 1966; Moore, Perez, and Gehring, 1968). A comparison of the complement fixation for S-100 in the original tissue extract and at various stages of purification showed that the protein was unaltered, at least in its immunological reactivity, during the purification procedure.

The complement fixation method of Wasserman and Levine (1961) was scaled down until we could detect 1×10^{-12} g of antigen, which is sufficiently sensitive to measure the amount of a given protein in a single neuron. When this microcomplement fixation method was utilized with serial dilutions of various rat tissue extracts, we found that S-100 is at least 1,000-fold more concentrated in brain than other tissues, and 14–3–2 is present in at least 100-fold concentration (Table 1).

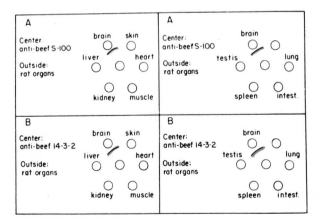

FIG. 1. Agar diffusion of anti-S-100 *(A)* and anti-14–3–2 *(B)* against rat organ extracts.

TABLE 1. *C^1-fixation by dilutions of rat organ extracts plus rabbit anti-beef-S-100 or anti-beef-14–3–2*

Organ extract dilutions	Brain	Liver	Kidney	Heart	Spleen	Muscle	Lung
S-100							
undiluted	+	+	+	−	−	+	−
10	++	−	−	−	−	±	−
30	++	−	−	−	−	−	−
100	++	−	−	−	−	−	−
300	++	−	−	−	−	−	−
1,000	++	−	−	−	−	−	−
3,000	++	−	−	−	−	−	−
10,000	±	−	−	−	−	−	−
30,000	−	−	−	−	−	−	−
100,000	−	−	−	−	−	−	−
14–3–2							
3	−	++	++	++	++	++	++
9	−	++	+	+	+	+	++
27	−	+	−	−	−	−	+
81	++	−	−	−	−	−	−
243	++	−	−	−	−	−	−
729	++	−	−	−	−	−	−
2,187	+	−	−	−	−	−	−

IV. EVOLUTIONARY CONSERVATION OF BRAIN-SPECIFIC PROTEINS

Agar diffusion of antibody to beef brain S-100 (Fig. 2) against brain extracts of various species showed a band of identity for all species tested, indicating that the antigens of these species were indistinguishable by this method. A band of identity for 14–3–2 was shown by all mammalian species, but the avian species showed some antigenic variation, as indicated by spurs on the precipitin bands, and no reaction could be demonstrated against fish or lower species (Fig. 2).

Further proof of species nonspecificity was obtained by immunoelectrophoresis. The S-100 and 14–3–2 proteins from different species had approximately the same electrophoretic mobility, as well as immunological reactivity, in the different vertebrate species. The 14–3–2 protein had a somewhat slower electrophoretic mobility than S-100, and its tendency to polymerize occasionally resulted in a double band.

Complement fixation curves have also been run for brain extracts of a number of species, using the antiserum to beef S-100, and there was a remarkable degree of cross-reactivity over a wide range of species, including mammals, birds, reptiles, and fish. Two-dimensional protein maps of

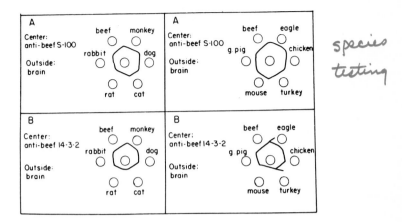

species testing

FIG. 2. Agar diffusion of anti-S-100 *(A)* and anti-14–3–2 *(B)* against brain extracts of different species.

brain extracts of a wide range of species, including some invertebrates such as squid and octopus, showed a great similarity of pattern, particularly the preponderance of small, acidic proteins in brain.

V. CELLULAR LOCALIZATION OF BRAIN-SPECIFIC PROTEINS

or, the localization in the cell type w/in the tissue...

After establishing the specificity and evolutionary conservation of these proteins, we began to investigate their localization to cell type within the tissue. This was much more difficult than we had initially anticipated. The first demonstration of the cellular localization of S-100 (Hydén and McEwen, 1966) indicated that the protein was probably of glial origin. This was also indicated later by the ability of C-6 astrocytoma cultures to synthesize the protein (Benda, Lightbody, Sato, Levine, and Sweet, 1968). *w/ degeneration*

In our laboratory, we initially attempted to determine cellular localization by inducing Wallerian degeneration of neuronal elements in the rabbit *tibia* tibial nerve. We observed that the S-100 level of the degenerating nerve *S-100 ↓* decreased virtually to zero (Perez and Moore, 1968), suggesting the protein *and* to be of neural origin. However, when we determined S-100 level in the *optic N.* optic nerve during Wallerian degeneration (Perez, Olney, Cicero, Moore, *S-100 ↑* and Bahn, 1970), we found that S-100 actually showed a slight increase, *while* whereas 14–3–2 levels decreased in phase with the histological course of *14-3-2 ↓* degeneration.

In view of these conflicting results, we next utilized a degeneration method in which cell bodies degenerate as well as nerve fibers (Cicero,

(cell bodies + nerve fibers degenerate)

Cowan, Moore, and Suntzeff, 1970). When the pia mater is stripped from one side of the rat cortex, the cortical layers degenerate and there is a retrograde degeneration of the neurons in the dorsal thalamus, since most of the axons of the neuronal cell bodies of this area go to the cortex. In agreement with our observations in the optic nerve, we found that S-100 levels increased slightly during the degeneration, probably as the result of *S-100* gliosis, whereas 14–3–2 levels rapidly decreased in phase with the de- *(glial* generation of cell bodies (Fig. 3). It thus appeared that S-100 was glial in origin and that 14–3–2 was a neuronal protein. *14-3- (neuro*

Direct confirmation of the localizations of these proteins has come from two approaches. The C-6 astrocytoma line produces large amounts of S-100 and very little or no 14–3–2, whereas several lines of human and mouse neuroblastoma produce large amounts of 14–3–2 and no S-100 (Benda et al., 1968; Moore and Goldstein, *unpublished observations*). We (Perez and Moore, *unpublished observations*) dissected single anterior horn and dorsal root ganglion cells from frozen dried sections, by the methods of Lowry, and measured the levels of S-100 and 14–3–2 using our microcomplement

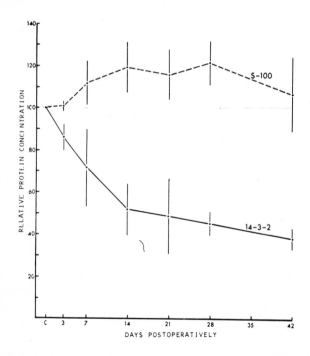

FIG. 3. Levels of S-100 and 14–3–2 in the rat dorsal thalamus following stripping of the pia mater from the cortex.

? neuropil collection of cell bodies

fixation assay. No S-100 could be detected in any of the nerve cells, but significant amounts were present in the surrounding neuropil. The 14–3–2 protein was present in both the cell bodies and the surrounding neuropil. In addition, immunofluorescence studies with S-100 antibody within the cerebellum show an intense fluorescence of the glial elements which surround the Purkinje cells (Simms and Moore, *unpublished observations*).

VI. DEVELOPMENTAL STUDIES

interesting!

Zuckerman, Herschman, and Levine (1970) observed a caudal-rostral appearance of S-100 in the human fetal brain. The spinal cord, medulla, pons, cerebellum, and midbrain began to produce detectable amounts of S-100 at 10 to 15 weeks of gestation, whereas S-100 levels in the frontal cortex did not rise until approximately 30 weeks of gestational age. Assays of S-100 in a number of areas of human brain in samples taken at autopsy indicated that the amount of protein increased linearly in most of the areas with age, with a three-fold increase from 2 to 80 years (Moore and Perez, 1968).

The clearest correlation with development has come from a study of both S-100 and 14–3–2 in the chick optic tectum (Cicero, Cowan, and Moore, 1970). This system is extremely well defined as to the kind of cell division, cell migration, laying down of layers, etc. during various stages of development. As shown in Fig. 4, the levels of both proteins remained low until immediately before hatching, at which time they rose rapidly and in parallel, reaching adult values 3 to 5 weeks after hatching.

Practically all cell division in the optic tectum is complete by 14 days of incubation, yet the levels of 14–3–2 and S-100 do not begin to increase appreciably until several days later. The same has been found recently in the spinal cord (Cicero and Provine, 1972), with the rapid rise in the two proteins occurring much later than histological maturation. This would suggest that the two proteins are correlated with functional rather than morphological development.

The period when S-100 and 14–3–2 begin to increase is also the time at which evoked potentials can be obtained in the tectum, and, in the cord, when spontaneous and uncoordinated limb movements are first observed. This is not to suggest a direct involvement of these proteins with these specific functions, but to emphasize that a number of the highly differentiated functions of the nervous system appear late in development, after morphological development of the nervous system appears to have reached maturity.

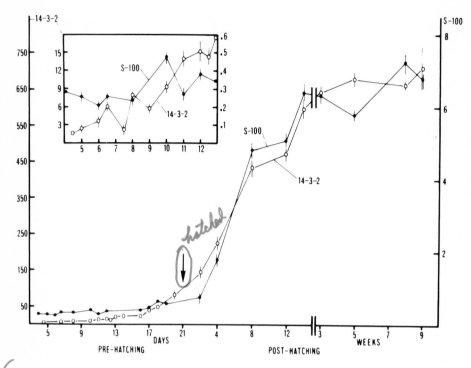

FIG. 4. Levels of S-100 and 14–3–2 in the chick optic tectum during the incubation and post-hatching periods. The inset shows days 5 through 12 on an expanded scale.

It is interesting to compare these results with observations made in tissue culture. S-100 is either not synthesized at all or is produced only in very small amounts during the growth period in astrocytoma (C-6) cell cultures (Benda et al., 1968). S-100 is synthesized in sizable amounts only when these cultures become confluent. These observations suggest that it is of great importance to study the mechanisms which control the bio-synthesis of these proteins. This can probably best be accomplished either in tissue culture or in cell-free systems, where it is possible to determine the level of control, i.e., at the level of transcription, translation, etc.

VII. CHEMICAL PROPERTIES OF S-100

Although the chemical studies that have been performed to date on S-100 have not yet elucidated its function, they have given us several

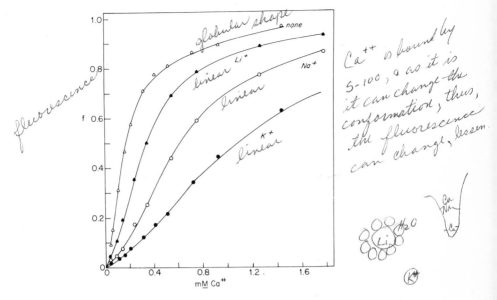

[handwritten annotations: "globular shape", "linear", "fluorescence", "Ca++ is bound by S-100, a as it is it can change the conformation, thus, the fluorescence can change, lessen."]

FIG. 5. Tryptophan fluorescence of S-100 as a function of Ca++ binding, and the antagonism of this effect by monovalent cations.

clues as to what to examine in searching for its function. These chemical studies are described in detail by Dr. Calissano in Chapter 2. He has found that S-100 undergoes a conformational change when it binds Ca++ (Calissano, Moore, and Friesen, 1969), an effect which is antagonized by monovalent cations (Fig. 5). This conformational change is reflected in a marked increase in the fluorescence of the single tryptophan in the S-100 molecule and by the exposure of a number of hydrophobic residues, including two of the three cysteine, one of the three tyrosine, and a number of phenylalanine residues. The occurrence of this conformational change has been confirmed by the observation that S-100 binds the fluorescent hydrophobic probe ANS in the presence of Ca++ but not in its absence.

These observations led us to examine the binding of S-100 to membranes under various conditions. We recently found that S-100 binds to synaptic membranes, and to other membranes such as myelin or even erythrocyte ghosts, only in the presence of Ca++ (Fig. 6), with maximum binding at 4 to 5 mM in the presence of 60 mM K+. This is higher than the Ca++ concentration required to produce the conformational change in the molecule

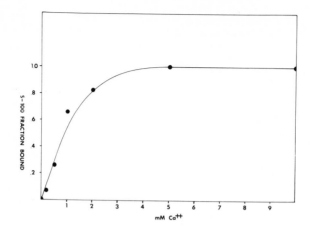

FIG. 6. Binding of S-100 to synaptic membranes as a function of Ca^{++} concentration.

(1 mM). However, these experiments were performed at 0°C, whereas the conformational studies were done at 25°C, and this difference may be due to a temperature effect.

We were then able to demonstrate that this binding is reversible (Table 2). Extraction with EDTA of a preparation of synaptic membranes with S-100 bound in the presence of Ca^{++}-containing medium removed all of the S-100. We have also found that the binding of S-100 to synaptic membranes is inhibited by the same divalent cations (K$^+$ and Na$^+$) that were previously shown (Fig. 5) to inhibit the conformational change in the molecule (Table 3).

TABLE 2. *Recovery of bound S-100 from synaptic membranes*

Incubation media		Extraction media		
mM Ca^{++}	Supernatant S-100	Ca^{++}	EDTA	Supernatant S-100
0	25.4	−	+	0
10	10.3	−	+	9.4
0	20.6	+	−	0
10	9.3	+	−	0

TABLE 3. *Effect of Na^+ and K^+ on Ca^{++}-dependent binding of S-100 to synaptic membranes*

Concn. (mM)			
Ca^{++}	Na^+	K^+	Bound S-100 (μg)
0	0	0	0
10	0	0	2.7
10	100	0	1.8
10	200	0	0.6
10	0	100	1.7
10	0	200	1.0

VIII. CONCLUSIONS

In conclusion, the original premise upon which our work has been based, i.e., that there are nervous system-specific, species-nonspecific proteins, has been shown to be correct. It remains, of course, to demonstrate what the specific functions of these proteins are. By a combination of biological and chemical approaches, as we and others have already begun to use, this problem will come nearer to solution.

REFERENCES

Benda, P., Lightbody, J., Sato, G., Levine, L., and Sweet, W. (1968): Differentiated rat cell strain in tissue culture. *Science,* 161:370.

Calissano, P., Moore, B. W., and Friesen, A. (1969): Effect of calcium ion on S-100, a protein of the nervous system. *Biochemistry,* 8:4318.

Cicero, T. J., Cowan, W. M., and Moore, B. W. (1970): Changes in the concentration of the two brain-specific proteins, S-100 and 14–3–2, during the development of the avian optic tectum. *Brain Research,* 24:1.

Cicero, T. J., Cowan, W. M., Moore, B. W., and Suntzeff, V. (1970): The cellular localization of the two brain-specific proteins, S-100 and 14–3–2. *Brain Research,* 18:25.

Cicero, T. J., and Provine, R. R. (1972): The levels of the brain-specific proteins, S-100 and 14–3–2, in the developing chick spinal cord. *Brain Research,* 44:294.

Hydén, H., and McEwen, B. (1966): A glial protein specific for the nervous system. *Proceedings of the National Academy of Sciences,* 55:354.

Moore, B. W. (1965): A specific nervous tissue protein. In: *Variation in Chemical Composition of the Nervous System as Determined by Developmental and Genetic Factors,* edited by G. B. Ansel, p. 81. Pergamon Press (Abstracts of International Neurochemical Conference) Oxford.

Moore, B. W. (1972): Chemistry and biology of two proteins, S-100 and 14–3–2, specific to the nervous system. In: *International Review of Neurobiology,* Vol. 15. Academic Press, New York.

Moore, B. W., and McGregor, D. (1965): Chromatographic and electrophoretic fractionation of soluble proteins of brain and liver. *Journal of Biological Chemistry*, 240:1647.

Moore, B. W., and Perez, V. J. (1966): Complement fixation for antigens on a picogram level. *Journal of Immunology*, 96:1000.

Moore, B. W., and Perez, V. J. (1968): Specific acidic proteins of the nervous system. In: *Physiological and Biochemical Aspects of Nervous Integration*, edited by F. D. Carlson, pp. 343–359. Prentice-Hall, Englewood Cliffs, N.J.

Moore, B. W., Perez, V. J., and Gehring, M. (1968): Assay and regional distribution of a soluble protein characteristic of the nervous system. *Journal of Neurochemistry*, 15:265.

Perez, V. J., and Moore, B. W. (1968): Wallerian degeneration in rabbit tibial nerve: Changes in amounts of the S-100 protein, *Journal of Neurochemistry*, 15:971.

Perez, V. J., and Moore, B. W. (1968): Wallerian degeneration in rabbit tibial nerve: Changes in amounts of the S-100 protein, *Journal of Neurochemistry*, 15:971.

Perez, V. J., Olney, J., Cicero, T. J., Moore, B. W., and Bahn, B. A. (1970): Wallerian degeneration in rabbit optic nerve: CNS cellular localization. *Journal of Neurochemistry*, 17:511.

Wasserman, E., and Levine, L. (1961): Quantitative microcomplement fixation and its use in the study of antigenic structure by specific antigen-antibody inhibition. *Journal of Immunology*, 87:290.

Zuckerman, J. E., Herschman, H. R., and Levine, L. (1970): Appearance of a brain-specific antigen (the S-100 protein) during human foetal development. *Journal of Neurochemistry*, 17:247.

Proteins of the Nervous System
Raven Press, New York © 1973

Specific Properties of the Brain-Specific Protein S-100

What's EDTA?

Pietro Calissano

I. THE INTERACTION OF S-100 WITH CATIONS

Early studies (Hydén and McEwen, 1966; Gombos, Vincedon, Tardy, and Mandel, 1966) demonstrated that more than one band of S-100 could be obtained under certain conditions of electrophoresis. In conjunction with Dr. Blake Moore, and utilizing his system of acrylamide gel electrophoresis, it was found that multiple S-100 bands appeared only when Ca^{++} was present in the buffer, whereas only a single band was obtained when EDTA was present in the system (Fig. 1).

The appearance of a multiple-band pattern in the presence of Ca^{++} could have been due to one of several possibilities. In order to determine whether Ca^{++} might induce an aggregation of the S-100 molecule, the elution profile on Sephadex and the sedimentation pattern on sucrose density gradients were determined in the presence and absence of Ca^{++}. No difference in either parameter was observed, and aggregation of S-100 in the presence of Ca^{++} was therefore excluded.

A second possible explanation was that Ca^{++} induced a conformational change in the protein and that the appearance of multiple bands was a reflection of several conformational states in equilibrium. If this hypothesis were correct, each band should in turn produce a multiple-band pattern when run separately on acrylamide gels, due to a shift in the equilibrium. However, there was no evidence of such interconversion of bands on electrophoresis, indicating that these were stable forms of S-100.

Still a third possibility was that there are small differences in the primary structure which are hidden in the absence of Ca^{++} and exposed in its presence by an induced conformational change. Such differences, when revealed, would result in multiple forms of S-100 having different electrophoretic mobilities. It was originally thought that S-100 was a single molecule of 22,000 to 24,000 daltons, but Dannies and Levine (1969) showed that the molecular weight shifts to 6,000 to 7,000 in the presence of sodium dodecyl sulfate, suggesting that the S-100 molecule contains several subunits. The hypothesis of a conformational alteration induced by Ca^{++} is still valid

13

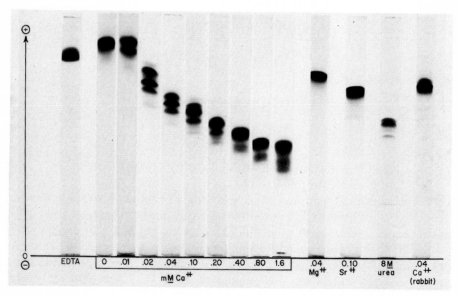

FIG. 1. Acrylamide gel electrophoresis patterns of S-100 as a function of Ca^{++} concentration. A single band is obtained when EDTA (0.1 mM) is present in the buffer, while up to five or six bands are obtained in the presence of Ca^{++}. Little effect on band pattern was induced by the addition of either Mg^{++} or Sr^{++}, whereas urea produced an effect somewhat similar to that of Ca^{++} (from Calissano, Moore, and Friesen, 1969).

whether or not the molecule contains multiple subunits, if the assumption is made that the various subunits possess binding sites with different affinities for Ca^{++}. This was later shown to be a correct assumption (see Figs. 6 and 7) and there are now known to be two separate sets of binding sites for Ca^{++}. Multiple combinations of subunits with different affinities for Ca^{++} would result in the appearance of multiple bands on electrophoresis.

II. THE INDUCTION OF CONFORMATIONAL CHANGES IN S-100 BY CA^{++}

In order to prove that Ca^{++} does induce a conformational change in the S-100 molecule, it was necessary to utilize more sensitive methods of analyzing such changes. Fluorescence measurement is highly sensitive to protein conformation and requires only small amounts of protein (Udenfriend, 1969). The fluorescence of a protein molecule at 360 mμ reflects the presence of the aromatic amino acids, primarily tyrosine and tryptophan. The addition of Ca^{++} increases the fluorescence of the S-100

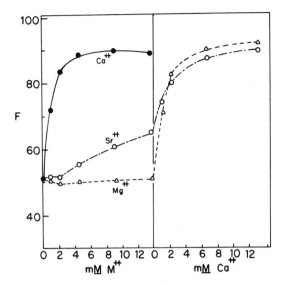

FIG. 2. The effects of divalent cations on the fluorescence (F) of S-100. Ca^{++} induced almost a twofold increase, Sr^{++} had only a slight effect, and Mg^{++} was ineffective. The lack of competition for Ca^{++} by Mg^{++} is indicated by identical increases in fluorescence in response to Ca^{++} both in the presence and absence of Mg^{++}.

molecule almost two-fold (Fig. 2). This effect is highly specific for Ca^{++}; Sr^{++} has only a slight effect, and Mg^{++} has no effect by itself and is unable to compete for Ca^{++}. This is highly significant, because Mg^{++} is the only divalent cation present in the nervous system in a concentration approaching that of Ca^{++}.

In contrast, monovalent cations are effective in competing against Ca^{++}, as indicated in Chapter 1 (Fig. 6). K^+ is most effective, and the affinity of S-100 for Ca^{++} is almost a linear function of K^+ concentration; for example, the affinity for Ca^{++} in 60 mM K^+ is 0.6 mM, although it is 0.1 mM in 10 mM K^+.

These fluorescence measurements indicated that the single tryptophan residue present in the S-100 molecule is involved in the effect of Ca^{++}. This experiment did not in itself prove that a conformational change in the molecule occurred in the presence of Ca^{++}, since the fluorescence of a molecule can be altered by simple quenching or by solvent perturbation following its interaction with effectors such as cations, substrates, or other molecules (Udenfriend, 1969).

While this investigation on the effect of Ca^{++} on S-100 was in progress, a study was published (Kessler, Levine, and Fasman, 1968) which showed no change in optical rotary dispersion (ORD) measurements of S-100 in the presence of Ca^{++} or EDTA. Such ORD measurements are often employed to detect large changes in the secondary structure of the protein. Small alterations in the tertiary structure of a protein as the result of binding ions or small molecules are sometimes reflected by a shift in the maximum of absorption of its aromatic residues to either lower or higher wave lengths (blue or red shift).

These changes can be detected with a differential spectrophotometer (Calissano, Moore, and Friesen, 1969). The use of such a system revealed a marked blue shift in the difference spectrum of S-100 in the presence of Ca^{++} and a slight red shift in the presence of K$^+$ (Fig. 3). The blue shift induced by Ca^{++} involves tryptophan (2,930 Å), as well as tyrosine (2,860 Å) and phenylalanine (2,780 and 2,720 Å) residues. This effect is approximately half that induced by guanidine-HCl.

These findings confirmed and extended the results of the fluorescence

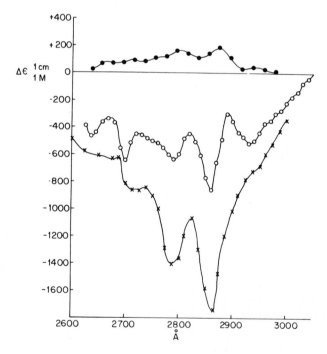

FIG. 3. Difference spectra of S-100 in 20 mM Tris-Cl pH 8.3. The reference cell contained S-100 in buffer and the sample cell contained S-100 in buffer plus: ● = 60 mM KCl; ○ = 4 mM CaCl$_2$; X = 6 M GU—HCl. Δε was calculated assuming a molecular weight for S-100 of 24,000.

studies, further supporting the exposure of tryptophan residues, and probably also of some tyrosine and phenylalanine residues, to the solvent in the presence of Ca^{++}. The effect of Ca^{++} is greater and opposite to that of K^+, confirming its antagonism to the Ca^{++} effect on fluorescence enhancement described above.

Titration of SH groups in a protein may also provide an indication of possible conformational changes. No titratable SH groups were present in the S-100 molecule in the absence of Ca^{++}, but increasing concentrations of Ca^{++} resulted in the appearance of 1.7 to 2.0 SH groups (Fig. 4). A third SH group became available for titration only when the molecule was completely unfolded in the presence of guanidine-HCl. Dannies and Levine (1971) have suggested that there may actually be four rather than three cysteine residues in the molecule. These titration data suggest that Ca^{++}

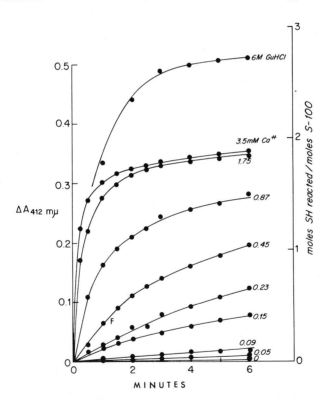

FIG. 4. The presence of titratable SH groups in the S-100 molecule in the presence of Ca^{++} and guanidine HCl. A maximum of two SH groups become available for titration with DTNB in the presence of Ca^{++}; a third group becomes available only when complete unfolding is induced by GuHCl.

binding by S-100 results in a conformational change which makes two of the three or four SH groups in the molecule available for titration. This observation of an unmasking of SH groups in the presence of Ca^{++} is probably the best available evidence in favor of a conformational change resulting from binding, because alterations in parameters dependent on the aromatic amino acids are frequently due to environmental changes other than true conformational changes in a molecule. The lack of any large change in the ORD spectrum, as indicated by Kessler et al. (1968) and confirmed by us, as well as a lack of change in the intrinsic viscosity of the protein (Calissano et al., 1969), indicate that the Ca^{++}-induced alteration probably does not lead to a large change in the shape of the molecule or in its secondary structure, but rather involves a small change in the tertiary structure.

Further evidence of a Ca^{++}-induced conformational change in the S-100 molecule was obtained from studies of proteolytic digestion under various ionic conditions (Fig. 5). Proteins are in general more easily digested by proteolytic enzymes when they assume relatively unfolded structures or when they are denatured than when they assume more compact globular structures. As shown in Fig. 5, the native S-100 molecule in the absence of Ca^{++} is digested at an extremely slow rate. The addition of Ca^{++} mark-

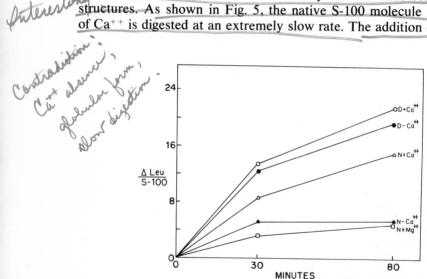

FIG. 5. The effects of Ca^{++} and Mg^{++} on the rate of proteolytic digestion of the S-100 molecule with chymotrypsin. Mg^{++} had no effect, whereas Ca^{++} (3.0 mM) induced approximately a threefold increase. Little enhancement of the digestive process was obtained when the S-100 molecule was unfolded by denaturation, further supporting a partial unfolding of the S-100 molecule in the presence of Ca^{++}. D and N refer to heat denatured and native S-100.

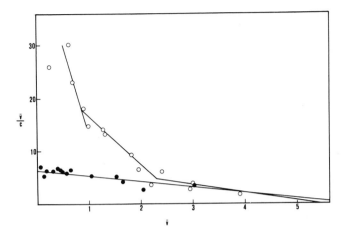

FIG. 6. Scatchard plot of the binding of Ca^{++} by the S-100 molecule in the presence (●——●) and absence (○——○) of K^+ (60 mM). The K_a for Ca^{++} is 10^{-3} M in the presence of K^+, whereas in the absence of K^+ there are two or three binding sites with an affinity of 3.0 to 6.0 × 10^{-5} M and six or seven sites with an affinity of 10^{-3} M.

edly increases this rate, but has little additional effect on the denatured molecule. Since chymotrypsin is known to specifically attack peptide bonds adjacent to aromatic amino acids, this observation further confirms the unmasking of these amino acids by Ca^{++}.

III. CA⁺⁺-BINDING SITES ON THE S-100 MOLECULE

Measurement of the binding of Ca^{++} to the S-100 molecule in the presence of K^+ indicates that the molecule contains six to eight binding sites, with an association constant of 10^{-3} M (Calissano et al., 1969). Since we knew from our earlier fluorescence studies that K^+ antagonized Ca^{++}, the binding was compared in the presence and absence of this ion. In the absence of K^+, at least two, and probably three, sets of binding sites with different affinities for Ca^{++} were revealed (Fig. 6). The disappearance of the high-affinity binding sites for Ca^{++} in the presence of K^+ provides a strong indication that K^+ competes for the high-affinity sites.*

It is justifiable at this point to make some hypotheses about these binding sites. If we assume that S-100 is comprised of several subunits, then we may assume that the high- and low-affinity binding sites are on different

---

* The investigation on the fluorescence of S-100, as well as its binding of Ca^{++} and liposomes, was performed in collaboration with Dr. Stefano Alemà.

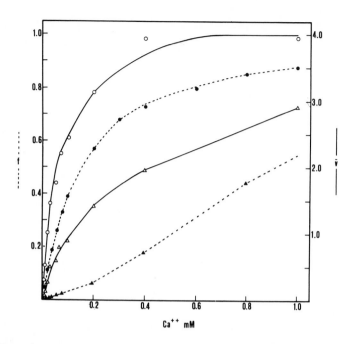

FIG. 7. The enhancement of S-100 fluorescence by Ca^{++} binding in the presence and absence of K^+. O——O The binding of Ca^{++} by S-100 in the absence of K^+. △——△ The binding of Ca^{++} in the presence of K^+. ●-----● The fluorescence of S-100 as a function of Ca^{++} concentration in the absence of K^+. ▲-----▲ The fluorescence of S-100 in the presence of K^+.

subunits. Figure 7 shows a correlation between the fluorescence enhancement of Ca^{++} and the binding of Ca^{++} by S-100 both in the presence and absence of K^+. At relatively high Ca^{++} concentrations, the inhibition by K^+ of both binding and fluorescence was only 20 to 30%, but the inhibition of both parameters at low Ca^{++} was two- to threefold greater in the presence of K^+. This confirms the results of the earlier binding experiments indicating that K^+ antagonizes the binding of Ca^{++} at the high-affinity binding sites. Since the 24,000 molecular weight S-100 has a single tryptophan which is primarily responsible for fluorescence changes, we may tentatively conclude that the subunit having this aromatic residue also has some of the high-affinity binding sites for Ca^{++} which are antagonized by K^+.

IV. THE INTERACTION OF S-100−CA^{++} COMPLEXES
WITH ARTIFICIAL MEMBRANES

The demonstration of a specific binding between S-100 and Ca^{++} or monovalent cations, characterized by different conformational states with certain hydrophobic residues masked or exposed to the solvent depending on the specific cation bound, suggested a possible interaction of the protein with a membrane. In order to test this hypothesis, we looked at the effects of S-100 in an artificial membrane system, rather than use biological membranes such as those from mitochondria or synaptosomes, which in addition to their complexity might be contaminated with S-100.

Bangham (1968) has developed a fairly simple method for the preparation of artificial lipid membranes in the form of small spheroids. We therefore looked at the effects of S-100 on the diffusion of cations across these membranes (Calissano and Bangham, 1971). This artificial membrane system is an ideal test system for any substance which is thought to interact with a membrane, since both the lipid composition and the test substance can be varied at will and examined under a variety of environmental conditions [for a review, see Bangham, 1968].

The rate of diffusion across the liposomal membrane is determined by incubating the liposomes, placed in a dialysis bag, in medium identical to that within the liposomes but without ^{86}Rb, followed by a determination of radioactivity released from the liposomes. The permeability of the liposomes is so low compared to that of the dialysis bag that the calculated diffusion rate represents the diffusion across the liposomes rather than that across the dialysis bag.

Figure 8 demonstrates the effect of S-100 on the diffusion of ^{86}Rb across the liposomal membrane. The protein had virtually no effect on the diffusion rate in the absence of Ca^{++}, whereas the addition of Ca^{++} resulted in a six- to eightfold increase in diffusion. The enhancement of diffusion by Mg^{++} is thought to be the result of Ca^{++} contamination of the phosphatidyl serine forming the membranes. Either Ca^{++} or S-100 alone had only a slight effect, and the addition of both produced a synergistic effect, i.e., Ca^{++} in some way activates the ability of S-100 to alter membrane permeability (Fig. 9).

A relatively large concentration of S-100 (up to 140 nm) was able to produce more than a 20-fold increase in diffusion. The increased rate of diffusion was greater after longer periods of incubation, suggesting a further interaction of the protein with the membrane lipid after the initial binding.

Many substances are now known to alter the permeability of artificial membranes (Bangham, 1968). If the effect of S-100 on membrane permeability were due to such a nonspecific effect, it should also increase the permeability of other solutes. Two types of liposomes were prepared, negatively charged liposomes consisting of phosphatidyl choline and phosphatidyl serine, and positively charged liposomes of phosphatidyl choline and stearil amine, containing ^{86}Rb and ^{14}C-glucose. S-100 induced an increase in the diffusion of ^{86}Rb from both types of liposomes, but had no effect on the diffusion of glucose in either case (Fig. 10). These studies have recently

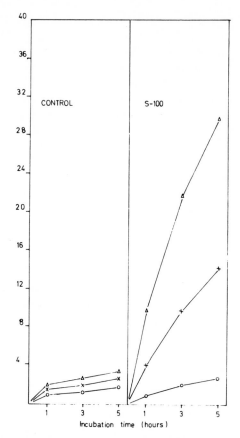

FIG. 8. The effect of S-100 on the diffusion of ^{86}Rb across liposomal membranes. O——O Diffusion in the presence of 0.1 mM EDTA. x——x Diffusion in the presence of 2.0 mM Mg[++]. △——△ Diffusion in the presence of 2.0 mM Ca[++].

been extended to other solutes, including ^{14}C-glutamate and ^{14}C-GABA. An effect on rubidium could always be demonstrated, but neither glutamate nor GABA diffusion was altered by the S-100.

It was also of interest to determine whether S-100 had a preference for certain types of liposomes. Liposomes were formed from various combinations of lipids, and the effects of S-100 on the diffusion of rubidium determined. A maximum diffusion increase in the presence of S-100 was obtained when phosphatidyl serine was present, and decreasing effects were seen in the order: stearil amine > sphingomyelin > phosphatidic acid > phosphatidyl choline.

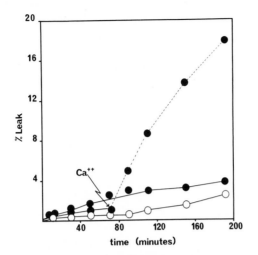

FIG. 9. The effect of Ca^{++} added to a mixture of liposomes plus S-100. After 70 min of incubation, 1.2 mM Ca^{++} was added to control (O——O) and S-100-containing (●——●) dialysis bags. Additional control and experimental bags were further incubated in 0.1 mM EDTA. The arrow indicates the addition of Ca^{++}, and the dashed line refers to the leak from bags containing S-100 subtracted from the leak of analogous control experiments.

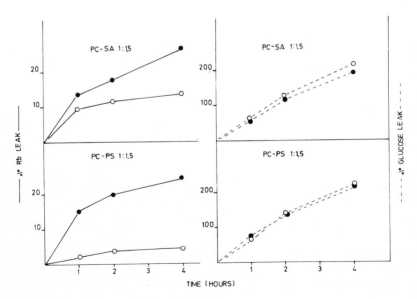

FIG. 10. Leak of ^{86}Rb (——) and ^{14}C-glucose (---) from negatively and positively charged liposomes. O = control, ● = S-100 (0.5 mg/ml).

These results were somewhat surprising in view of the fact that both S-100 and phosphatidyl serine are negatively charged, and stearil amine is positively charged and would therefore be expected to interact more strongly with S-100. Indeed, stearil amine was found to bind two orders of magnitude more S-100 than phosphatidyl serine. The lack of a correlation between the extent of binding of S-100 and its ability to interact in such a way as to lead to an increase in membrane permeability indicates that the effect of S-100 on permeability is specific.

Since Ca^{++} is known to bind to phosphatidyl serine, and we had already demonstrated Ca^{++} binding by S-100, it appeared possible that the diffusion of Ca^{++} across liposomal membranes might be enhanced by S-100. In parallel experiments we measured the efflux of K^+ and the influx of Ca^{++} into the liposomes, and found that the presence of S-100 did increase Ca^{++} influx as well as K^+ efflux (Fig. 11).

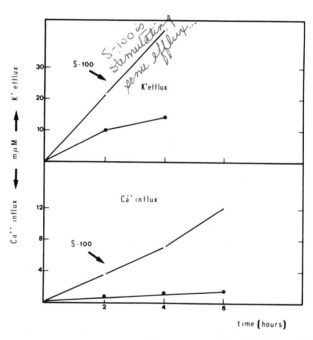

FIG. 11. Efflux of K^+ and influx of Ca^{++} into liposomes in the presence of S-100. Experimental conditions were identical to those described for Figs. 8–10. The influx of Ca^{++} was determined by incubating liposomes with 0.8 mM cold Ca^{++} plus trace amounts of $^{45}Ca^{++}$. Samples of the suspension were removed at intervals and placed on a Sephadex G-25 column equilibrated with the same buffer used for the incubation but with 1 mM EDTA added. The amount of $^{45}Ca^{++}$ eluted with the liposomes was assumed to be bound or trapped by them.

As indicated earlier, the effect of S-100 on membrane permeability increased after longer periods of incubation, suggesting an interaction with the membrane subsequent to binding. This was further supported by attempts to remove S-100 from the liposomes after different periods of incubation. The binding of the protein was reversible initially, but with increasing periods of incubation a progressively higher amount of the S-100-liposome complex was not separated on a Sephadex column containing EDTA.

V. A MODEL OF S-100-LIPOSOME INTERACTIONS

We have demonstrated that S-100 interacts with monovalent and divalent cations and that these specific interactions are accompanied by a relatively specific Ca^{++}-dependent interaction with membranes. Based on these observations, it is possible to propose a hypothesis about the way in which the S-100 molecule may function in this system, which may or may not reflect its function *in vivo*. Since 1 mM Ca^{++}, 60 mM K^+, and S-100 are present outside the liposomes, and only 60 mM K^+ is present inside, then the binding of Ca^{++} will be strongly favored over that of K^+ in the external medium. The formation of a $Ca^{++}-$S-100 complex is characterized by a change in the conformation of the S-100 molecule such that hydrophobic residues are exposed to the solvent. This exposure should make the molecule less soluble and induce its binding to the liposomal membranes. If a small portion of the S-100 molecule penetrates the membrane, it will enter a region where Ca^{++} is not present. Under these conditions, K^+ will compete for Ca^{++} and displace it, with a net result of Ca^{++} transported across the membrane. The displacement of Ca^{++} by K^+ would result in the assumption of a new conformation with only a low affinity for the membrane, and the K^+-S-100 complex will once again enter the external medium, K^+ will be released by the competition of Ca^{++}, and this entire process will be repeated. The differential movement of ions can be explained on the basis of multiple sites with different affinities. At the present state of our investigations, it is difficult to explain the observed increased strength of binding between S-100 and liposomes with time of incubation. This finding would be of great interest if it can be confirmed in *in vivo* experiments. *Yes!*

VI. CONCLUSION

Two major findings have emerged from these experiments on the properties of the S-100 molecules. The interaction of the S-100 protein with Ca^{++} and monovalent cations is accompanied, first, by a specific change in its conformation, and second, strictly dependent on the conformational change, by a specific interaction of the protein with a lipid membrane. Further investigations will tell us whether the increased permeability resulting from such interaction is simply a "by-product" of this event or whether it mimics, at least to some extent, an *in vivo* situation.

REFERENCES

Bangham, A. D. (1968): Membrane models with phospholipids. *Progress in Biophysics and Molecular Biology,* edited by J. A. V: Butler and D. Noble, pp. 31–87.

Calissano, P., and Bangham, A. D. (1971): Effect of two brain specific proteins (S-100, 14.3.2) on cation diffusion across artificial lipid membranes. *Biochemical and Biophysical Research Communications,* 43:504.

Calissano, P., Moore, B. W., and Friesen, A. (1969): Effect of calcium ion on S-100, a protein of the nervous system. *Biochemistry,* 8:4318.

Dannies, P., and Levine, L. (1969): Demonstration of subunits in beef brain acidic protein (S-100). *Biochemical and Biophysical Research Communications,* 37:587.

Dannies, P. S., and Levine, L. (1971): Structural properties of brain S-100 protein. *Journal of Biological Chemistry,* 246:6276.

Gombos, G., Vincedon, G., Tardy, J., and Mandel, P. (1966): Hétérogéneité électrophorétique et preparation rapide de la fraction proteique S-100. *Comptes Rendus de l'Academie des Sciences* (Paris), 263:150.

Hydén, H., and McEwen, B. (1966): A glial protein specific for the nervous system. *Proceedings of the National Academy of Sciences,* 55:354.

Kessler, D., Levine, L., and Fasman, G. (1968): Some conformational and immunological properties of a bovine brain acidic proteins (S-100). *Biochemistry,* 7:758.

Udenfriend, S. (1969): *Fluorescence Assay in Biology and Medicine,* Vol. II, edited by B. Horecker and N. O. Kaplan. Academic Press, New York.

Proteins of the Nervous System
Raven Press, New York © 1973

Myelin-Specific Proteins

Edwin H. Eylar

I. INTRODUCTION

Although myelin might be expected to resemble a type of plasma membrane because the myelin wrapping of the axon is essentially an extension of either oligodendroglial cell or the Schwann cell plasma membrane, in reality it is markedly different (Table 1). The lipid-protein ratio of myelin is much higher than that of the usual plasma membrane, and the myelin-lipid composition differs in its relatively low content of gangliosides and triglyceride and its high content of cerebrosides, cerebroside sulfate, and the galactosyldiglycerides. The latter may be specific to myelin (1). In contrast to the large number of protein components found in the plasma membrane, including glycoproteins, myelin has only two major proteins.

TABLE 1. *A comparison of the chemical composition of CNS bovine myelin and plasma membranes*

		Plasma membrane		
Constituents	CNS myelin	HeLa cell	L cell	Red cell
Composition				
% Protein	21	60	60	63
% Lipid	78	40	40	37
Lipid (weight %)				
Cholesterol	28	24	21	28
Phospholipid	42	43	59	61
Neutral lipid	0	33	20	0
Cerebroside	25	—	0	11
Cerebroside sulfate	5	0	0	—
Monogalactosyl diglyceride	+	0	0	0
Gangliosides	Trace	+	+	+
Glycoprotein	—	+	+	+
Enzymes	1–2		Many	
Protein components	A1 protein 30% Proteolipid 50%		> 15	

The only enzyme which appears localized in myelin is the 2′,3′-cyclic nucleotide phosphohydrolase (2); plasma membranes contain many enzymes and proteins. These differences in composition probably reflect the fairly static insulating role of myelin as opposed to the plasma membrane as a dynamic, transporting system.

Figure 1 shows sodium dodecylsulfate (SDS) gel electrophoresis patterns obtained from rabbit brain, spinal cord, and sciatic nerve myelin. The two major protein components of CNS myelin—the proteolipid (50%), described in the chapter by Dr. Folch-Pi, and the A1 protein (30%)—together account for approximately 80% of the total myelin protein of brain or spinal cord (4). For all other components, including the double bands referred to as Wolfgram protein (5), questions arise about their origin; i.e., are they

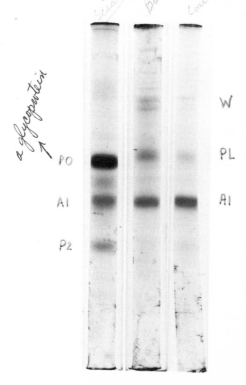

FIG. 1. Electrophoresis of myelin (from top to bottom) in SDS using 7% cross-linked polyacrylamide gels. From left to right, gel patterns of rabbit sciatic nerve, brain, and spinal cord myelin are shown as prepared by a modification of the procedure of Autilio and Norton (3). The A1 protein, P2 protein, and the P0 proteins are clearly seen in sciatic myelin; the Wolfgram (W), proteolipid (PL), and A1 protein bands are marked in the CNS myelins.

true myelin constituents or are they derived from membranes contaminating the myelin preparation? Direct evidence has not been presented to discriminate between possible impurities in the myelin preparations and possible minor components, which generally show a higher molecular weight (Fig. 1), particularly in peripheral nerve.

The A1 protein is also found in peripheral nerve myelin and was previously termed the P1 protein (6). Direct identification of the A1 protein in sciatic nerve myelin was made by amino acid sequence determination (7). The presence of the A1 protein in peripheral nerve was probably missed by other workers (8) because they used myelin from bovine sources, which has relatively less A1 protein than the rabbit material.

More significant perhaps is the presence in peripheral nerve myelin of another basic protein, referred to as the P2 protein, which is *not* found in CNS myelin (6). The P2 protein is smaller than the A1 protein with a molecular weight of 12,000 compared to 18,400 for the latter. The dominant protein of peripheral nerve (55% total protein) has a molecular weight of

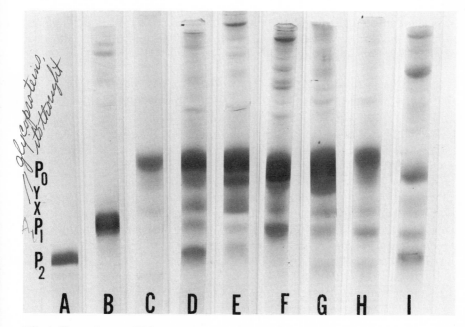

FIG. 2. Discontinuous SDS gel electrophoresis patterns of peripheral nerve myelin from various species are shown as found by Greenfield et al. (9): *(A)* P2 protein; *(B)* A1 protein; *(C)* P0 protein; *(D)* beef intradural root; *(E)* rabbit sciatic nerve; *(F)* guinea pig sciatic nerve; *(G)* human sciatic nerve; *(H)* rat sciatic nerve; *(I)* mouse brain. For myelin, 100 μg defatted material was applied; the bands were stained with fast green.

nearly 30,000, and was designated by us as the P0 protein. It is insoluble in aqueous solvents but is not of the proteolipid type since it is insoluble in chloroform-methanol as well.

Until recently, there have been relatively few studies made of peripheral myelin due to the difficulty of isolation; direct extraction of myelin proteins from intact peripheral nerve is not efficient because of abundant connective tissue. These problems are minimized in rabbit sciatic nerve, in contrast to human or equine sources, because peripheral myelin is easily obtained in relatively high purity. Figure 2 shows the discontinuous SDS gel electrophoresis profile of peripheral nerve myelin obtained from many species as shown by Greenfield et al. (9).

In every case the P0 protein predominates, but the relative proportions of the A1 (P1) and P2 basic proteins vary greatly; in guinea pig sciatic nerve it is almost entirely A1 protein but in bovine peripheral myelin, the P2 protein dominates. These data suggest that the A1 and P2 proteins may have the same structural role in the myelin membrane. It should be noted that between the P0 and P1 proteins, two protein bands referred to as X and Y bands can be distinguished to varying degrees. Many trace components of higher molecular weight are seen above the P0 protein; whether they are intrinsic myelin components is questionable.

II. THE RELATIONSHIP OF THE A1 PROTEIN TO EXPERIMENTAL ALLERGIC ENCEPHALOMYELITIS

The initial goal of our work was to find and purify the agent in CNS tissue responsible for encephalomyelitis (EAE) and to study it using conventional methods of protein chemistry. We focused our attention on basic protein because the early work of others (10, 11) had shown that protein material rather than lipids or proteolipid was probably responsible for the induction of EAE, an inflammatory demyelinating disease of CNS tissue which usually leads to paralysis and death (4). From time to time, many components from nervous system tissue have been reported to induce EAE, but these were probably contaminated with basic protein. It is now generally agreed that the basic protein, which we refer to as the A1 protein (12), is the factor in nervous system tissue and in myelin that is responsible for this autoimmune disease.

EAE is probably the most widely studied autoimmune disease, because it is one of the few such diseases for which the antigen is known. It is possible to isolate the A1 protein in soluble form in large quantities (13), which is not true for many membrane proteins. When we began our work, there was much disagreement concerning the purity, number, and composition of basic proteins in CNS tissue. The problem was thus mainly one of protein purification; i.e., it was essential to isolate the factor in order to obtain unambiguous immunologic data that could be related to human demyelinating diseases for which EAE is considered to be a model (12).

Although it has some similarities to multiple sclerosis, EAE, an acute and usually fatal disease, differs from this chronic condition in some respects. It is similar to the post-rabies vaccine encephalitis that was discovered soon after the development of the rabies vaccine by Pasteur. The rabies virus used for innoculation is sometimes contaminated with the nervous system tissue in which it is grown, and such contamination can lead to an EAE-like disease, particularly in South America where vaccination is relatively frequent because of bites from rabid bats.

We were able to purify the A1 protein by column chromatography on CM-cellulose, Cellex-P, or Amberlite IRC 50 (14). It appears homogeneous by gel electrophoresis (at various pH's or in SDS) and by ultracentrifugation. It is a single polypeptide chain with a molecular weight of 18,500, and it constitutes 30% of total CNS myelin (4). Except for additional, smaller, basic protein present in the rat and mouse myelin (15), the A1 protein appears to be the only basic protein present in CNS myelin for most species. The relative ease of degradation of this protein by proteolytic enzymes (16) is responsible for much of the early controversy regarding its size and localization. Proteolysis may occur either *in situ* in the myelin (13) or during acid extraction by cathepsins (10).

The A1 protein is highly encephalitogenic; as little as 0.1 μg can induce mild infiltration of mononuclear cells into white matter. In guinea pigs, 5 μg or more induces severe histologic lesions, weakness, paralysis, and death. A similar response is seen in monkeys at much higher doses (17). The severity of the immunopathologic response often increases with increasing amounts of tubercle bacillus used in the Freund's adjuvant as part of the inoculum. EAE is a classical autoimmune disease, which can be transferred from one animal to another by lymph node cells, presumably lymphocytes (18). Figure 3 shows the type of lesions produced in this condition. Such lesions may be seen in animals that are without clinical symptoms when small quantities of Al protein (less than 5 μg) have been used, even as small as 0.1 μg (13).

A similar histological picture is seen in the peripheral nervous system * EAN (PNS) in experimental allergic neuritis (EAN), which is induced with peripheral nerve myelin. A hallmark of EAN, produced in the monkey with sciatic nerve myelin, is severe cellular infiltration and demyelination in the dorsal root ganglia, particularly as shown in Fig. 4.

The lesions in monkeys in this case are restricted solely to the peripheral

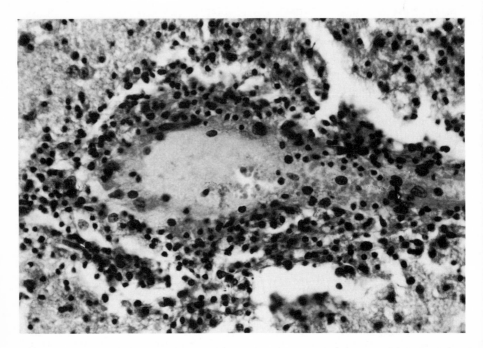

FIG. 3. A typical section from the white matter of the centrum semiovale of a monkey with clinical signs of EAE produced by the human A1 protein given in CFA intradermally in the foot pad 15 days earlier. Extensive cellular infiltration and perivascular cuffing are seen; the darkly stained nuclei of the invading cells (mononuclear with some polymorphonuclear) stand out.

nervous system (19). Since peripheral myelin is known to contain the identical A1 protein (7) which induces EAE when isolated, the failure to observe EAE lesions in this case suggests that the encephalitogenic sites of the A1 protein are masked in peripheral myelin. EAN can also be induced in monkeys by the P2 protein (6), a protein exclusively localized to peripheral myelin, a fact that suggests that it is this protein which is the focus for immune attack in EAN. Since EAN mimics the human polyneuritis or Guillain-Barré disease, as stressed by Arnason (20), the P2 protein may have particular relevance to this human disease as well.

III. CHEMICAL PROPERTIES OF THE A1 AND P2 PROTEINS

The amino acid composition of the A1 protein is shown in Table 2. The three basic amino acids, lysine, histidine, and arginine, comprise approxi-

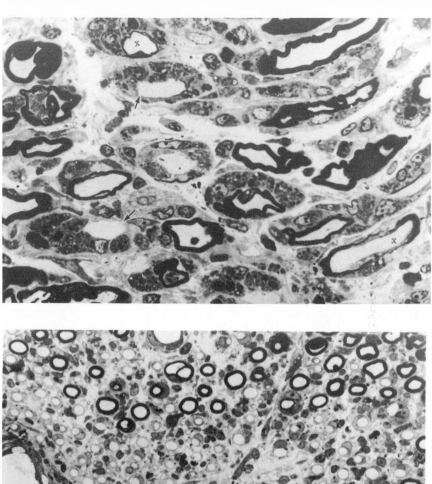

FIG. 4. The upper plate shows a typical acute lesion of the dorsal root ganglia of a monkey with EAN in which many myelin-loaded macrophages are seen next to naked axons *(arrows)* or partially demyelinated axons *(x)*. Epon section stained with toluidine blue, × 448 [after Wisniewski et al. (43)]. The lower plate shows a typical chronic lesion; a large perivascular demyelinated plaque in a monkey with EAN. The absence of myelin-loaded macrophages is noted. Two micron epon section stained with toluidine blue, × 280.

mately 25% of the total protein. There is a sizable percentage of proline and glycine, one tryptophan, two methionine, and no half-cystine residues. It is not a glycoprotein, and does not appear to contain any lipid.

TABLE 2. *Amino acid composition of the A1 protein and P2 proteins*

Amino acid	Moles %	
	Bovine A1	Rabbit P2
Lysine	7.65	10.8
Histidine	5.88	1.9
Arginine	10.59	5.9
Aspartic	6.47	8.3
Threonine	4.12	8.8
Serine	11.18	6.9
Glutamic	5.88	10.3
Proline	7.06	3.8
Glycine	14.71	10.8
Alanine	8.24	6.7
Valine	1.77	5.9
Methionine	1.20	1.6
Isoleucine	1.77	4.2
Leucine	5.88	7.3
Tyrosine	2.35	1.9
Phenylalanine	4.71	4.3
Tryptophan	0.59	0.8

The moles % for the bovine A1 protein are calculated from the amino acid sequence reported in reference 22; the analyses of the P2 protein are from ref. (6).

Unlike most globular proteins, particularly small basic molecules such as lysozyme, cytochrome *c,* and ribonuclease, the A1 protein has a highly unfolded conformation, with an axial ratio of approximately 10:1 in 0.3 M NaCl, as shown by viscosity studies (21). It is this observation that explained its unusual behavior on gel filtration, and suggested that its antigenic sites might, like those of unfolded synthetic polypeptides, be defined as small discreet regions of the polypeptide chain. The molecule contains no significant secondary structure, can be heated at 95°C for 1 hr or treated with 8 M urea, typical conditions for denaturing proteins, with no loss of immunologic activity (EAE induction or interaction with antibody); it is extremely labile in the presence of very small amounts of proteolytic enzymes. These data show that the A1 molecule is essentially "denatured" or unfolded, as it is isolated. Thus the properties of the A1 molecule are essentially maintained in derived peptides.

The amino acid composition of the P2 protein is compared with the A1 protein in Table 2. Although both proteins are basic, the ratio of lysine, histidine, and arginine differs markedly as do the glutamic and proline residues. The P2 protein appears to be a unique, single polypeptide chain of 12,000 molecular weight (6) with an unknown conformation. By analogy to the A1 protein, with its lack of cyst(e)ine, it might be suspected that the P2 protein also is highly unfolded. It does, however, appear to have some secondary structure, possibly as much as 50% β-structure as shown by comparison with polylysine (6).

Since the A1 molecule is highly unfolded, its amino acid sequence assumes special significance by analogy with synthetic polypeptides. The complete amino sequence of bovine and human A1 proteins was determined by the Edman degradation method (22) using isolated tryptic and peptic digests (Fig. 5). Unlike the histones, where basic and nonpolar residues are segregated into different portions of the molecule, there is a fairly general distribution of these residues in the A1 protein. In view of its unfolded conformation, this suggests that the protein is designed for maximal interaction with other myelin components. At least some of this interaction must be in the form of electrostatic bonding to the negatively charged groups on the myelin lipids. Palmer and Dawson (24) have shown that the A1 protein interacts with phosphoinositides, and recent studies by London et al. (25) have demonstrated preferential cerebroside sulfate-A1 protein interaction.

In addition to its unusual composition, myelin differs from most cellular membranes in having a smooth, unpitted surface produced by freeze-etching techniques. The absence of strongly basic proteins from plasma membranes, in general, suggests that the A1 protein might be responsible in part for the less complex myelin structure. Are there features of the A1 protein sequence which relate specifically to its role as a major structural protein in addition to its general basic character? A region exists near the midpoint of the molecule which has rare structural features that may directly subserve the role of the A1 protein in the myelin membrane. First, the A1 protein is the only known protein that can serve as an acceptor for the polypeptide N-acetylgalactosaminyl transferase (from submaxillary glands); the enzyme glycosylates the A1 protein giving a ^{14}C-N-acetylgalactosamine-A1 protein product (26). Two radioactive peptides were eventually isolated which showed that the single threonine residue at position 98 was the target for the reaction.

The question arises whether the A1 protein, which contains no sugar when isolated, is glycosylated at some stage during myelin formation and then

```
              ( )                        (His-Gly)                      Thr
N-Ac-Ala-Ser-Ala-Gln-Lys-Arg-Pro-Ser-Gln-Arg-Ser-Lys-Tyr-Leu-Ala-Ser-Ala-Ser-Thr-Met-
              ( )       5                (His-Gly)               15        Thr    20

                                                                        Ile
Asp-His-Ala-Arg-His-Gly-Phe-Leu-Pro-Arg-His-Arg-Asp-Thr-Gly-Ile-Leu-Asp-Ser-Leu-Gly-Arg-
              25              30              35                        Ile

          Gly                                      Ser
Phe-Phe-Gly-Ser-Asp-Arg-Gly-Ala-Pro-Lys-Arg-Gly-Ser-Gly-Lys-Asp-Gly-His-His-Ala-Ala-Arg-
          45              50              52              60
    Ala                                   Ser ( )
Thr-Thr-His-Tyr-Gly-Ser-Leu-Pro-Gln-Lys-Ala-Gln-Gly-His-Arg-Pro-Gln-Asp-Glu-Asn-Pro-
65                   70                   Ser ( )          80                   85

Val-Val-His-Phe-Phe-Lys-Asn-Ile-Val-Thr-Pro-Arg-Thr-Pro-Pro-Pro-Ser-Gln-Gly-Lys-Gly
              90                   95              100                   105
                                                      Arg
Arg-Gly-Leu-Ser-Leu-Ser-Arg-Phe-Ser-Trp-Gly-Ala-Glu-Gly-Gln-Lys-Pro-Gly-Phe-Gly-Tyr-
    Thr-Val              115              120                   125

                                              Phe         Val
Gly-Gly-Arg-Ala-Ser-Asp-Tyr-Lys-Ser-Ala-His-Lys-Gly-Leu-Lys-Gly-His-Asp-Ala-Gln-Gly-Thr-
    130         Ala         135              140              Ala 145

Leu-Ser-Lys-Ile-Phe-Lys-Leu-Gly-Gly-Arg-Asp-Ser-Arg-Ser-Gly-Ser-Pro-Met-Ala-Arg-Arg-COOH
150              Leu    155              160              165                   170
```

FIG. 5. The complete amino acid sequence of the bovine A1 protein is shown with the substitutions occurring in the human and rabbit A1 proteins shown above and below the bovine sequence respectively. The human and bovine sequences were determined by Edman degradation of tryptic and peptic peptides (22, 22a); the rabbit sequence was obtained by comparison of tryptic peptides (7).

deglycosylated. There are a few proteins in addition to mucins in which the GalNAc-threonine moiety exists naturally, most notably in rabbit IgG; as in the A1 protein, the key threonine residue resides in a sequence rich in proline, which suggests that the amino acid sequence of this peptide segment forms a site universally recognized by the transferase in these proteins as well as in many mucin-type glycoproteins, including membrane glycoproteins. A three-dimensional model of this region of the A1 molecule shows that conformational restrictions imposed by the four proline residues (res. 96–101) induce a sharp bend. Thus the A1 molecule can be reasonably represented, not by a random coil, but by an open double-chain structure as shown schematically in Fig. 6.

Another unusual feature of this region is the presence of a modified arginine residue at position 107. This residue exists in approximately 20%

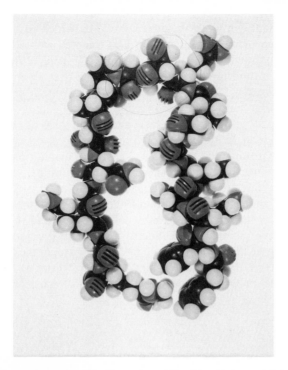

FIG. 6. A possible conformation for the region of the A1 protein containing the proline-rich region and the methylarginine locus at position 107 *(large arrow):* Phe-Phe-Lys-Asn-Ile-Val-Thr-Pro-Arg-Thr-Pro-Pro-Pro-Ser-Gln-Gly-Lys-Gly-Arg (Methyl). The two phenylalanine side chains occur directly across from the methylarginine residue in this conformation.

of the molecules as dimethylarginine; in most of the rest, it exists as mono-methylarginine. We isolated these arginine derivatives from the A1 protein following digestion with pronase and leucine aminopeptidase (27); our results were confirmed later by Baldwin et al. (28). The peptide linkage containing the dimethylarginine appears to be trypsin resistant; several tryptic peptides were isolated from this region in which the methylated Arg-Gly linkage was intact (22). These methylated derivatives may be an important structural feature since they appear in all mammalian A1 proteins as well as in chicken and turtle A1 proteins (27). Since methylation makes the arginine residue 107 more energetically acceptable for a nonpolar environment, it is possible that this residue interacts cross-chain with the two phenylalanine residues brought into proximity by the proline-rich bend (Fig. 6), or that it interacts with lipids of the myelin membrane.

A logical model can be formulated for myelin which reasonably incorporates the known properties of myelin and the A1 protein and proteolipid components as shown in Fig. 7. Caspar and Kirshner (29) have shown by X-ray diffraction and neutron-scattering studies that myelin fits closely to the classical Davson-Danielli concept in which protein and water appear to be located external to the bimolecular leaflet of lipid. The hydrophilic A1 protein is most probably, therefore, located on the outer side of the membrane where it can interact electrostatically with the negatively charged lipid phosphate groups and sulfatides. There are, in addition, five regions of eight to 10 residues that lack positively charged groups, which could conceivably reach into the deeper nonpolar lipid region. The proteolipid, however, is a more ideal membrane-type protein in the terminology of Singer; based on its size (23,000 molecular weight) and the lack of pits in the freeze-etching pictures of myelin, it is likely that it extends partially into the bimolecular leaflet, when it can interact hydrophobically. No protein appears to extend through the leaflet the way it does in the erythrocyte membrane. The proposed model is energetically feasible. The extrinsic

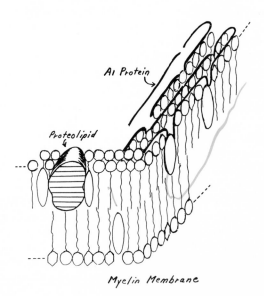

FIG. 7. A schematic model of CNS myelin is shown in which the proteolipid and the A1 protein are positioned within the framework of the bimolecular leaflet. The proteolipid is shown as an internal, compact protein in the convention of Singer where it interacts hydrophobically with lipids within the leaflet into which it extends deeply. The A1 protein is shown as an external protein in its open, double-chain conformation interacting mainly with charged groups of the lipid membrane.

nature of the A1 molecule is indicated by its ease of extraction with strong salt solutions, its role in EAE, and its interaction with antibody while in intact myelin. The A1 protein is thus very different from the conventional types of membrane proteins, such as the proteolipids. Its major role may be, in fact, to stabilize the myelin membrane by preventing the fluidity that is now recognized as an important feature of plasma membranes. Such a role for the A1 protein would be most compatible with the role of myelin as a static insulator of the axon. It is probable that in peripheral nerve myelin the A1 and P2 proteins serve the same function since the ratio of these proteins varies so markedly in comparison to myelin from various animal species (Fig. 2).

IV. IMMUNOLOGICAL STUDIES WITH THE A1 PROTEIN AND A1 PEPTIDES

The available immunologic data strongly support the concept that EAE and EAN are not mediated by antibodies, but by sensitized cells, possibly the T lymphocytes. It was found from the studies of Johnson et al. (30) that the injection of A1 protein is followed by sensitization of lymphocytes in the appropriate lymph node. It is probable that these cells migrate to the brain and release factors upon encounter with the A1 protein which call in and activate macrophages, the cells responsible for demyelination. Wisniewski and co-workers (31) have found that demyelination of peripheral nerves does occur in the rabbit during the course of the nonfatal, chronic EAE which is more typical in the rabbit than the more acute, fatal response seen in many species. This suggests that peripheral nerve involvement will occur in EAE if the animal survives long enough. This finding is reconciled by our finding that peripheral myelin contains the A1 protein (7).

These studies have shown that the Schwann cell is probably not a focus of immunopathologic attack in EAE in the rabbit since remyelination eventually occurs. The macrophages which strip myelin from segments of the axons do not attack the plasma membrane of these cells (20), suggesting either that the plasma membrane does not contain the A1 protein or that it is present in masked form. This is supported by preliminary data using fluorescent antibody techniques, which show a marked fluorescence in peripheral nerve myelin with the antibody to the A1 protein, but none in Schwann cells.

Our strategy in characterizing the A1 protein has emphasized peptides derived either from chemical or enzymatic cleavage of peptide bands (32). One of the best enzymes for this purpose is bovine cathepsin D, which shows a marked preference for cleavage at Phe-Phe linkages. In the A1 protein, however, hydrolysis occurs only at Phe-Phe linkage at res. 43–44 and not at res. 89–90, indicating that the latter is protected or masked (33). This action of cathepsin D, therefore, yields two peptides only, referred to as CD1 and CD2, which were purified by fractionation on Cellex P and have proven useful for immunological studies.

Peptide CD1, containing residues 1–43, contains a major antigenic site since it displaces 80% of the ^{125}I-labeled A1 protein from rabbit antibody in the radioimmune assay based on the Farr procedure (33). Although the avidity of CD1 is much less than that of A1 (about 50 times the concentration required for 50% displacement of label), use of labeled CD1 showed that the activity was intrinsic and not due to an impurity. Peptide CD1 was only slightly less active than A1 protein in displacing the labeled peptide for antibody. As discussed later, Peptide CD1 also has a minor site which is slightly encephalitogenic in monkeys (see Table 3).

TABLE 3. *Peptides from the A1 protein having immunogenic activity*

Peptide	Residues	Activity
CD1	1–43	Antigenic site for rabbit antibody. Minor encephalitogenic site active in the monkey.
T18	116–122	Major encephalitogenic site in guinea pigs and rabbits.
SP	116–122 (synthetic)	Encephalitogenic in guinea pigs and rabbits, not in monkeys.
R	43–89	Encephalitogenic in rats and rabbits, very weakly in monkeys, not in guinea pigs.
L	1–116	Antigenic site for antibody.
T	117–170	Highly encephalitogenic in monkeys, but not in guinea pigs.
P14	133–170	Major encephalitogenic site active in monkeys.

Our major goal in these studies has been to localize and define the encephalitogenic regions of the A1 protein. In 1968 (34), we found for the first time that a 14-residue peptic peptide (Peptide E) from the region of the single tryptophan possessed the capacity to induce EAE identical in all ways to that induced by the A1 protein. This result strongly suggested that lymphocytes sensitized to Peptide E were able to respond to this same peptide region within the A1 molecule, further supporting the concept that the protein assumes a highly unfolded structure such that the conformation of a peptide region within the intact molecule is essentially maintained in the peptide. However, we cannot assume that the conformation of the A1 protein in solution is necessarily similar to that in the myelin membrane, although it is obvious that the tryptophan region in the A1 molecule of intact myelin must be both accessible and of similar conformation to the isolated A1 protein and Peptide E since each of these is capable of eliciting EAE. The sensitized lymphocytes mediating the disease show strict requirements for the arrangement of amino acids in the tryptophan region as shown by studies of a series of synthetic polypeptides (35). In this study, we first found that the minimum length of the encephalitogenic tryptophan region was nine residues as found in the tryptic peptide T18 (res. 114–122) as shown in Table 3. Removal of the COOH-terminal Lys or the NH_2-terminal Phe from the nonapeptide leads to inactivation (36). The lysine residue appears essential because it cannot be replaced, except by arginine (which occurs naturally in the human A1 protein sequence), which suggests that a basic residue must be present at position 122 for encephalitogenic activity. The COOH-terminal phenylalanine is not essential, since it can be replaced by valine, which suggests that the amino group must not approach too closely to the essential tryptophan residue (36).

A large group of synthetic polypeptides were synthesized by the Merrifield technique to ascertain the specific residue requirements for disease induction. In summary, at least three residues (35) appear crucial over the nine-residue span: tryptophan, glutamine, and the basic residue (lysine or arginine). These residues cannot be replaced without serious loss of activity. The glutamine residue (#121) cannot be deamidated, in fact, without inactivation.

There is abundant evidence that the nonapeptide tryptophan region is the major encephalitogenic site active in the guinea pig (12). The isolated or synthesized peptide is approximately equal to the A1 protein on a molar basis in its ability to induce EAE. The A1 molecule becomes virtually nonencephalitogenic when the single tryptophan residue is modified by reaction (37) with 2-hydroxy-5-nitrobenzyl bromide (HNB-A1 protein). As shown in Fig. 8, amino acid analyses of the A1 proteins from many mammalian species showed virtually no alteration in the sequence of this region, with the exception of the permissible replacement of lysine with arginine; all of these proteins show equal encephalitogenic activity when tested in the guinea pig. The only exception to this constancy of sequence and encephalitogenic activity was found in the chicken A1 protein where histidine replaces the essential glutamine as shown in Fig. 8; the A1 protein from this species is nonencephalitogenic on a clinical basis and produces only minor histological signs of EAE. Thus the correlation between amino acid sequence in the tryptophan region and activity established with the synthetic peptides is preserved on a phylogenetic basis.

Further evidence that the tryptophan region is the major encephalito-

Phylogenetic Variation in the Tryptophan Region of the A1 Protein

Species	Sequence of Tryptic Peptide T19
Bovine, Rabbit, Guinea Pig, Horse, Monkey, Pig, Sheep, Dog	Phe⊥Ser–Trp–Gly–Ala–Glu–Gly–Gln– Lys – Pro–Gly–Phe–Gly–Tyr⊥Gly–Gly–Arg
Human, Rat	Phe–Ser–Trp–Gly–Ala–Glu–Gly–Gln– Arg –Pro–Gly– etc.
Chicken	Phe–Ser–Trp–Gly–Gly–Glu–Gly– His – Lys – Pro– [3 Gly, Tyr, Ser, Phe] – Lys

FIG. 8. The amino acid sequence of the tryptophan region is shown for various animal species. Only in the sequence of the chicken peptide are significant changes found, particular His for Gln (#121). Only the chicken peptide is relatively nonencephalitogenic in the guinea pig.

genic site active in guinea pigs comes from data on Peptides L (res. 1–116) and T (117–170). These peptides are derived from the A1 protein (32) by the action of BNPS-skatole, an oxidizing agent, which cleaves the COOH-tryptophanyl peptide linkage at high concentration. These peptides were isolated in high yield and purity by chromatography on a Cellex-P column (32). As expected, these peptides are virtually nonencephalitogenic. It must be noted that each peptide, however, does induce a cell-mediated response as shown on the delayed-type skin test. Thus it appears that other immunogenic sites *do exist* in the A1 molecule but which are not encephalitogenic. Bergstrand (38), using the migration inhibiting factor (MIF) test, demonstrated in this regard several immunogenic sites in the A1 molecule. His data confirm our earlier studies with the T and L peptides, and with the HNB-A1 protein, the latter being nonencephalitogenic but nonetheless fully capable of eliciting cell-mediated immunity equal to the A1 protein as shown by the MIF test, and the release of lymphokines from lymphocytes of preimmunized guinea pigs (39).

The picture that emerges from our immunologic studies with the nonapeptide and the HNB-A1 protein suggests that, although many sites are present in the A1 molecule which elicit cell-mediated immunity, only the nonapeptide region is active in the guinea pig since it is this site alone in the intact myelin which is able to interact with sensitized lymphocytes mediating the disease. Direct evidence (40) was found for the identical conformation of the tryptophan region in the peptide and in the intact A1 molecule; lymphocytes from animals immunized with the nonapeptide respond to the A1 protein as shown by uptake of ^{3}H-thymidine and release of lymphokine. Since antibody to the nonapeptide was not found, these results provide additional strong data that EAE is mediated by sensitized lymphocytes (probably T lymphocytes) rather than antibody.

The remarkable encephalitogenic activity of the tryptophan region does not extend broadly across species, however. It is a potent inducer of EAE in rabbits as well as guinea pigs as shown by the activity of the tryptic peptide T18, but it is inactive in monkeys (17). We have lately emphasized studies on EAE induction in rhesus monkeys because it is likely that the disease-inducing site(s) would be most relevant to human demyelinating diseases. The first clue that the tryptophan region was inconsequential in the monkey came from the undiminished activity of the HNB-A1 protein. The major disease-inducing site active in the monkey was localized in Peptide T, a 53-residue peptide (Table 3). This site was further delineated by the finding that peptic Peptide P14, a 35-residue peptide from the COOH-terminal region, was *as active* on a molar basis as the A1 protein. Peptide P14 must contain, therefore, the major encephalitogenic site active in the monkey, and is at least 10-fold more active than Peptide CD1 and also Peptide R (res. 44–89), a peptide which has been claimed to have mild activity in the monkey and the rabbit (41). A species variation exists, therefore, in response to encephalitogenic determinants, and may be a reflection of species differences in both the immune response and/or the ultrastructure of myelin. The disease-inducing site in the monkey does assume special significance with regard to human demyelinating diseases, particularly since we have now shown that EAE can be permanently suppressed in monkeys with either the A1 protein (42) or Peptide T even after severe clinical signs have appeared.

REFERENCES

1. Inoue, T., Deshmukh, D., and Pieringer, R.: *J. Biol. Chem.*, 246:5688 (1971).
2. Kurihara, T., and Tsukada, Y.: *J. Neurochem.*, 15:827 (1968).
3. Autilio, L., Norton, W., and Terry, R.: *J. Neurochem.*, 11:17 (1964).
4. Eylar, E. H.: In: *Functional and Structural Proteins of the Nervous System*, edited by A. Davison, P. Mandel, and I. Morgan. Plenum Press, New York, pp. 215–240 (1972).
5. Wolfgram, F., and Kotorii, K.: *J. Neurochem.*, 15:1281 (1968).
6. Brostoff, S., Burnett, P., Lampert, P., and Eylar E.: *Nature New Biol.*, 235:210 (1972).
7. Brostoff, S., and Eylar, E. H.: *Arch. Biochem. Biophys.*, 153:590 (1972).
8. Wolfgram, F., and Kotorii, K.: *J. Neurochem.*, 15:1291 (1968).
9. Greenfield, S., Brostoff, S., Eylar, E. H., and Morell, P.: *J. Neurochem.*, 20:1207 (1973).
10. Nakao, A., Davis, W., and Einstein, E. R.: *Biochim. Biophys. Acta*, 130:163 (1966).
11. Laatsch, R., Kies, M., Gordon, S., and Alvord, E.: *J. Exp. Med.*, 115:777 (1962).

12. Eylar, E. H.: In: *Multiple Sclerosis,* edited by F. Wolfgram, G. Ellison, J. Stevens, and J. Andrews, Academic Press, New York, pp. 449–486 (1972).
13. Eylar, E. H., Salk, J., Beveridge, G., and Brown, L.: *Arch. Biochem. Biophys.,* 132:34 (1969).
14. Oshiro, Y., and Eylar, E. H.: *Arch. Biochem. Biophys.,* 138:392 (1970).
15. Martenson, R., Deibler, G., and Kies, M.: *Biochem. Biophys. Acta,* 200:353 (1970).
16. Hashim, G., and Eylar, E. H.: *Arch. Biochem. Biophys.,* 129:635 (1969).
17. Jackson, J., Brostoff, S., Lampert, P., and Eylar, E. H.: *Neurobiology,* 2:83 (1972).
18. Paterson, P. Y.: *J. Exp. Med.,* 111:119 (1960).
19. Wisniewski, H., Prineas, J., and Raine, C.: *Lab. Invest.,* 21:105 (1969).
20. Arnason, B., Asbury, A., Astrom, K., and Adams, R.: *Trans Amer. Neurol. Assoc.,* 93:133 (1968).
21. Eylar, E. H., and Thompson, M.: *Arch. Biochem. Biophys.,* 129:468 (1969).
22. Eylar, E. H., Brostoff, S., Hashim, G., Caccam, J., and Burnett, P.: *J. Biol. Chem.,* 246: 5770 (1971).
22a. Eylar, E. H.: *Proc. Nat. Acad. Sci.,* 67:1425 (1970).
23. Carnegie, P.: *Biochem. J.,* 123:57 (1971).
24. Palmer, F., and Dawson, R.: *Biochem. J.,* 111:629 (1969).
25. London, I.: *Biochem. Biophys. Acta,* in press.
26. Hagopian, A., Whitehead, J., and Eylar, E.: *J. Biol. Chem.,* 246:2519 (1971).
27. Brostoff, S., and Eylar, E. H.: *Proc. Nat. Acad. Sci.,* 68:765 (1971).
28. Baldwin, G., and Carnegie, P.: *Biochem. J.,* 123:69 (1971).
29. Kirchner, D., and Caspar, D.: *Ann. N.Y. Acad. Sci.,* 195:309 (1972).
30. Johnson, A., Wisniewski, H., Raine, C., Eylar, E., and Terry, R.: *Proc. Nat. Acad. Sci.,* 68:2694 (1971).
31. Wisniewski, H., Terry, R., Whitaker, J., Cook, S., and Dowling, P.: *Arch. Neurol.,* 21:269 (1969).
32. Burnett, P., and Eylar, E. H.: *J. Biol. Chem.,* 246:3425 (1971).
33. Brostoff, S., and Eylar, E. H.: *Biochemistry, in press.*
34. Eylar, E. H., and Hashim, G.: *Proc. Nat. Acad. Sci.,* 61:644 (1968).
35. Eylar, E. H., Caccam, J., Jackson, J., and Robinson, A.: *Science,* 168:1220 (1970).
36. Westall, F., Robinson, A., Caccam, J., Jackson, J., and Eylar, E. H.: *Nature,* 168:1220 (1970).
37. Eylar, E. H., and Hashim, G.: *Arch. Biochem. Biophys.,* 131:215 (1969).
38. Bergstrand, H.: *Eur. J. Biochem,* 21:116 (1971).
39. Spitler, L., von Muller, C., Fudenberg, H., and Eylar, E. H.: *J. Exp. Med.,* 136:156 (1972).
40. Bailey, P., and Eylar, E. H.: *To be published.*
41. Kibler, R., Re, P., McKneally, S., and Keeling, M.: *J. Biol. Chem.,* 247:969 (1972).
42. Eylar, E. H., Jackson, J., Rothenberg, B., and Brostoff, S.: *Nature,* 236:74 (1972).
43. Wisniewski, H., Brostoff, S., Carter, H., and Eylar, E. H.: *Lab. Invest., in press.*

Proteins of the Nervous System
Raven Press, New York © 1973

Proteolipids

Jordi Folch-Pi

I. INTRODUCTION

During the development of a method for the extraction and purification of lipids from the central nervous system (Folch, Ascoli, Lees, Meath, and LeBaron, 1951), it was observed that a chloroform:methanol (CM) mixture (2:1 v/v) extracted some protein material from central nervous system (Folch and Lees, 1951). This material was not removed from the extract upon repeated washing with water. Its presence was noted when the extract was taken to dryness by evaporation of the solvents, and the re-sulting residue proved to be only partly soluble in the CM mixture that had been used in the original extraction of the tissue. The portion of the residue that was insoluble in CM was also found to be insoluble in water and in all of a large number of aqueous solutions and organic solvents that were tested. The insoluble material contained 14% N, 1.76% S, and between 0.2 and 0.4% P. Upon adequate acid hydrolysis, more than 91% of its N could be recovered chromatographically as free amino acids, i.e., the insoluble material was mainly protein in nature.

It was assumed that this protein material was extracted from the tissue as a protein-lipid complex, and that the latter moiety conferred to the com-plex its characteristic lipid-like solubility in CM mixtures and insolubility in water. The only protein-lipid complexes described prior to that time had been blood plasma lipoproteins, which were soluble in water and destroyed or dissociated by organic solvents. To emphasize the marked difference in solubility properties between plasma lipoproteins and the recently dis-covered brain protein-lipid complexes, the latter were designated as *proteo-lipids*.

The amino acid composition of proteolipids is rather unusual, with a high content of sulfur and nonpolar amino acids, and a comparatively low content of acidic and basic amino acids (Table 1). Proteolipids proved to be resistant to the usual animal proteolytic enzymes. They are extracted from tissues by CM 2:1, v/v, mixtures in amounts which are consistent for comparable tissue samples. A subsequent extraction with the same solvent mixture fails to yield additional amounts of proteolipids, i.e., the extrac-tion appears to be quantitative in the first extraction. Alternatively, the

45

absence of additional proteolipids in second and subsequent extracts might indicate an "insolubilization" of any possible unextracted proteolipids by the changes brought about by the first extraction:dehydration, the removal of lipids and many small molecule solutes, etc.

TABLE 1. *Amino acid composition of proteolipid apoprotein (PLA) from different tissues*

		Tissue and PLA preparation						
		Central gray matter		Heart		Liver		Kidney
Amino acid	Central white matter	71-VII	72-VI	72-III	72-VII	72-V	72-IX	72-IV
			(Moles/100 moles recovered in hydrolysate)					
Arginine	2.6	2.39	2.62	2.41	3.26	3.34	3.15	2.99
Histidine	1.8	1.65	1.90	1.91	1.61	1.73	1.48	1.82
Lysine	3.8	3.86	3.70	3.31	3.26	3.90	3.08	3.80
Aspartic	4.0	4.78	4.84	6.29	6.78	6.12	6.57	5.98
Glutamic	5.8	6.07	5.76	5.22	5.69	6.03	5.70	5.69
Half Cystine	4.0	2.39	1.74	–	0.36	0.27	0.80	–
Methionine	1.9	2.39	2.78	5.35	4.65	3.90	3.68	3.94
Serine	8.5	5.61	5.70	6.03	6.29	6.03	6.76	6.21
Threonine	8.5	7.54	7.36	6.69	6.67	5.85	6.30	5.98
Proline	2.8	3.86	4.52	5.29	4.96	5.48	5.43	5.25
Glycine	10.3	10.58	10.23	8.90	9.11	9.09	9.44	9.71
Alanine	12.5	12.06	12.04	10.05	10.28	10.02	10.38	10.80
Valine	6.9	7.27	7.15	5.82	6.11	6.87	6.69	6.58
Leucine	11.1	11.60	11.88	14.59	13.09	14.20	13.60	14.09
Isoleucine	4.9	5.71	5.60	7.50	6.60	6.40	6.43	6.86
Tyrosine	4.6	4.69	4.58	3.41	3.67	3.53	3.47	3.43
Phenylalanine	7.9	7.54	7.55	7.23	7.15	7.24	7.03	6.86

The amount of proteolipids in extracts may be estimated in a number of ways: 1) by determining the amount of solutes that become insoluble in CM upon removal of the solvents by vacuum distillation; this procedure must be repeated three times, if a quantitative result is sought; 2) by estimating total protein (by one of its modifications); 3) by estimating the amount of amino acids released by acid hydrolysis, and computing from it the amount of protein by the use of an empirical factor (Folch and Lees, 1951). 4) For the purposes of monitoring the presence of proteolipids, the extinction coefficient at 278 nm provides an indicator which is fairly quantitative, especially for comparative purposes, and which has the advantage of simplicity and sensitivity.

II. DISTRIBUTION OF PROTEOLIPIDS

Although especially abundant in central nervous tissue, proteolipids are present in a wide variety of animal and vegetable tissues. Bovine tissues were found to contain the following amounts of proteolipid protein (mg/g fresh tissue weight): heart, 3.5; kidney, 2.0; lung, 0.95; skeletal muscle (biceps), 0.4; smooth muscle (uterus), 0.6. In spinach chloroplasts proteolipids represent 2 to 4% dry weight (Zill and Harmon, 1961). All values reported are only indicative, because the yields obtained may often have been incomplete.

In the central nervous system proteolipids are especially abundant in brain white matter, where they have been shown to be mainly myelin components (Autilio, 1966). They are absent or present in very small amounts in fetal brain (Folch, 1955), and their appearance and progressive accumulation is concurrent with myelination.

In a study of 28 anatomical areas of the human nervous system, Amaducci (1962) observed marked and consistent differences from one anatomical area to another (Table 2). The highest concentration was found in corpus callosum and centrum ovale, where proteolipids constitute 2.5 to 2.8% of fresh tissue weight. In cerebral gray matter they are present in one-fifth to one-tenth their concentration in brain white matter. In spinal cord,

TABLE 2. *Distribution of proteolipids in the human nervous system*

Cerebral white matter		Cerebral cortex	
Corpus callosum	24.0	frontal	2.6–3.3
Corona radiata		sensorimotor	4.1–4.7
anterior	24.0	parietal, inferior	2.1–2.4
posterior	24.0	temporal	2.4–2.9
Cerebellar white		occipital	5.4–6.0
matter	21.0	Cerebellar cortex	3.6–4.8
Optic pathway,		Caudate	5.9
mainly chiasm	18.6	Pulvinar	8.1
Spinal cord		Thalamus	11.6–14.1
anterolateral columns		Mesencephalon	15.8
cervical	16.0	Pons	18.9
thoracic	12.9–14.8	Medulla oblongata	16.5
lumbar and sacral	7.5–10.9	Vermis cerebelli	8.6
posterior columns		Anterior spinal roots	3.3–4.5
cervical	15.3	Posterior spinal roots	4.5
thoracic	13.2	Sciatic nerve	1.1
lumbar and sacral	14.5	Brachial plexus	0.3

Results expressed as mg proteolipid protein/g fresh tissue.
From L. Amaducci (1962).

proteolipids exhibit a rostrocaudal decrease in concentration, and in peripheral nerve they are present at very small concentrations. Hence, although in central white matter they are mainly myelin components, their concentration does not exactly parallel the concentration of myelin, an observation that suggests that the protein composition of myelin shows quantitative differences in various anatomical areas.

Proteolipids in the central nervous system are found in structures other than myelin (Lapetina, Soto, and de Robertis, 1968). In heart muscle they are mainly components of mitochondria (Joel, Karnovsky, Ball, and Cooper, 1958; Murakami, Sekine, and Funahashi, 1962). Proteolipids have generally been found in association with membranous structures. It is therefore justified to think of them principally as membrane components.

III. STUDY OF CENTRAL WHITE MATTER PROTEOLIPIDS

In brain white matter, proteolipids represent almost exclusively myelin protein. Indeed, with the isolation of myelin it was found that myelin was soluble in CM (Laatsch, 1963; Autilio, Norton, and Terry, 1964), and it was inferred that all central myelin protein was proteolipid. However, a number of observations soon indicated that the solubility of myelin in CM was misleading and that proteins other than proteolipids were present in myelin. Thus, Lees (1968) demonstrated that CM will dissolve proteins other than proteolipids when brain tissue homogenates are freed of diffusable electrolytes. Also, it was known that isolated myelin produced allergic encephalomyelitis when injected into animals with the necessary adjuvants, indicating that myelin contained the antigenic protein (Laatsch, 1963). Since this was known to be a basic protein that was quite different from proteolipids, it was clear that myelin contained at least the antigenic basic protein in addition to classical proteolipids. This and other observations have shown that myelin contains at least three types of protein: 1) the classical proteolipids of Folch and Lees (1951), 2) the antigenic basic protein responsible for the experimental allergic encephalomyelitis, and 3) the proteolipid of Wolfgram (1966), which is quite different from the classical proteolipid of Folch and Lees.

These three proteins can be separated from isolated myelin by a very simple method that has been developed in our laboratory by Gonzalez-Sastre (1970). The method is based on the observations that Wolfgram's proteolipid is insoluble in neutral CM mixtures, and that the encephalitogenic basic protein is insoluble in CM in the presence of electrolytes. In this method, myelin isolated by one of the standard methods of subcellular fractionation is dissolved in CM. The solution is then centrifuged at approximately $1,000 \times g$ for 10 min or until clear. The small amount of insoluble residue collected represents 2 to 3% of the dry weight of myelin, i.e., 10 to 15% of the total protein present. The supernatant is then diluted by addition of 5% of its volume of 0.5 M KCl, and the precipitate formed is collected by centrifugation. We thus have divided myelin into three fractions: the original CM fraction (I), the subsequent fraction insoluble in CM:KCl mixture (II), and the final supernatant (III). These three fractions have been analyzed both chemically and by polyacrylamide gel electrophoresis. Fraction I has the electrophoretic mobility and the amino acid composition of Wolfgram's proteolipid; II has the mobility and the amino acid composition of the basic antigenic protein; and III has a mobility and amino acid composition indistinguishable from those of the classical proteolipids. The respective amounts of these three fractions as percent of total myelin protein are Wolfgram's proteolipid: 15 to 17%; basic protein: 30%; classical proteolipids: 50 to 55%. These values are consistent with results obtained by other researchers using different methods (Eng, Chao, Gerstl, Pratt, and Tavaststjerna, 1968).

A large amount of work has gone not only into the purification of proteolipids proper, i.e., the separation of the protein-lipid complex from adventitious lipids, but also into the preparation of the protein moiety free of lipids, i.e., the proteolipid apoprotein. Proteolipids can be concentrated by solvent fractionation, by differential centrifugation, by dialysis in organic solvents, by gel permeation, or by a combination of these procedures. The specific procedures that have been developed are 1) the "fluff" method of Folch and Lees (1951), which was first used for the separation of proteolipid-enriched fractions from the tissue CM extract. The extract is overlaid with at least fivefold its volume of water. Eventually, a "fluff" accumulates at the interface, which can be collected by freezing. From this fluff, by solvent fractionation, two preparations are obtained, proteolipids A and B. Proteolipid C is obtained from the chloroformic solution underlying the fluff by solvent fractionation. 2) The emulsion-centrifugation procedure (Folch, Webster, and Lees, 1959) is based on the difference between the specific gravity of protein and that of lipids. The lipid and proteolipid mixture recovered from a washed lipid extract is emulsified in 30-fold its weight of water; by centrifugation, proteolipids are collected quantitatively at the bottom (crude proteolipid), leaving the majority of lipids in emulsion in the supernatant. A "concentrated proteolipid" preparation is obtained from the pellet by solvent fractionation. 3) Free lipids diffuse through the dialysis membrane in organic solvents, whereas the proteolipids are retained. At the completion of dialysis, the retentate contains proteolipids freed of the greater part of lipids. 4) In gel permeation, as in dialysis, the proteolipids are separated from free lipids because of their larger molecular size. Using polystyrene gel, Autilio (1966) was able to separate proteolipids from isolated myelin. Later, Mokrasch (1967) obtained a highly enriched preparation of proteolipids by combining precipitation with ethyl ether with permeation on Sephadex LH20. Finally, Soto, Pasquini, Placido, and La Torre (1969) used Sephadex LH20 in the purification of proteolipids from white and gray matter. They were able to separate a distinct fraction from the latter which exhibited many of the properties postulated for an acetylcholine receptor, and for which the function of physiological receptor is being claimed (de Robertis, Fiszer, and Soto, 1967).

Since these procedures were not always designed to yield proteolipids of the highest possible protein content, the different products obtained show a wide range of variation in lipid composition. The preparations with the highest protein content, obtained by dialysis or by gel permeation, still contain approximately 15% lipids or more. These lipids, which are the most firmly bound to the protein, are mainly, if not exclusively, phosphatidylserine, sulfatides, and polyphosphoinositides, i.e., they are acidic lipids. They appear to be bound to the protein moiety by ionic linkages. They can be removed in part by chromatography on silicic acid (Matsumoto, Matsumoto, and Folch-Pi, 1964) or on a Dowex 1-X2 (Mokrasch, 1967), both procedures yielding products with approximately 95% protein. To remove the lipids completely, however, it is necessary to submit the proteolipid to dialysis in CM acidified by the addition of concentrated HCl to a final HCl concentration of 0.04 N. A protein is then obtained which contains only traces of some lipids, with the exception of 2 to 4% covalently bound fatty acids (see below). This is the proteolipid apoprotein.

The chromatography of proteolipids on silicic acid has been carried out by Matsumoto et al., (1964) with preparations obtained by the emulsion-centrifugation procedure. Typical conditions are a 10-mm inner diameter column packed with 4 g of silicic acid and loaded with approximately 70 mg of a preparation containing 60% protein. The column is eluted with a discontinuous gradient of CM:H$_2$O mixtures of increasing polarity, starting at 85% choloform and ending with CM (1:1, v/v) containing 12% 0.05 N HCl. Free lipids appear at 85 and 75% chloroform, and three protein peaks appear at 75, 70, and 50% chloroform (acidified). No difference is found among the three protein peaks in amino acid composition and in the nature of the up to 5% lipids that each contains, which are mainly polyphosphoinositides.

The preparation of maximally delipidated apoprotein was first carried out by Tenenbaum and Folch-Pi (1966). It consisted in dialyzing a washed lipid extract against CM (2:1, v/v) for 7 days, with daily changes of the

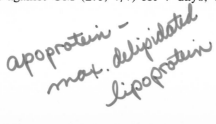

diffusate, followed by dialysis for 7 more days against CM:HCl (2:1:0.04 N) followed by dialysis against a series of outer phases in which water gradually replaced the organic solvents, until they were completely eliminated. The final retentate contained a "water-soluble proteolipid protein."

IV. PROPERTIES AND COMPOSITION OF CENTRAL WHITE MATTER PROTEOLIPIDS

The different proteolipid preparations obtained by the foregoing procedures are freely soluble in CM mixtures and insoluble in water and in aqueous solutions. In the biphasic system CM:H_2O (8:4:3, v/v), they will concentrate quantitatively in the lower chloroformic phase, and will be completely absent from the upper methanol:water phase (with the exception of the last protein peak eluted from silicic acid column; approximately one-fifth of the protein partitions into the upper phase). The retention of the original solubility properties throughout the gradual removal of lipids forces the conclusion that the characteristic solubilities of proteolipids must be explained in terms of the conformation of the protein moiety. Studies of some of these preparations by optical rotatory dispersion (ORD) show that proteolipids are characterized by a high content of α-helix which remains unchanged throughout the procedure of gradual delipidation (Sherman and Folch-Pi, 1970; Zand, 1968). Upon removal of the last traces of lipids, the resulting apoprotein is soluble in water, although still retaining its solubility in organic solvents. The newly acquired solubility in water is paralleled by a decrease of the α-helix content to below the detectable limits ($<10\%$), i.e., there is a conformational change which apparently makes available to the medium the hydrophilic groups of the protein which in the starting proteolipid must have been buried inside the molecular structure.

The solutions of proteolipids in CM (2:1, v/v) are quite stable; they keep for years without developing turbidity or precipitates, even at room temperature. They can be taken to dryness by evaporation of the solvent without loss of solubility of the proteolipids in the residue, provided the evaporation takes place at 40°C or lower, and provided no biphasic system develops in the course of the evaporation. The formation of a biphasic system results in partial or total insolubilization of the proteolipid protein unless corrected immediately by addition of the proper solvent (usually methanol). A similar result is obtained by exposing the proteolipid solution in a biphasic system to slight alkalinity in the presence of ions; for example, in the biphasic system CM:H_2O (8:4:3, v/v) at pH 8.8, proteolipids will become insoluble to an extent which is proportional to the logarithm of the ionic strength, between 0.001 and 1.0 M NaCl. The same result is obtained with Na_3 or K_3 citrate solution (Webster and Folch, 1961).

All proteolipid preparations are resistant to the action of pepsin, trypsin, papain, and erepsin. This resistance is not due to the presence of lipids, because it persists in the apoprotein. The only enzyme that attacks proteolipids is pronase, although the extent of this susceptibility has not been thoroughly explored. However, Lees, Messinger, and Burnham (1967) have reported that trypsin attacks proteolipids in the presence of Triton X-100.

The amino acid composition of the protein moiety of the various proteolipids appears to be the same in all preparations, whereas the lipid "moiety" varies according to the procedure of preparation. Fractionation by solvents, emulsion-centrifugation, permeation on Sephadex LH20, and dialysis in CM separate from the protein cholesterol the bulk of cerebrosides, sulfatides, and phospholipids; hence these lipids are bound to the protein, if at all, only by labile bonds that are easily disrupted. Most remaining phospholipids are removed by chromatography on silicic acid, leaving only polyphosphoinositides and small amounts of sulfatides. A similar removal of lipids is attained with Dowex 1×2, although no information is available on the exact nature of the lipids still remaining. Finally, the highest degree of delipidation is obtained with dialysis in CM:HCl, which proves that the most tightly bound lipids must be bound through ionic linkages.

The composition of the different preparations, up to and including the apoprotein, shows that the amino acid pattern of proteolipids is not affected by the previous procedures of purification. The amino acid pattern has the following characteristics: 1) There is a relative scarcity of basic and acidic amino acids; arginine, lysine, and histidine account jointly for less than 10% of amino acids in the hydrolysate, and aspartic and glutamic amount jointly to approximately 10%. 2) There is a relative abundance of the so-called nonpolar amino acids, i.e., amino acids that, when combined in a peptide chain, offer only nonpolar groups to the medium; leucine, isoleucine, valine, glycine, proline, phenylalanine, and alanine amount to 57 to 58% of amino acids. If tryptophan is added, about 60% of amino acids are nonpolar. The relatively high concentration of tryptophan is indicated by the high absorption at 280 nm. 3) There is a relative abundance of methionine and half-cystine, as is to be expected from the high concentration of sulfur in proteolipid protein (1.76%). In a study of the conditions necessary for the preparation of the carboxymethyl cysteine derivatives of proteolipids, Lees, Leston, and Marfey (1969) have shown that the protein contains both sulfhydryl and disulfide groups, but the sulfhydryl groups are difficult to demonstrate. They are available for reaction with alkylating agents only in the presence of sodium dodecyl sulfate (SDS), and a portion of them react slowly. Approximately one-third of the half-cystine residues exist in the sulfhydryl form when exposed to SDS; the remainder occur in disulfide linkages which must be reduced before alkylation can occur.

V. PREPARATION OF A STABLE CENTRAL WHITE MATTER PROTEOLIPID APOPROTEIN

The apoprotein prepared by Tenenbaum and Folch-Pi (1966) proved too unstable for careful chemical and physical studies. It was obtained in the form of an aqueous solution containing only 0.1% protein. The protein precipitated at neutral pH, and when recovered by lyophilization proved either insoluble in water or soluble only below pH 5. On standing, either the original solution or the reconstituted solutions developed precipitates. The protein remained soluble in CM. As already stated, ORD measurements showed it to have no measurable α-helix content, compared to the high helicity of the starting proteolipid.

In an attempt to obtain more stable apoprotein preparations, the procedure was reinvestigated. The result of this study is a new procedure which yields a consistent and stable preparation of proteolipid apoprotein, upon which extensive studies have been carried out. The details of the development of this procedure have been discussed in some detail elsewhere (Folch-Pi, 1971). In summary, central white matter is homogenized with fivefold its volume of CM, 1:1, v/v, and one-half its volume of aqueous 2 M KCl. The lower phase in the resulting biphasic system contains essentially all of the tissue lipids and proteolipids, including the polyphosphoinositides. The upper phase contains gangliosides, nonproteolipid protein, and low molecular weight tissue components.

The system is resolved by centrifugation, and the lower phase collected, placed in dialysis bags, and dialyzed against several changes of 10-fold its volume of CM 2:1, preferably in the dark and at 4°C. When two-thirds of the starting total solutes have dialyzed out, dialysis is continued against CM:HCl 800:100:3, v/v until at least 85% of the solutes in the starting lower phase have been removed. Dialysis is then continued further for at least five changes of neutral CM, or until the solutes in the outer fluid amount to 0.05% or less of the starting solutes, whichever is longer. The length of time required to reach these levels of dialysis varies from sample to sample of dialysis tubing; it can take as little as 2 days to reach diffusion of two-thirds of the starting solutes and 4 days to reach more than 85%, increasing to twofold or threefold these lengths of time.

The dialysis in acid medium is prolonged until at least 85% of the solutes in the original lower phase have been removed, because after removal of the acidic lipids the proteolipid protein may form complexes with sphingomyelin upon return to a neutral medium. These sphingomyelin-protein complexes are not dissociated by additional dialysis either in acidified or neutral CM. Empirically, it has been found that these complexes are not formed if the removal of lipids is continued to the point at which at least 85% of the original solutes has been removed.

The final retentate is usually clear and contains about 5 mg apoprotein per ml. Upon evaporation, it yields the apoprotein as a residue which has a characteristic glass-like appearance. By comparison, apoprotein samples that have not been maximally delipidated will give a whitish residue.

VI. PREPARATION OF THE WATER-SOLUBLE APOPROTEIN

The apoprotein recovered from the retentate is freely soluble in CM and in many other organic solvents, and it is completely insoluble in water. In order to render it water soluble, it is necessary to make it pass from solution into CM into solution in water by placing the CM solution in, or under, a stream of nitrogen, which removes chloroform preferentially (Folch-Pi, 1971). When approximately four-fifths of the weight of the solution has thus been removed, water is added to the concentrate until cloudiness develops, or until a volume of water equal to the concentrate has been added. Passage of nitrogen is continued until the weight of the solution has again been reduced by half; the concentrate is again diluted with an equal volume of water, and the passage of nitrogen continued until the weight of the solution has once again been reduced by half. At this stage, the solution is essentially free of chloroform and methanol, and can be kept for further study as an aqueous solution of apoprotein. It can also be taken to dryness in a vacuum desiccator. The glass-like residue is freely soluble both in water and CM, although some time of contact between residue and solvent may be required and, in the case of CM, the addition of 1 or 2% water to the mixture may be necessary to bring about complete solution. The residue retains these solubilities for as long as we have kept it, which is several weeks. Aqueous solutions up to 3 to 4% can be easily prepared. Above 4% concentration, the aqueous solutions show increasing viscosity, and they become essentially gels at 5 to 6%.

It must be emphasized that only the maximally delipidated apoprotein is soluble in water. The presence of very small amounts of residual lipids result in incomplete insolubility in water. For instance, the sphingomyelin-protein *de novo* complexes are quite insoluble in water.

The aqueous solutions of apoprotein are indefinitely stable at neutral or slightly acid pH. They appear to be markedly, if not totally, resistant to bacterial contamination. In our experience, solutions stored at 4°C but with frequent stays at room temperature, and also frequently opened for the taking of samples, have remained sterile for as long as they have been kept, which in some cases has been as long as 18 months.

At pH 7.5 and above, aqueous solutions of apoprotein develop a turbidity which disappears at higher pH's but persists upon acidification. Aqueous solutions brought rapidly to 0.1 N NaOH or higher alkali concentrations develop a transient turbidity followed by complete clarification. This turbidity is so transient as to go unnoticed unless special attention is paid to its appearance and disappearance. The solutions in 0.1 N NaOH or higher remain clear for at least several days, but upon acidification a massive precipitate is formed which collects readily, leaving a supernatant that shows only negligible absorption at 280 nm, i.e., the apoprotein appears to have precipitated out quantitatively. This insolubilization of the apoprotein, exposed to 0.1 N NaOH, in aqueous acid develops over a period of approximately 2 hr.

The apoprotein is insolubilized, just as proteolipids are, by taking to dryness from biphasic solutions and by exposure to low alkalinity in the presence of ions. Thus, when a solution of apoprotein in CM (2:1, v/v) is diluted with one-fifth its volume of 0.1 M sodium citrate, the bulk, if not all, of the protein is precipitated out of solution and collects as an insoluble residue at the interface. This residue is completely insoluble in all aqueous solutions and organic solvents that have been used, including 5% SDS. It has the same chemical composition as that of the apoprotein, including the amount of covalently bound fatty acids. Treatment of the residue with CM:HCl fails to extract any of the bound fatty acids. Hence, it appears that exposure to alkali may render the apoprotein completely insoluble without any release of its bound fatty acids.

Although no systematic study has been made of the influence of salts on the solubility of the apoprotein in water, it has been observed that it is precipitated out of solution by NaCl at about 0.27 M concentration. The precipitation is reversible, and the apoprotein goes back into solution upon elimination of or decreasing the concentration of NaCl.

VII. PHYSICAL PROPERTIES OF THE APOPROTEIN

Apoprotein in aqueous solution exhibits one main peak and a much smaller second peak, both in the ultracentrifuge and by moving boundary electrophoresis at both pH 7.0 and 5.0 (Figs. 1 and 2). In both analyses, the main peak represents at least 90% and the second peak 10% or less of the material in solution (Folch-Pi, 1971).

Under various conditions of polyacrylamide gel electrophoresis, several

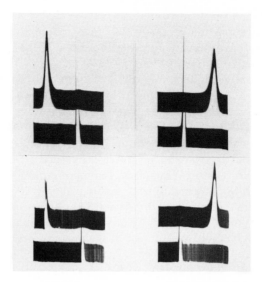

FIG. 1. *(Top):* Electrophoretic pattern of a 1.2% solution of proteolipid apoprotein 68-XIV 22°C H⁺ in acetate buffer, pH 5.0 $r/2 = 0.1$. The ascending boundary is on left; the descending boundary in on the right. The scanning exposures below are initial boundaries; scanning exposures above, after 44 m electrophoresis. *(Bottom):* Electrophoretic patterns of a 1.1% solution of proteolipid apoprotein 68-XIV 22°C H⁺ in phosphate buffer, pH. 7.0, $r/2 = 0.1$. The ascending boundary is on the left; the descending boundary is on the right. The scanning exposures below are initial boundaries; scanning exposures above, after 80 m of electrophoresis.

workers have reported single bands for proteolipid apoprotein, using either isolated myelin (Gonzalez-Sastre, 1970), partly purified proteolipids (Thorun and Mehl, 1968), or apoprotein preparations (Braun and Radin, 1969). In our experience, gel electrophoresis has given far from satisfactory results. Penetration of the apoprotein in the gel was only obtained originally by using gel concentrations below 5% or by increasing cross-linking. Better penetration was later obtained by using phenol-formic acid, water, and SDS, but the extent of the penetration does not permit drawing any final conclusions as to the physical homogeneity or heterogeneity of the preparation.

In summary, although proteolipid apoprotein has been judged by many to be homogeneous from past physical evidence, we recently concluded tentatively that the available evidence does not permit any statement beyond saying that proteolipid apoprotein shows a high tendency to aggregate, and that more work is necessary, particularly in gel electrophoresis, before the question of its homogeneity or heterogeneity is settled.

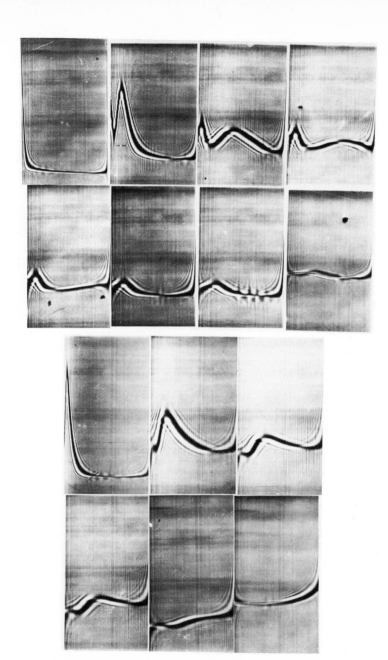

FIG. 2. Ultracentrifuge patterns of a 1.2% solution of proteolipid apoprotein preparation 68-XIV 22°C H⁺ in Na acetate buffer, pH 5.0, $r/2 = 0.1$ run at 26,000 rpm. *Top row:* left to right, 0, 8, 28, and 44 min. *Second row:* left to right, 60, 92, and 124 min at 26,000 rpm, and then 14 min more at 56,000 rpm.

Ultracentrifuge patterns of a 1.1% solution of proteolipid apoprotein 68-XIV 22°C H⁺ in phosphate buffer, pH 7.0, $r/2 = 0.1$ run at 24,000 rpm. *Third row:* left to right, 0, 8, and 16 min running time. *Bottom row:* left to right, 20 and 30 min running time, and then 36 min more at 52,000 rpm.

The apoprotein shows an absorption peak at 278 nm. Its $E_{1\%}^{1cm}$ at 278 nm is 13.6, which is lower than the values reported in other studies (Tenenbaum and Folch-Pi, 1966). The higher values may reflect contamination and, in some cases, the lack of correction for turbidity.

VIII. RELATIONSHIP BETWEEN THE SOLUBILITIES OF THE PROTEOLIPID APOPROTEIN AND ITS CONFORMATION

The apoprotein occurs in two forms, a lipophilic form soluble in organic solvents and a hydrophilic form soluble in aqueous media. It can pass from one form to the other reversibly under proper conditions. To pass from the lipophilic to the hydrophilic form, it is necessary to follow the procedure described in Section VI. The reverse passage is much easier, and the apoprotein dried from aqueous solutions can be dissolved directly into CM, although the addition of a small amount of water may be necessary.

It is not known what exact changes occur with these reversible changes in solubility, but it is fair to assume that in the lipophilic apoprotein the lipophilic groups predominate at the surface of the molecule, whereas in the hydrophilic apoprotein it is the hydrophilic groups that predominate at the molecular surface. Optical rotatory dispersion and circular dichroism measurements on solutions of apoprotein in different solvents (Table 3)

TABLE 3. *Optical rotatory dispersion analysis of typical proteolipid apoprotein (results obtained on sample 68-XIV-22A)*

Solvent	Conc. (%)	b_0^a	% α-helix computed from [m′] 233 nm[b]	a_0
CHCl$_3$-MeOH	1.14	66	65	+131
ClCH$_2$CH$_2$OH	0.92	60	61	+ 97
F$_3$CCH$_2$OH	0.61	90	93	+ 69
H$_2$O	0.32	38	37	− 73
H$_2$O[c]	0.35	16	17	−136
MeOH[d]	0.71	33	41	−289
CHCl$_3$-MeOH 60% lipid	0.81	69	66	+164

[a] $b_0 = -630$ for 100% α-helix; $\lambda_0 = 212$ nm.
[b] [m′] 233 nm $= -13,000$ (deg. cm^2/decimole) for 100% α-helix and $-1,700$ (deg. cm^2/decimole) estimated for 0% α-helix.
[c] Prepared in presence of excess MeOH.
[d] When MeOH solution diluted with CHCl$_3$ to make 2:1, C-Me, the 233 trough shifts from 231 to 235, mμ, the helix becomes 33%. The MeOH seems to be a mixture of α-helix plus some other conformation that is not reversible.

demonstrate that conformational changes do occur, but without defining their nature. Zand (1968) reported originally that proteolipid was characterized by a high content of α-helix, whereas the "water-soluble" protein of Tenenbaum and Folch-Pi (1966) showed no measurable α^π-helix. Sherman and Folch-Pi (1970) confirmed Zand's observations on proteolipids and extended them to show that the α-helix content did not change in the course of the gradual delipidation of the proteolipid to the apoprotein stage. However, they found that in sharp contrast with the absence of measurable α-helix of the "water-soluble" apoprotein of Tenenbaum and Folch-Pi, the present apoprotein retained approximately one-half of the α-helix content of the CM soluble apoprotein, and that this change in conformation was reversible. The apoprotein regained its former α-helix content when placed back into solution in CM. This change appeared to be repeatedly reversible, and a given sample of apoprotein could be changed back and forth repeatedly from its CM soluble form into its water soluble form with the corresponding changes in α-helix content.

Sherman and Folch-Pi (1970) found that the reversibility of this change in conformation can only be preserved if exposure to water-methanol mixtures or pure methanol is kept to a minimum. Methanol apparently changes the conformation of the apoprotein irreversibly. This produces an apoprotein with a reduced α-helix content which is soluble in methanol and which, if it goes into solution in CM at all, will do so without regaining its former α-helix content. In water, this apoprotein will form only very dilute solutions which gradually yield a precipitate that is insoluble in all the solvents tested. Presumably, it is this effect of methanol that is responsible for the instability and the low α-helix content of the water-soluble apoprotein of Tenenbaum and Folch-Pi.

The contrast between the stability of solutions of apoprotein in organic solvents and in water, and the ease with which the apoprotein can be obtained as an almost universally insoluble residue (short of chemical breakdown) by such simple means as drying from biphasic solutions, exposure to low alkaline pH in the presence of ions, or exposure to methanol, suggests that the apoprotein is apt to undergo a number of changes in conformation, some reversible and some irreversible. None of these changes appear to change the chemical composition of the apoprotein.

IX. CHEMICAL COMPOSITION OF THE PROTEOLIPID APOPROTEIN

The apoprotein does not show any spots on thin-layer chromatography for lipids even when samples as large as 5 to 10 mg are taken. It contains traces of P (0.01 to 0.04%) and of carbohydrate (<0.1% as galactose). Its

P is released by treatment with 0.1 N NaOH at room temperature for 16 hr as water soluble organic P, i.e., it is not phosphoprotein P. The water solution shows no absorption at 260 nm, which indicates that the P is not a nucleic acid derivative. As discussed below, this P most likely represents traces of phospholipids. The carbohydrate present is mainly galactose, and most likely corresponds to residual sulfatides and cerebrosides. In summary, the apoprotein is neither a phosphoprotein, a glycoprotein, nor a nucleoprotein.

The most striking feature of the chemistry of the apoprotein is the presence of from 2.0 to 3.2% fatty acids. These fatty acids (Sherman and Folch-Pi, 1970) show a consistent pattern of approximately 60% palmitic, 25% oleic, and 10% stearic acids, with 5% other acids (Table 4). Stoffyn and Folch-Pi (1971) have established conclusively that these fatty acids are esterified since they do not react with diazomethane, which shows that they are not free acids, and they react with sodium borohydride to produce the corresponding alcohols, which shows that they are bound by ester linkages.

TABLE 4. *Fatty acids combined in proteolipid apoprotein (PLA)*

PLA preparation[a]	Total fatty acids as % of weight of PLA (a)	Composition of fatty acid mixture as % of values in column *a*						P in PLA %
		14:0	16:0	16:1	18:0	18:1	20:0	
White matter PLA								
69-XVII	2.0	—	56.0	—	9.7	27.0	n.d.	0.01–0.04
69-XIX	3.2	—	62.0	—	9.1	23.0	n.d.	"
69-XXI	3.2	—	62.0	—	8.6	26.0	n.d.	"
70-III-2	3.0	—	58.5	—	10.6	25.4	n.d.	"
70-XII	2.45	—	60.0	—	9.1	26.0	n.d.	"
Gray matter PLA								
71-VII	3.88	15.1	49.2	3.1	14.1	18.5	n.d.	0.077
72-VI	3.30	4.4	54.0	5.3	11.1	25.2	n.d.	0.042
Heart PLA[b]								
72-III	0.40							0.033
72-VII	0.52							0.042
Kidney PLA[b]								
72-IV	0.56							0.017
Liver PLA								
72-V	2.45	6.7	26.2	—	37.3	26.6	n.d.	0.015
72-IX	2.17	6.6	32.9	5.9	20.2	24.6	n.d.	—

[a] All these preparations contained about 0.1% carbohydrate, as galactose. As galactolipids, this would account for about 0.15% fatty acids but this is unlikely because of the absence of fatty acids 20:0 or longer.

[b] The amounts of fatty acids present in *Heart* and in *Kidney PLA* can readily be attributed to phospholipids, since in a diacylphosphoglyceride, fatty acids amount to 18-fold the concentration of P, on a weight basis.

These fatty acid residues do not belong to any recognizable lipid. An exhaustive analysis of the apoprotein for possible lipid moieties with which these fatty acids might be bound shows that the amounts of P, ethanolamine, choline, sphingosine, inositol, galactose and other sugars, sialic acid, and glycerol present in the apoprotein are individually and jointly unable to account for from less than one-tenth to no more than one-fourth of the fatty acids present. In summary, it is necessary to conclude that these esterified fatty acids in the apoprotein must be esterified on the polypeptide chain itself, except for the remote possibility that they are constituents of an as yet unidentified lipid. Such a hypothetical lipid would be singularly devoid of the most common moieties of lipids known at the present time.

The apoprotein exhibits an amino acid composition indistinguishable from that of either the crude or partly purified proteolipids. It preserves intact the resistance to most proteolytic enzymes that is characteristic of the proteolipids. Because the least abundant residue is 2 methionines per mole of protein, the apoprotein appears to have 125 residues, giving a possible molecular weight of approximately 12,000 daltons.

The apoprotein dried to constant weight in high vacuum, in the presence of NaOH, produces an aqueous solution with a pH of approximately 3.5. Apparently the apoprotein is obtained as a fully, or almost fully, protonated anion. Titration of two apoprotein preparations between pH 3.5 and 7.17 requires 1 μmole of NaOH for each 3.58 mg of apoprotein. Braun and Radin (1969) report the use of 1 μmole of HCl for each 2 mg of apoprotein between pH 6.0 and 3.0. Although the two sets of values are not strictly comparable, it is obvious that the apoprotein of Braun and Radin exhibited a larger number of titratable acid groups than do our preparations. A possible explanation for this discrepancy is that their procedure involved a much more prolonged exposure to acid than our own, with the result that some glutamine residues may have been deamidated to glutamic acid.

X. THE QUESTION OF THE HOMOGENEITY OF THE WHITE MATTER PROTEOLIPID APOPROTEIN AND ITS MOLECULAR SIZE(S)

As already stated, under certain conditions of operation proteolipid protein exhibits a single band on polyacrylamide gels, indicating a physical homogeneity in each particular case. However, especially with the use of SDS and various denaturing agents, the same preparations of PLA will exhibit more than one band, although there is usually a main band present. In summary, the question of the homogeneity of PLA therefore remains to be proven. In view of the marked tendency of PLA to aggregate, the physical heterogeneity indicated by various bands might well represent different degrees of aggregation of a single monomer. This leads to the problem of the molecular size of PLA. Thorun and Mehl (1968), using gel electrophoresis on a polyacrylamide density gradient, obtained a value of 34,000 to 36,000 for the molecular weight of their proteolipid preparation. In 1971 Eng, using a 10% acrylamide gel and phosphate buffer in 0.1% SDS, reported a molecular weight of 22,000 to 23,000 for his preparation. This molecular size has also been observed by Waenheldt and Mandel (1972) and by Agrawal, Burton, Fishman, Mitchell, and Prensky (1972). The latter group has, of course, shown the presence of a different protein of the proteolipid type in the range of 20,500.

Speculating on the size of a possible monomer, Folch-Pi in 1959 computed from the amino acid composition of proteolipids a possible monomeric molecular size of approximately 12,500, based on two methionines as the least abundant constituent amino acid. In 1971 Folch-Pi reported that a portion of the proteolipid is dialyzable through cellophane membranes, presumably impermeable to molecules above a size of 12,000. This dialyzable fraction accounts for a greater or smaller fraction according to the relative permeability of the cellulose membrane used. Paradoxically, the more permeable the membrane, the smaller the fraction of proteolipid protein that diffuses through it. In addition, this diffusion of proteolipid protein occurs only at the very beginning of the dialysis procedure, and then ceases completely, so that a second dialysate does not contain any protein. This behavior suggests that a major or minor fraction of the total proteolipid in the original tissue extract may be maintained in a diffusable monomeric form of dispersion by a factor or factors. This factor (or factors) is changed or eliminated during the dialysis process, and the proteolipid changes to an aggregate, undialyzable form with its removal.

The following recent observations appear to support this sequence of events. A CM extract is submitted to dialysis until diffusion of protein through the membrane ceases. At this moment the retentate is collected and replaced in the dialysis bag by a fresh portion of the same CM extract. The diffusion of protein starts again in a manner comparable to the course observed with the original portion of extract, i.e., the permeability of the membrane to protein does not appear to have changed. At the same time, the original retentate is placed in a fresh dialysis bag, cut from the same roll as the first one. No diffusion of protein is observed, i.e., the protein remaining in the retentate after diffusion of protein ceases is truly undialyzable. Finally, if a diffusate-containing protein is submitted to dialysis, it is observed that little or none of the protein proves dialyzable, i.e., the protein that had originally diffused out has become undialyzable.

If, indeed, proteolipid protein possesses a monomer size of 12,500, the values obtained by Eng (1971) and by Thorun and Mehl (1968) would represent a dimer and a trimer, respectively.

In another approach to the problem of molecular size of PLA, D. R. Whikehart and M. Lees *(personal communication)* have determined the amino and carboxyl end groups of various preparations of central white matter proteolipids. The results (Table 5) show that bovine PLA exhibits two N-terminal end groups, glycine and glutamic acid, in the approximate molar proportions of 3:1. The corresponding C-terminal amino acids are phenylalanine and glycine. The yields obtained are low for the molecular sizes indicated by polyacrylamide gel electrophoresis. However, the presence of two N-terminal and two C-terminal amino acids indicates heterogeneity.

TABLE 5. *N-terminal amino acids of proteolipid apoprotein (PLA) from different bovine tissues*

	N-terminal amino acid expressed as nanomoles per mg of protein		
PLA sample	Aspartic acid[a] (or asparagine)	Glutamic acid[a] (or glutamine)	Glycine
70-IX White matter PLA	trace[b]	5.8	16.8
	trace[b]	6.9	16.5
70-XII White matter PLA	trace[b]	6.9	21.2
dialyzable	trace[b]	6.8	19.0
71-VII Gray matter PLA[c]	3.2	1.8	8.3
72-III, Heart PLA[c]	34.2	n.d	n.d.
72-IV, Kidney PLA[c]	15.8	n.d.	n.d.
72-V, Liver PLA[c]	14.5	n.d.	n.d.

[a] The procedure followed does not differentiate between the acids and the corresponding amides.
[b] Trace indicates amounts below 1 nanomole per mg of protein.
[c] Average of two determinations.
n.d. = not detectable.
D. R. Whikehart and M. Lees, *personal communication.*

XI. STUDY OF PLA FROM CENTRAL GRAY MATTER AND FROM NON-NEURAL SOURCES

By the same procedure used with central white matter, Folch-Pi and Sakura (1973) have obtained PLA from central gray matter, heart, kidney, and liver. The study of their chemical and physical properties shows interesting differences among the different PLA's, within a framework of common properties. Thus the amino acid compositions, given in Table 1, show for all PLA's the same abundance of nonpolar amino acids and S-amino acids and the same relative poverty in polar amino acids. However, non-neural PLA's show little or no half-cystine, with a proportionate increase in methionine. They show less glycine, alanine, and tyrosine, and more aspartic acid, proline, leucine, and isoleucine than white matter PLA. Gray matter PLA shows a composition intermediate between that of white matter and of non-neural tissues. PLA from non-neural tissues shows only aspartic acid as N-terminal and lysine as C-terminal amino acids. The most marked chemical difference among the different PLA's is the presence of covalently bound fatty acids in white matter, gray matter, and liver PLA, and their absence from heart and kidney PLA (Table 4). Physically, all PLA's share the ability to change conformation reversibly according to the polarity of the solvent medium (Table 6). In addition, in the course of the preparation, the CM extracts from the different tissues showed the same diffusion of protein during the first stage of dialysis in CM that had been first observed with central white matter CM extracts. Finally, in polyacrylamide gels the various PLA have exhibited single bands or several bands according to conditions of operation.

In summary, the marked chemical and physical similarities among all PLA's studied suggest a common role in the respective membrane structures.

TABLE 6. *Changes in α-helix content of proteolipid apoprotein (PLA) from different bovine tissues according to the polarity of the solvent medium: Reversibility of such changes*

		α-helix content of PLA		
ORD/CD no.	Source of PLA	In CM 2:1 (original dialysis retentate)[a]	In water (prepared from the retentate)[b]	In CM (by dilution of the aqueous solution)
	White matter			
108	71-VI-1	67%	22%	69%
116	71-VI-2	67%	41%	—
—	—	66%	37%	66%
131	Gray matter	58%	37%	(80%)
129	Heart	68%	26%	60%
130	Kidney	58%	22%	54%
127	Liver	61%	22%	—

[a] From ORD measurements [m'] 233 nm.
[b] From CD measurements [θ] 208 nm.

Addendum

Work carried out by Folch-Pi and Sakura (1973) since the presentation of this review shows that the heterogeneity observed on polyacrylamide gels by different PLA's increases with the addition of SDS and of denaturing and of reducing agents during the electrophoresis. The effect is especially marked with non-neural PLA's, which exhibit as many as 10 bands in presence of SDS and 8 M urea. The molecular size of these bands ranges from 6,000 upward, with main components at 30,000. Central white matter PLA shows a main band at 24,000 and minor bands at 12,000 and 20,000, the latter presumably corresponding to the protein described by Agrawal et al. (1972). The presence in all PLA's of protein bands at 12,000 lends support to the dialyzability of varying proportions of proteolipid protein, and to their change to a polyaggregated state during dialysis.

REFERENCES

(✱) deaggregating agents...

Agrawal, H. C., Burton, R. M., Fishman, M. A., Mitchell, R. F., and Prensky, A. L. (1972): Partial characterization of a new myelin protein component. *Journal of Neurochemistry,* 19:2083–2089.

Amaducci, L. (1962): The distribution of proteolipids in the human nervous system. *Journal of Neurochemistry,* 9:153–160.

Autilio, L. (1966): Fractionation of myelin proteins. *Federation Proceedings,* 25:764.

Autilio, L., Norton, W. T., and Terry, R. D. (1964): The preparation and some properties of purified myelin from the central nervous system. *Journal of Neurochemistry,* 11:17–27.

Braun, P. E., and Radin, N. S. (1969): Interaction of lipids with a membrane structural protein from myelin. *Biochemistry,* 8:4310–4318.

Eng, L. F. (1971): Molecular weights of the major myelin proteins. *Federation Proceedings,* 30:1248.

Eng, L. F., Chao, F.-C, Gerstl, B., Pratt, D., and Tavaststjerna, M. G. (1968): The maturation of human white matter myelin. Fractionation of the myelin membrane proteins. *Biochemistry,* 7:4455–4465.

Folch, J. (1955): Composition of the brain in relation to maturation. In: *Biochemistry of the Developing Nervous System,* edited by H. Waelsch. Academic Press, New York.

Folch, J., Ascoli, I., Lees, M., Meath, J. A., and LeBaron, F. N. (1951): Preparation of lipid extracts from brain tissue. *Journal of Biological Chemistry,* 191:833–841.

Folch, J., and Lees, M. (1951): Proteolipids, a new type of tissue lipoproteins. Their isolation from brain. *Journal of Biological Chemistry,* 191:807–817.

Folch, J., Webster, G. R., and Lees, M. (1959): The preparation of proteolipids. *Federation Proceedings,* 18:228.

Folch-Pi, J. (1959): Études récentes sur la chimie du cerveau et leur rapport avec la structure de la gaine myelinique. *Exposes Annuels de Biochimie Medicale,* 21:81–95.

Folch-Pi, J. (1971): Nature of the dialyzable brain white matter proteolipid. Third Intern. Meet. Intern. Soc. Neurochem. Abst.:239.

Folch-Pi, J., and Sakura, J. D. (1973): Proteolipid apoprotein (PA) from bovine non-neural tissues. *Federation Proceedings,* 32:624.

Folch-Pi, J., and Stoffyn, P. J. (1972): Proteolipids from membrane systems. *Annals of the New York Academy of Sciences,* 195:86–107.

Gonzalez-Sastre, F. (1970): The protein composition of isolated myelin. *Journal of Neurochemistry,* 17:1049–1056.

Joel, C. D., Karnovsky, M. L., Ball, E. G., and Cooper, O. (1958): Lipid composition of the succinate and reduced diphosphopyridine nucleotide oxidase system. *Journal of Biological Chemistry,* 233:1565.

Laatsch, R. H. (1963): Fractionation of myelin constituents by a two-phase system. *Federation Proceedings,* 22:316.

Lapetina, E. G., Soto, E. F., and De Robertis, E. (1968): Lipids and proteolipids in isolated subcellular membranes of rat brain cortex. *Journal of Neurochemistry,* 15:437.

Lees, M. B. (1966): Influence of sucrose on the extraction of proteolipids from brain and other tissues. *Journal of Neurochemistry,* 13:1407–1420.

Lees, M. B. (1968): Effect of ion removal on the solubility of rat brain proteins in chloroform-methanol mixtures. *Journal of Neurochemistry,* 15:153–159.

Lees, M. B., Leston, J. A., and Marfey, P. (1969): Carboxymethylation of sulfhydryl groups in proteolipids. *Journal of Neurochemistry,* 16:1025–1032.

Lees, M. B., Messinger, B. F., and Burnham, J. (1967): Tryptic hydrolysis of brain proteolipid. *Biochemical and Biophysical Research Communications,* 28:185–190.

Matsumoto, M., Matsumoto, R., and Folch-Pi, J. (1964): The chromatographic fractionation of brain white matter proteolipids. *Journal of Neurochemistry,* 11:829–838.

Mokrasch, L. C. (1967): A rapid purification of proteolipid protein adaptable to large quantities. *Life Sciences,* 6:1905–1909.

Murakami, M., Sekine, H., and Funahashi, S. (1962): Proteolipid from beef heart muscle. Application of organic dialysis to preparation of proteolipid. *Journal of Biochemistry,* 51:431–435.

de Robertis, E., Fiszer, S., and Soto, E. F. (1967): Cholinergic binding capacity of proteolipids from isolated nerve-ending membranes. *Science,* 158:928.

Sherman, G., and Folch-Pi, J. (1970): Rotatory dispersion and circular dichroism of brain proteolipid protein. *Journal of Neurochemistry,* 17:597–605.

Soto, E. F., Pasquini, J. M., Placido, R., and La Torre, J. L. (1969): Fractionation of lipids and proteolipids from cat grey and white matter by chromatography on an organophilic dextran gel. *Journal of Chromatography,* 41:400–409.

Stoffyn, P. J., and Folch-Pi, J. (1971): On the type of linkage binding fatty acids present in brain white matter proteolipid apoprotein. *Biochemical and Biophysical Research Communications,* 44:157–161.

Tenenbaum, D., and Folch-Pi, J. (1966): The preparation and characterization of water-soluble proteolipid protein from bovine brain white matter. *Biochimica et Biophysica Acta,* 115:141–147.

Thorun, W., and Mehl, E. (1968): Determination of molecular weights of microgram quantities of protein components from biological membranes and other complex mixtures. Gel electrophoresis across linear gradients of acrylamide. *Biochimica et Biophysica Acta,* 160:132–134.

Waehneldt, T. V., and Mandel, P. (1972): Isolation of rat brain myelin, monitored by polyacrylamide gel electrophoresis of dodecyl sulfate-extracted proteins. *Brain Research,* 40:419–436.

Webster, G. R., and Folch, J. (1961): Some studies of the properties of proteolipids. *Biochimica et Biophysica Acta,* 49:399–401.

Wolfgram, F. (1966): a new proteolipid fraction of the nervous system. *Journal of Neurochemistry,* 13:461–470.

Zand, R. (1968): Solution properties and structure of brain proteolipids. Biopolymers, 6:939–953.

Zill, L. P., and Harmon, E. A. (1961): Chloroplast proteolipid. *Biochimica et Biophysica Acta,* 53:579–581.

Proteins of the Nervous System
Raven Press, New York © 1973

Studies of Nervous System Proteins

Diana Johnson Schneider

I. INTRODUCTION

A number of contributors to this symposium presented recent data on the various brain specific proteins and on proteins which play crucial roles in nervous system function. These data are presented in this chapter in summary form, and it is hoped that they will provide the reader with a general view of the many possible approaches to the study of nervous system proteins.

II. SPECIES-SPECIFIC NERVOUS SYSTEM PROTEINS

A. *Aplysia* Nerve Proteins

Berry, Arch, and Wilson have extensively studied the abdominal ganglion of the sea hare *Aplysia*, which contains unipolar neurons many of whose cell bodies are 50 to 1,000 μ in diameter. Their large size, pigmentation, relative constancy of position, and appearance have made it possible to map the location, electrical behavior, and connectivity of approximately 30 of the neurons (Frazier, Kandel, Kupfermann, Waziri, and Coggeshall, 1967). It is possible to remove single cells from the ganglion and to perform various biochemical analyses using scaled-down versions of standard methods.

It is thus possible to examine biochemical parameters in single neurons whose electrophysiology and pharmacology have been described, and whose electrical behavior can be measured and manipulated with a fair degree of precision. Recent studies of protein function, synthesis, and regulation have been based primarily on the identification of patterns of neuronal protein synthesis and content by electrophoresis on sodium dodecyl sulfate (SDS)-polyacrylamide gels. This technique was scaled down from standard methods by Wilson (1971), and is capable of resolving ^{3}H-leucine-labeled proteins in the 10,000- to 100,000-dalton range in extracts of single neurons.

The neurons of the isolated *Aplysia* abdominal ganglion may be divided into two classes, one of which is electrically silent unless driven synaptically

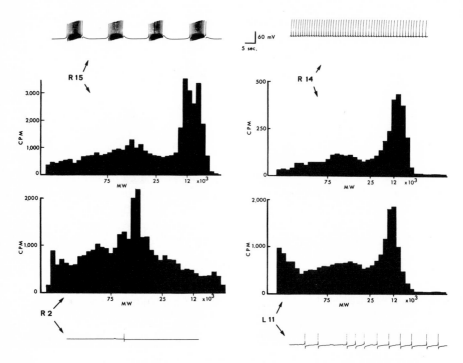

FIG. 1. Intracellular recordings and protein synthetic patterns from prominent neurons in the *Aplysia* abdominal ganglion. Ganglion labeling, protein extraction, and electrophoresis were as reported by Wilson (1971). Label was ^{14}C-leucine for R_{14}, ^{3}H-leucine for others. R_{14} and L_{11} were run on the same gel; note difference in peak position. Labeling times: R_{15}, 19 hr; R_2, 5 hr; R_{14} and L_{11}, 12 hr.

by an interneuron or by stimulation of a nerve; neurons of the second class exhibit an endogenous regular or bursting pacemaker activity, which may in some cases be modulated by synaptic input. Wilson (1971) found marked differences in the labeling patterns of these two basic types of neurons (Fig. 1). Of particular interest was the observation that all pacemaker cells had a large peak in the labeling pattern at about 12,000 daltons, although this component was absent in nonpacemaker cells. Furthermore, the low molecular weight peak was not the same in all pacemakers. Its migration rate was the same in R_{15} and L_{11}, but another rate was found for R_3 through R_{14}. In contrast to a pacemaker cell such as R_{15}, the silent giant cell R_2 synthesizes a broad spectrum of proteins.

When cells were labeled for 24 hr with ^{3}H-leucine and dissected into nucleus, cytoplasm, and a fraction containing glia, membranes, and remnants of cytoplasm (method modified from Lasek and Dower, 1971), R_2

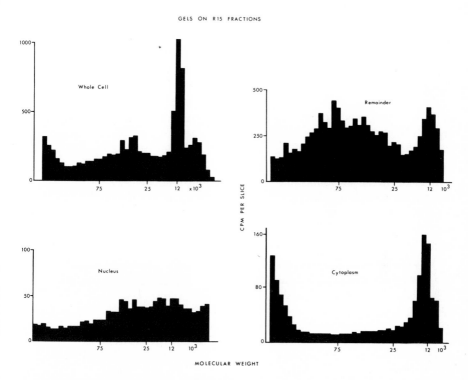

FIG. 2. Protein synthetic patterns of fractions of R_{15}. Cells were labeled 20 to 24 hr with ^{3}H-leucine, dissected, and treated as in Wilson (1971). Individual fractions are from cells from different animals. Note presence of free leucine (first few slices on left) in cytoplasm and whole cell only.

and R_{15} showed different distributions of label. Most of the labeled protein in R_2 was found in the membrane-containing fraction, with smaller amounts of most of the proteins in the cytoplasm. A small degree of incorporation into diffuse low molecular weight material was found in the nucleus. In R_{15}, the nuclear fraction resembled that of R_2; the low molecular weight material was the major cytoplasmic component, and most of the higher molecular weight label was in the remaining fraction (Fig. 2).

Most of the pacemaker cells are believed to be neurosecretory on the basis of their content of large dense-cored vesicles. The presence of the 12,000-dalton material primarily in the cytoplasm suggests that it might be involved in neurosecretion rather than in the generation of pacemaker activity, in which case it would be expected to be localized within the cell membrane. However, the possibility that this substance serves as a precursor to a membrane component cannot as yet be eliminated.

The 12,000-dalton peak from R_{15} was further localized to the particulate fraction of the cytoplasm. It was not released at low ionic strength, suggesting that this protein is unlikely to be neurosecretory material or chromogranin-like. Further studies are needed to determine if it is a vesicle constituent.

Berry, Peterson, and Kernell have demonstrated that synaptic stimulation of R_2 increases its incorporation of ^{3}H-uridine into RNA by 75 to 100%, and Kernell and Peterson (1970) further showed that direct intracellular stimulation did not increase incorporation. Neither uridine uptake nor the percentage of intracellular label converted to UTP was altered under conditions of increased incorporation (Berry and Cohen, 1972). However, no detectable change in the pattern of protein synthesis was observed up to 3 hr after intense synaptic activation (Wilson and Berry, 1972), suggesting that any regulation of protein function in response to stimulation must occur at the enzymatic level.

An effect of neuronal activity on the synthesis of a nerve-specific protein has been demonstrated for the 6,000-dalton neurosecretory peptide of the bag cells, a homogeneous group of small neurons located at the base of the ganglionic connectives. This peptide, which induces egg laying when injected into a recipient animal, is released into the medium when the bag cells are stimulated electrically or in response to elevated external K^+ (Arch, 1972a), and this release is blocked in low Ca^{++}–high Mg^{++} solutions (Arch, 1972b). This material appears to be bound within cytoplasmic vesicles.

The 6,000-dalton material arises from a 25,000-dalton precursor, which is cleaved into two 6,000-dalton peptides and a 12,000-dalton fragment. The synthesis of 12,000- and 6,000-dalton material is increased 35 to 40% relative to that of other proteins following massive release of the protein (Fig. 3). This increase is not due to more rapid or complete degradation of the precursor, so that it would appear that functional demand can influence protein synthesis in these cells.

B. Specific Proteins of the Cephalopod Nervous System

Utilizing the bidimensional fractionation techniques described in Chapter 1 by Moore, Giuditta, Moore, Prozzo, and Packard (1971) detected several acidic brain-specific proteins in the optic lobe of two cephalopods, *Octopus vulgaris* and *Loligo vulgaris.* The octopus brain protein having the higher electrophoretic mobility was purified via multiple chromatography. The protein has a molecular weight of approximately 12,000, and an amino acid composition of which 36% of the residues are glutamic and aspartic acids.

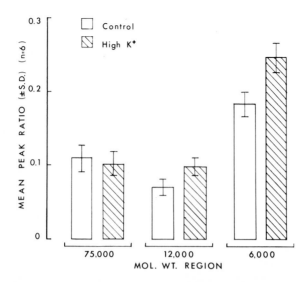

FIG. 3. Stimulated synthesis of bag cell-specific proteins. Bag cells were incubated 4 hr in elevated potassium medium (high K+) or in normal potassium (control), then labeled 2 hr in normal potassium with ³H-leucine. This was followed by a 70-min chase, extraction, and electrophoresis as in Arch (1972b). Ordinate gives the ratio of counts in a particular molecular weight region to the total counts in the gel. Counts at 12,000 and 6,000 daltons after a 15-min chase were subtracted from those at 70 min to eliminate the contribution of material not arising from the 25,000-dalton precursor.

Immunological studies indicated that the protein is at least 10-fold more concentrated in the optic lobe than in other organs. Strong cross-reactions were demonstrated for extracts from the nervous system of other molluscs, including squid, sepia, snail, abalone, and *Aplysia*. No cross-reaction could be demonstrated with beef S-100 or 14–3–2.

A similar brain-specific acidic protein has been purified from the optic lobes of *Loligo vulgaris* and *Sepia officinalis* (Alemà, Calissano, Rusca, and Giuditta, 1973). Alemà has found the protein to have a molecular weight of 12,000 daltons, with two Ca^{++} binding sites per molecule having a $K_{diss} = 2.5 \times 10^{-5}$ M at physiological concentrations of KCl. The protein was found to be largely confined to the nervous system (Table 1).

In order to study eventually the role of purified proteins in suitable biological systems, Giuditta and Prozzo *(in preparation)* have analyzed by acrylamide gel electrophoresis the protein patterns of different lobes of the octopus brain and of different compartments of the stellate nerve and ganglion of the squid, and have found marked differences in protein pattern in these different regions.

TABLE 1. *Distribution of the protein in some organs and in different regions of the nervous system of cuttlefish and squid*

Species	Organ or N.S. district	µg/mg TSP [*]	mg/g.w.w.	n[**]
Sepia off.	Optic lobe	5.1	0.317	(4)
	Hepatopancreas	0.05	0.004	(2)
	Muscle	undetectable		(2)
	Gills	undetectable		(1)
Loligo vulg.	Optic lobe	7.57	0.251	(4)
	Stellate ganglion			
	a) giant-fiber lobe	28.50	0.989	(3)
	b) neuropile	4.55	0.075	(3)
	c) cortical layer	3.53	0.072	(3)
	Stellate nerve			
	a) axoplasm	60.1	2.437	(3)
	b) sheath	51.7	0.170	(3)
	c) small fibers	5.27	0.048	(3)
	Kidney	1.6	0.098	(2)
	Hepatopancreas	0.06	0.006	(1)
	Gills	0.13	0.003	(1)
	Muscle	undetectable		(1)'
	Sistemic heart	undetectable		(1)
	Branchial heart	undetectable		(1)

[*]TSP = total soluble proteins (see Methods).

[**]n refers to the number of specimens examined.

C. Human Brain-Specific Protein

Warecka described studies of a human brain-specific protein, first isolated by Warecka and Bauer (1966, 1967), which can be prepared by a method similar to that of Moore (1965a). Its specificity to human brain has been demonstrated immunologically. Its electrophoretic migration in the α_2 area, PAS staining in agar, and cleavage by neuraminidase indicated that it is an acidic α_2-glycoprotein. This was confirmed by affinity chromatog-

TABLE 2. Results of immunological and histological studies in 25 fetal and 10 infantile brains

Length of Fetus cm	Weight of Fetus g	Weight of Brain g	Age			Immunoelectrophoresis of Extracts of Fetus Brain Tested with Anti-Brain-Serum			Antibodies against Brainspecific Protein	Histological Examination	Number of Cases Examined
			Weeks	Months	Years	Serum Proteins	Organ Proteins	Brainspec. Proteins			
0,8	1,5		3-4			+	–	–	no material	no material	1
7,0	21,8	3,80	8-9			+	+	–	–	Neuroblast	1
9,0	23,6	4,02	10-11			+	+	–	–	Gliablast	1
12,0	35,0	7,70	12-13			+	+	–	not tested		1
16,0	103,2	15,45	16-18			+	+	–	–	Neuroblast Glioblast (nerv cells) (macroglia)	2
37,0	1082,0	174,00	24-28			+	+	–	+	myelination glia in the cerebrum, thin myelin sheaths in the pons	9*)
46,0	1700,0	250,00	32-36			+	+	–	+	myelination glia in the cerebrum, thin myelin sheaths in the midbrain	8**)
54,0	3445,0	330,00	40-42 birth			+	+	–	+	myelination glia, myelin and differentiation of glia	2
		750,00		3-4		+	+	±	+	myelination glia, myelin and differentiation of glia	2
		1200,00			1-5	+	+	+	+	brain full developed	8

*)five of these survived up to three days, **)five of these survived up to 17 days.

In those collectives, in which more than one brain was examined, the length and weights are concerned as an average.

raphy isolation and SDS-polyacrylamide gel electrophoresis (Brunngraber, Susz, and Warecka, *in preparation*). The glycoprotein is composed of two subunits, with molecular weights of 50,000 and 12,000.

The introduction of affinity chromatography for preparation of the protein permitted the preparation of a homologous antibody, although a double line is observed following electrophoresis and immunodiffusion. It is not yet known whether this is due to the presence of two subunits or whether the protein is split during the isolation procedure.

Several lines of evidence suggested a glial origin of the protein. This was confirmed by the separation of neuronal perikarya and glia (Warecka, Müller, Vogel, and Tripatzia, 1972). The protein was further localized to the microsomes and postmicrosomal supernatant by differential and density-gradient centrifugation. The glial origin of the protein was further indicated by the correlation of the appearance of the protein during development with myelination. Preliminary immunofluorescence data also demonstrated a glial localization (Simon and Warecka, *in preparation*). The specific fluorescence was restricted to glia, and probably exclusively to oligoden-droglia.

Studies in human fetuses (Warecka and Müller, 1969) showed the protein to appear between gestational weeks 24 and 28 (Table 2), which is also the period when myelination glia can be detected histologically (Roback and Scherer, 1935). These data also revealed a sequential appearance of human serum proteins, common organ proteins, and brain-specific proteins during ontogenesis (Table 3).

Extracts of adult brain contain two brain-specific proteins, whereas fetal brain contains only one. Antiserum to the adult brain-specific protein reacts

TABLE 3. *Approaches to the study of human brain-specific protein*

LENGTH (CM)	AGE (WEEKS)	PROTEINS	NEUROELEMENTS
0.8	3 – 4	ANTIBODIES AGAINST SERUM – PROTEINS	GLIOBLAST NEUROBLAST
7	8 – 9	ANTIBODIES AGAINST ORGAN – PROTEINS	GLIOBLAST NEURO-BLAST + (MACROGLIA, NERVOUS CELLS)
37	24 – 28	ANTIBODIES AGAINST BRAIN – SPECIFIC GLYCOPROTEINS	MYELINATIONGLIA

only with adult brain tissue, whereas antiserum to the fetal protein cross-reacts with the adult protein. These data have been confirmed by Delpech, Delpech, Clement, and Laumonier (1972).

III. REGIONALLY SPECIFIC NERVOUS SYSTEM PROTEINS

A. Olfactory Bulb-Specific Protein

Margolis has examined various brain regions in the mouse for the presence of regionally specific proteins. A protein band that appeared to be restricted to the olfactory bulb was observed in 14% polyacrylamide gel electrophoretic patterns of mouse brain soluble protein extracts. This protein was isolated and purified to homogeneity from the olfactory bulb by ammonium sulfate fractionation, DEAE-cellulose chromatography, and isoelectric focusing. The protein has a minimal molecular weight of approximately 20,000, an isoelectric point of 4.7, and seems not to be a glycoprotein. Its amino acid composition (Table 4) shows a twofold excess of acidic over basic residues and lacks cysteine.

TABLE 4. *Amino acid composition of the mouse olfactory bulb protein*

Amino acid	Moles per 20,000 g			
	1	2	3	4
Lysine	12.7	11.5		
Histidine	1.3	1.4		
Arginine	8.1	8.4		
Aspartate	19.4	19.1	17.4	
Threonine	7.8	7.6		
Serine	9.1	7.6		
Glutamate	26.4	25.7	26.0	
Proline	7.2	6.7	5.7	
Glycine	11.9	9.4	13.2	
Alanine	11.6	9.9		
Cysteine	—	—	0.3	
Valine	7.7	8.1	7.3	
Methionine	2.9	2.9	3.0	
i-Leucine	5.0	5.0		
Leucine	17.6	17.9		
Tyrosine	2.0	2.0		
Phenylalanine	6.1	6.1		
Tryptophan				1.8

1, 2—22-hr hydrolysis at 110°C in constant boiling HCl of the electrophoretically homogeneous protein.
3—performic acid oxidation of 90% homogeneous protein.
4—value determined spectrophotometrically.

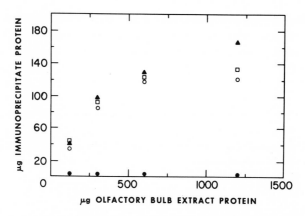

FIG. 4. Effect of preabsorption of mouse olfactory bulb (MOB) protein antiserum with various mouse tissue extracts on the immunoprecipitation titration against MOB extracts. Antiserum (1.5 ml) preabsorbed with 150 mg of lyophilized soluble extract: olfactory bulb (●); whole brain following removal of olfactory bulb (□); liver (○); bovine serum albumin (▲).

The regional specificity of this protein was demonstrated by immunoprecipitation; only extracts of the olfactory bulb were able to react with antibody against the protein (Fig. 4). The reactive protein appears to represent approximately 0.5 to 1% of the total soluble protein of the mouse olfactory bulb. There is a significant amount of the protein present at birth, and a marked increase after this time.

TABLE 5. *Strain survey of mob protein levels in female mouse olfactory bulbs*

μg immunoprecipitate protein	
mg extract protein	Strain
0–200	
200–400	SEA/GnJ, DBA/2J, LP/J, 129/J, C3H/HeJ, DBA/1J*, C3HeB/FeJ*
400–600	BUB/BnJ, PL/J, Au/SsJ, C58/J*, Ttf/t⁶*, SM/J, AKR/J, C57L/J, TP/R1, ot¹*, RF/J, RIII/2J, C57BL/6J, C57BL/KsJ*, CBA/CaJ*, LB/J, P/J*, DBA/2DeJ*, C57BL/6J-cʲ*, CF-1, C57BL/6J-T²ʲ*, MWT*
600–800	BALB/cJ, C57BL/10J, CBA/J, SJL/J, MA/J*, C57Br/cdJ, A/J, A/HeJ, SWR/J, BDP/J*, I/LnJ*, ST/bJ*
800–1,000	CE/J, SEC/1ReJ

* Not tested for electrophoretic variant.

When different mouse strains were compared, no differences in electrophoretic mobility of the protein were observed between strains, and the level of the protein remained fairly constant (Table 5). Since olfaction is heavily involved in modulating various behaviors, particularly sexual behaviors, it was thought that the olfactory bulb-specific protein might be responsive to endocrine condition. However, there were no sex differences in level within a given strain, and the level was not significantly altered by hypophysectomy, gonadectomy, or adrenalectomy.

Olfactory receptor cells make their first synapse within the olfactory bulb. When a radioimmunoassay method was utilized to examine the distribution of the specific protein within the olfactory areas, it was localized in the olfactory bulb, the nasal olfactory epithelium, and the vomeronasal organ. A cross-reaction could be obtained in these same regions of the hamster and rat but not of other species, suggesting either that the protein is found only in rodents or that the antiserum is very specific. Immunoprecipitation of protein labeled with ^{3}H-amino acid indicated that only those two tissues containing the receptor cells synthesize the protein (Fig. 5). The protein is present in, but not synthesized by, the bulb, suggesting that it arrives there by axoplasmic flow. The absence of the protein from the tongue and lung indicates that it is not generally found in chemoreceptor cells nor in respiratory epithelium, respectively.

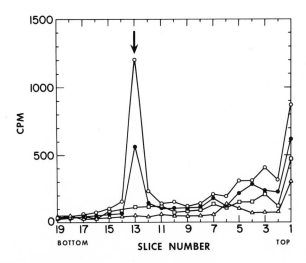

FIG. 5. SDS-polyacrylamide gel electrophoresis patterns of the ^{3}H-labeled immunoprecipitates from extracts of olfactory epithelium (○), Jacobson's vomeronasal organ (●), lung (□), and tongue (△) following incubation with ^{3}H-amino acids *in vitro*. Carrier nonradioactive bulb extract was added to the lung and tongue extracts. The arrow indicates the location of the MOB protein.

In collaboration with B. Hartman (Washington University, St. Louis), preliminary histological examination with fluorescent antibody has shown that the distribution of the protein is unique and is consistent with its localization to the sensory receptor cells. This unique localization to a single neuron within a fairly well-known pathway will be used to study its function. These olfactory receptor cells are of particular interest because they do not originate from the embryonic neural crest, but are one of the few neuronal types which directly synapse in the brain but originate from the periphery. This protein is an example of selective genetic expression by a specific differentiated neuron.

B. The Glial Fibrillary Acidic Protein

A water-soluble protein which has been designated glial fibrillary acidic protein (GFAP) has been isolated by Eng from human pathologic tissues rich in fibrous astrocytes, i.e., plaques from multiple sclerosis (MS) brains (Eng, Gerstl, and Vanderhaegen, 1970; Eng, Vanderhaegen, Bignami, and Gerstl, 1971). The protein isolated from MS plaques by ammonium sulfate precipitation and isoelectric precipitation is more than 95% GFAP, and a fraction containing 60 to 70% GFAP can be obtained from normal white matter by the same procedure. Further purification in good yield has been hampered by the tendency of the protein to aggregate. The GFAP contains high levels of aspartic and glutamic acid, alanine, and leucine, no cysteine, and negligible amounts of lipid and carbohydrate. It does not bind to concanavalin, has no Na^+, K^+, Mg^{++}, Ca^{++}-activated ATPase or actomyosin ATPase activity, and does not bind to DEAE-Sephadex as strongly as neurotubule protein.

The protein migrates as two bands with an average molecular weight of 43,000 by SDS electrophoresis, but is excluded by Sephadex G-100 and G-200. Sedimentation velocity studies in the analytical ultracentrifuge suggest that it is a globular protein, and sedimentation equilibrium analyses indicate that the native molecular weight is over 100,000. The use of the bifunctional reagent, dimethyl suberimidate (Davies and Stark, 1970), and SDS gel electrophoresis has shown that freshly prepared soluble GFAP occurs in solution primarily in the monomer form of 43,000 daltons; however, the protein aggregates to 120,000 to 160,000 daltons on standing in the cold for 24 hr. The latter results are consistent with the data obtained by column chromatography and ultracentrifugation, which suggest that the protein occurs in solution (24 hr or more) as an oligomer with molecular weights in excess of 100,000.

Cyanogen bromide peptide maps of the protein analyzed on SDS gels showed that 50% of the protein has degraded to a fraction with a molecular weight of 20,000 to 21,000, with the remainder occurring in two fractions less than 13,000. The protein separates into two closely migrating bands in SDS electrophoresis at pH 7, but these bands are well separated in the urea-Tris-glycinate buffer system at pH 8.3 (Bryan and Wilson, 1970). Amino acid compositions of the two fractions show similar high proportions of aspartic and glutamic acid, alanine, and leucine. The N-terminal amino acids of the two proteins as determined by dansylation are alanine and leucine.

Specific antibodies against the water-soluble GFAP have been produced in the rabbit. Rabbit anti-GFAP serum cross-reacts with extracts of human brain tissue, both normal and pathological (old MS plaques, leucotomy scars, and fibrillary astrocytoma). No cross-reaction was observed with other organs and tissues, peripheral nerve included (Uyeda, Eng, and Bignami, 1972). The GFAP is not species specific; cross-reaction occurs between anti-human GFAP serum and brain extracts of rabbit, guinea pig, rat, and dog. With anti-GFAP serum, astrocytes are selectively stained with the indirect immunofluorescence technique in both normal and pathological (gliosed) brain tissue (Bignami, Eng, Dahl, and Uyeda, 1972).

Based on amino acid composition, molecular weight, and electrophoretic mobility in three different acrylamide gel systems, it was thought that the GFAP was also the main protein in the water-insoluble MS plaque fraction. It was suggested that the water-soluble GFAP was the nonaggregated subunits whereas the water-insoluble GFAP was the glial filaments observed in astrocytes (Bignami et al., 1972). When buffer containing 0.5% Sarkosyl (dodecyl sarcosine) was used to dissolve microtubule antigens for immunologic studies (Fulton, Kane, and Stephens, 1971), the water-insoluble GFAP was found to react specifically with serum from rabbits immunized with the water-soluble GFAP. Using 0.5% Sarkosyl buffer to solubilize the proteins, the contents of the protein in the water-soluble and -insoluble proteins of MS plaques were determined and found to correspond to that obtained chemically. Antibody against the water-insoluble GFAP prepared in guinea pigs was found to react specifically with the water-soluble and -insoluble GFAP. The protein did not react with antiserum to rat antigen alpha (kindly provided by Dr. G. Bennett), antiserum to S-100 (kindly supplied by Dr. H. Herschman), or antiserum to chick neurotubule protein. Antisera to the GFAP produced in the guinea pig or rabbit did not react with purified chick and human neurotubule protein or with S-100 protein.

C. Visual System-Specific Protein in the Pigeon

Retinal ablation (Cuénod, Sandri, and Akert, 1970) or depression of both fast and slow axoplasmic flow by the intraocular injection of colchicine

(Boesch, Marko, and Cuénod, 1972) in the pigeon are rapidly followed by the development of enlarged optic nerve terminals (Cuénod, Sandri, and Akert, 1972). Cuénod, Marko, and Niederer (1973) have examined the subcellular fractions of the optic lobe contralateral to an ablated retina to determine if this histologic change was accompanied by a change in protein composition. No changes were found in the synaptosome-enriched fraction, as indicated by SDS-polyacrylamide gel electrophoresis. However, the fraction which sediments between 1.4 and 1.6 M sucrose shows the disappearance of one protein band 3 weeks after retinal ablation.

The decrease in this protein can be detected by 7 days after ablation, and it is labeled within 1 day following intraocular injection of ^{3}H-proline, indicating that its levels are maintained via the fast axoplasmic transport mechanism. The bands corresponding to this protein were not found following SDS-polyacrylamide gel electrophoresis of the same subcellular fraction from pigeon telencephalon or spinal cord, suggesting that it is specific for pigeon optic nerve.

IV. NERVOUS SYSTEM PROTEINS OF WIDE PHYLOGENETIC DISTRIBUTION

A. The S-100 Protein

Although many chemical and biological studies of the acidic glial-specific protein S-100 have been carried out, little knowledge is currently available concerning either its exact structure or function. There is a growing body of evidence which indicates that the S-100 protein fraction from brain is not a single homogeneous protein species but rather a heterogeneous mixture of polypeptide chains possessing similar physiochemical properties. The initial work of Gombos, Vincedon, Tardy, and Mandel (1966) indicated that S-100 was electrophoretically heterogeneous, and this has been verified subsequently (Vincedon, Waksman, Uyemura, Tardy, and Gombos, 1967; Uyemura, Vincedon, Gombos, and Mandel, 1971). The observations of Calissano, Moore, and Friesen (1969) that a set of distinct protein species could be separated from "homogeneous" bovine S-100 preparations by electrophoresis in the presence of low concentrations of Ca^{++} or 8 M urea would be easily explained if heterogeneity exists. Stewart (1972) recently demonstrated that bovine brain homogenates contain proteins of different native molecular weights which cross-react with anti-bovine S-100 antisera, and was able to subfractionate the smallest size class (19,500 to 21,000 daltons) into a number of distinct species. Antiserum prepared against one of these distinct species cross-reacted with all others, even the other molecular weight size classes (43,000 and 71,000 daltons). [Unfortunately, because no chain weight determinations were carried out on the various size classes, varying aggregation states cannot be ruled out.]

Dannies and Levine (1969) have shown that S-100 is probably a trimeric molecule consisting of three 7,000 dalton subunits, and have indicated (Dannies and Levine, 1971) that at least one of these subunits is different from the others, containing the single tryptophan residue present in the 21,000-dalton protein.

Vanaman and his co-workers have attempted to elucidate the primary and quaternary structure of the S-100 protein and its possible relationship to other acidic proteins of the nervous system. In order to minimize possible proteolytic degradation of S-100 during preparation, they have devised a new preparation scheme which is rapid yet applicable to large amounts of material. The preparation scheme consists of: (1) preparation of a brain homogenate supernatant in Tris-acetate, pH 6.5; (2) absorption of basic and neutral proteins on CM-Sephadex C-50 using a batch process; (3) concentration of the acidic protein fraction by absorption, then step elution using DEAE-Sephadex A-50; (4) separation of this acidic fraction on DEAE-Sephadex A-25 with a shallow salt gradient at pH 7.5; and (5) gel filtration chromatography on Sephadex G-100. The entire procedure can be completed in 4 days. More importantly, the S-100 fraction is separated from the bulk protein very rapidly. This procedure also purifies to homogeneity another very acidic brain protein (called post-S-100 protein), which resembles S-100 in physicochemical properties but is apparently unrelated to it.

The S-100 protein fraction from bovine or porcine brain was prepared by the above procedure and compared to that obtained by the procedure of Dannies and Levine (1971). All preparations of S-100 cross-reacted with rabbit antibovine S-100 antiserum (provided by Dr. L. Levine, Department of Biochemistry, Brandeis University), gave single broad bands migrating faster than bromphenol blue on analytical gel electrophoresis as described by Calissano et al. (1969), and had similar amino acid compositions. All preparations showed gross heterogeneity when examined on pH 3 to 6 analytical isoelectric focusing gels in 6 M urea (Fig. 6), with a minimum of four major bands, as opposed to post-S-100 protein which gave only a single sharp band. Figure 7 shows the resolution, on 15% acrylamide urea-SDS gels, of two distinct species in the S-100 fractions from various preparations having apparent chain weights of 6,900 and 5,000 daltons. Again, the presence of two distinct sizes of polypeptide chains in the S-100 fraction is independent of the source of S-100 or the method of preparation. Post-S-100 protein has a chain weight of 19,200.

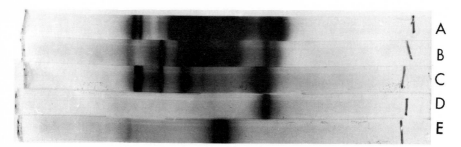

FIG. 6. Analytical isoelectric focusing gels of various S-100 preparations. 7.5% Acrylamide–0.1% bisacrylamide with pH 3 to 6 ampholines in 6M urea. The pin indicates the pH 3 end of the gel. A: bovine S-100 prepared as described in the text; B: bovine S-100 prepared by the method of Dannies and Levine (1971); C: porcine S-100 prepared as described in the text; D: porcine post-S-100 protein; E: standard bovine α-lactalbumin.

The post-S-100 protein is totally devoid of cysteine and tryptophan as compared to S-100, which has four cysteines and one tryptophan. The amino acid composition of the Ca^{++} binding phosphoprotein of Wolff and Siegel (1972) bears a striking resemblance to S-100 on a mole percent basis. The molecular weight of this phosphoprotein is 11,500 daltons, which agrees well with the sum of the chain weights which Vanaman has found in the

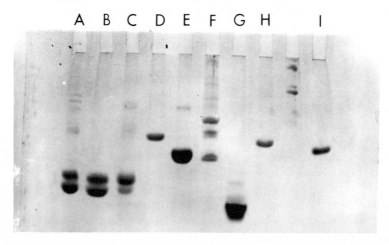

FIG. 7. Urea-SDS gel electrophoresis of S-100 and post-S-100 protein preparations. 15% Acrylamide–0.2% bisacrylamide, 0.1% SDS, 0.1M NaPi, 0.01M 2-mercaptoethanol, 6M urea, pH 7.1. A: bovine S-100 as in 6 A, above; B: as in 6 B; C: as in 6 C; D: as in 6 D; E: cytochrome C; F: avian myeloblastosis virus; G: insulin B-chain; H: sperm whale myoglobin; I: bovine α-lactalbumin.

S-100 protein fraction. Current studies are in progress to examine further possible relationships between these two protein species.

All preparations of S-100 thus far obtained possess blocked amino termini as judged by both the dansyl technique and by use of the automatic Edman method. Detailed quantitative and qualitative analysis of the tryptic peptides obtained from oxidized porcine S-100 has revealed that trypsin digestion of S-100 produces 14 to 16 short peptides isolatable in very low yields. In contrast, one or two major insoluble core peptides contain 95% of the cysteic acid present in the S-100 starting material. The major peptide in this fraction has glutamic acid or glutamine at its amino terminus. Similar results have been obtained using reduced ^{14}C-S-carboxymethyl bovine S-100. These preliminary findings strongly suggest, although they do not demonstrate unequivocally, that the S-100 fraction obtained from brain using the purification procedures described above is heterogeneous, consisting of a major core polypeptide with varying lengths of partially degraded chain attached.

F. Michetti, N. Miani, G. DeRenzis, A. Caniglia, and S. Correr have obtained evidence indicating that the S-100 protein is an integral constituent of the chromatin acidic protein fraction. Nuclei were obtained from rabbit cerebral cortex (Løvtrup-Rein and McEwen, 1966), and the nuclear proteins were fractionated into soluble and deoxyribonucleoprotein (DNP) fractions (Steele and Busch, 1963; Wang, 1967). As shown in Table 6, S-100 is present in both nuclear protein fractions. Although the nuclear S-100 constitutes only 0.55% of the total soluble S-100 present in the cytosol, the concentration of S-100 in the cytosol is not more than 10-fold greater than that in the nucleus. That the nuclear S-100 is not the result of contamination is indicated by the insignificant amount present in the nonsonicated suspension and the high DNA/RNA ratios of this suspension. Furthermore, addition of fluorescein-labeled S-100 antibody to these nuclei showed an intense fluorescence within all large nuclei but a weak fluorescence within smaller nuclei. The nucleolar core within the large nuclei exhibited only a weak fluorescence. Virtually no antibody reaction was observed using liver nuclei.

The possibility that S-100 was transported into the nuclei was tested utilizing ^{125}I-S-100 (Rosa, Scassellati, Pennisi, Riccioni, Giagnoni, and Giordani, 1964). Ca^{++} or Mg^{++} was required in order to obtain significant uptake into isolated nuclei. In agreement with the initial findings, salt fractionation released labeled S-100 into both the soluble and DNP fractions (Table 7). An additional release of DNA-related S-100 was obtained following DNase treatment, but further treatment with RNase released only a small additional amount, suggesting that the protein is not primarily

TABLE 6. *S-100 and DNA in fractions of isolated nuclei and in the cytosol of rabbit brain cortex (μg or mg/g wet wt)*

Fraction	S-100 μg	DNA μg	S 100/Protein μg/mg	DNA/RNA mg/mg
Nuclear suspension	trace	281.7	—	25
Soluble protein fraction 0.14 M-NaCl	0.211	0	0.634	—
Deoxyribonucleoprotein fraction 2 M-NaCl	0.107	213.1	0.330	150
Cytosol 150,000 g_{av} supernatant	139.500	0	5.070	—

The values are the average of seven experiments. The nuclear yield was 40.2 ± 5 per cent.

TABLE 7. *In vitro uptake of [^{125}I]-S-100 into fractions of isolated nuclei of rabbit brain cortex*

Fraction	[^{125}I]-S-100 recovery%	Specific activity cpm×10^{-3}/mg DNA	cpm×10^{-3}/mg prot.
Nuclear suspension	100.0	135.1	26.5
Soluble protein fraction 0.14 M-NaCl	43.5	—	45.2
Deoxyribonucleoprotein fraction 2 M-NaCl	19.0	66.9 ·	13.9
DNase extract	10.7		
RNase extract	2.7		
Residual or "nucleolar" fraction	24.6		

related to RNA in the residue. A consistent amount of S-100 remains in the residual fraction, generally thought to consist of nuclear membrane fragments and nucleoli (Busch, 1967). It is therefore assumed that the labeled ^{125}I-S-100 interacts with components of these structures through forces that are not disrupted by ionic strength and DNase.

The uptake of labeled S-100 by liver nuclei followed the same general pattern as that seen in brain nuclei, but to only one-tenth the specific activity. These studies indicate that the S-100 protein is an integral constituent of the chromatin acidic protein, and its presence here suggests that it may be involved in genomic regulation within neural tissue. This possibility is currently being examined by studying the effect of the protein on RNA synthesis.

B. The 14–3–2 Protein

The identity of antigen α, first described by Bennett and Edelman (1968), with the 14-3-2 protein of Moore has been determined following a series of studies with antibodies to the two proteins. The appearance of this protein during ontogeny in the rat has now been examined by Bennett using microcomplement fixation. Only 2% of the total adult level is present on day 17 of gestation. This level increases threefold by the time of birth on day 21, at which time highest levels are found in the spinal cord and cortical levels

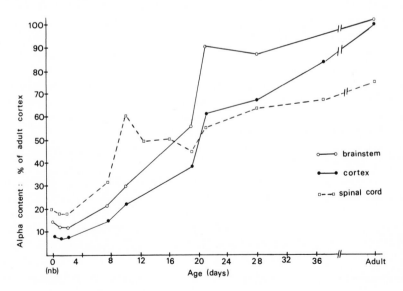

FIG. 8. Change in antigen alpha content of rat brain regions with age.

are quite low. A gradual increase occurs in all areas, with spinal cord levels essentially reaching their adult value by day 12 and brainstem reaching 90% adult level by 20 days; cortex reaches 80% of its adult level by day 36 (Fig. 8). Levels in the dorsal root ganglion and sciatic nerve are much lower than those seen in the CNS.

V. BRAIN-SPECIFIC SOLUBLE SIALOGLYCOPROTEIN

Glycoproteins are widely distributed in virtually all tissues. They are present in all brain regions, with highest levels in those areas which are rich in neuronal cell bodies, and are predominantly membrane bound. In brain, 30% of the sialic acid is incorporated into glycoprotein, occurring as the terminal sugar moiety. Van Nieuw Amerongen, Van den Eijnden, Heijlman, and Roukema (1972) have isolated an apparently brain-specific soluble sialoglycoprotein from the cortical gray matter of calf brain.

Following a two-step pH precipitation of the soluble cell fraction, the supernatant was concentrated and sialic acid-rich protein fractions were eluted with Tris-HCl buffer from a Biogel P-300 column. The fraction which is soluble in 70% ethanol following a two-step ethanol precipitation contains the sialoglycoprotein, which has been designated as GP-350, because it can be eluted from DEAE-cellulose columns with 350 mM NaCl at pH 7.0. The protein has a molecular weight of approximately 11,600 daltons and contains only one sialic acid residue per molecule (A. Van Nieuw Amerongen and P. A. Roukema, *personal communication*).

Approximately 3% of the protein and at least 20% of the sialic acid of the original soluble cell fraction is comprised of the isolated sialoglyco-protein, indicating that it represents at least 390 μg of protein and 14 μg of sialic acid per gram of wet cortical gray matter. The purity of the GP-350 protein was indicated by the presence of only one protein and carbohydrate band in 7.5% acrylamide gels at pH 8.9 and 7.5 and one band in 15% gels. The GP-350 protein is present in all brain areas. The highest levels were found in those regions which are relatively rich in ganglia, such as caudate nucleus, cerebellar gray and pons, with the lowest levels in cerebral gray and white matter and in corpus callosum. Amino acid analysis of the protein showed that 26.1% of the amino acid residues were glutamic and aspartic acids and their amides. An O-glycosidic bond of galactosamine to serine or threonine is alkali labile; an N-glycosidic bond of glucosamine to aspara-gine is alkali stable. Alkaline sodium borohydride treatment resulted in a loss of serine and threonine and a loss of two-thirds of the galactosamine content, whereas the glucosamine content was unaltered, indicating that the

O-glycosidic linkages in the molecule involve galactosamine and serine and/or threonine. The O-glycosidic linkages comprise only 15 to 20% of all peptide-carbohydrate linkages in brain glycoproteins, and only microtubular protein has been found to have such linkages (Margolis, Margolis, and Shelanski, 1972).

Another unusual feature of the molecule is the presence of 4% glucose in the carbohydrate moiety of GP-350. This glucose did not appear to be the result of contamination with glycolipids or glycogen, and the glucose does appear to be a true structural component of the molecule.

A sialoglycoprotein representing the fastest migrating band of the soluble fraction of human, sheep, and rat brain has also been detected, and the human and rat brain sialoglycoprotein has been found to have very similar properties to that of calf brain. DEAE-cellulose column analysis indicates that the protein is absent from calf kidney, liver, and blood serum.

Subcellular distribution studies indicated that GP-350 is present in the soluble cell fraction and in the synaptosomal membrane fraction, whereas it is absent from the purified nuclei, mitochondria, myelin, and the microsomal fraction. The brain specificity and the cellular localization of the protein will be investigated further using immunological techniques.

VI. THE ANALYSIS OF COMPLEX PROTEIN MIXTURES

A quantitative method for the analysis of complex protein mixtures, termed crossed immunoelectrophoresis, has been applied to soluble rat brain proteins by Bock, Mellerup, and Rafaelson (1972) and to synaptosomal extracts by Bock and Jørgensen. The protein mixture is first electrophoresed on agarose-coated glass plates at pH 8.6, then the gel strip with the protein bands is cut out of the first dimension gel and placed on a second glass plate. The rest of this plate is covered with gel containing antibodies against either water extractable rat brain proteins or rat synaptosomal proteins. The proteins of the first dimension electrophoresis are then electrophoresed into the antibody-gel, forming precipitation lines for each of the different proteins. The area enclosed by a specific line is proportional to the amount of the corresponding protein originally applied. It is possible by absorption *in situ* (Bock, 1972) to distinguish brain-specific proteins from nonspecific proteins. By means of this technique, Bock has identified five brain-specific proteins in rat brain extracts, four of which are common to the synaptosomal extracts. It has been possible to detect approximately 60 different proteins in the rat brain system and about 30 different proteins in the synaptosomal system.

VII. THE SYNTHESIS OF BRAIN PROTEINS

A. The Synthesis of Tubulin

Cell-free protein synthetic systems are potentially well suited to the study of regulation of specific proteins since they permit a sequential variation of the many parameters which may regulate this process *in vivo*. With the exception of some recent reports (Raeburn and Baxter, 1971; Zomzely-Neurath, York, and Moore, 1972), little is known about the cell-free synthesis of specific proteins or their regulation in the nervous system. The importance and relative abundance of microtubular protein in the nervous system (see Chapters 10 and 11) make it a logical protein for such investigation. Raeburn and Baxter (1971, 1972, *Personal Communication*), have recently demonstrated the incorporation of ^{14}C-labeled amino acid substrates into soluble protein fractions that possess many of the properties of colchicine-binding microtubular protein.

Ribosomal and pH 5 enzyme fractions were incubated with a standard incubation mixture of ^{14}C-amino acids and cofactors modified from Tewari and Baxter (1969). The newly synthesized ^{14}C-labeled protein was released from the polyribosomes, isolated from the high-speed supernatant fraction, and analyzed for ^{14}C-labeled colchicine-binding protein.

It was possible to demonstrate the binding of more than 25% of the ^{14}C-labeled soluble protein with ^{3}H-colchicine. Some unlabeled colchicine-binding protein from a post-microsomal supernatant fraction was used as a carrier. When this mixture was chromatographed on DEAE-Sephadex A-50, the elution patterns of ^{14}C-labeled supernatant protein coincided with that of protein-bound ^{3}H-colchicine (Fig. 9). Gel filtration on Sephadex G-200 showed coincidence of a ^{14}C-labeled protein peak with ^{3}H-colchicine-binding protein and indicated a molecular weight for the ^{3}H-colchicine-binding protein of 120,000, which is in good agreement with the value obtained by Weisenberg, Borisy, and Taylor (1968) for porcine microtubular protein.

Isoelectric focusing (Fig. 10) demonstrated a coincidence of two peaks of protein-bound ^{3}H-colchicine with two peaks of ^{14}C-labeled material, with isoelectric points of 5.3 and 4.2. This is in agreement with the observation (James and Austin, 1970) that two ionic species of colchicine-binding microtubular proteins are formed *in vivo* in the chicken sciatic nerve.

Incubation of the ^{14}C-labeled supernatant protein with carrier microtubular protein, ^{3}H-colchicine, and vinblastine sulfate under conditions

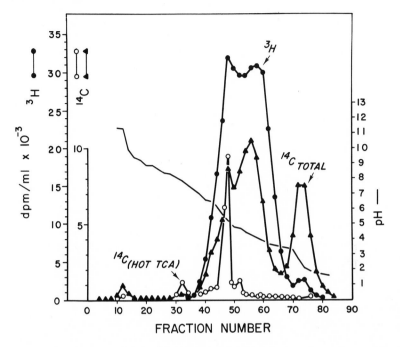

FIG. 9. DEAE-Sephadex A-50 chromatography of ^{14}C-labeled supernatant protein and ^{3}H-colchicine-binding protein. The ribosomal cell-free system was incubated with ^{14}C-leucine and the resulting ^{14}C-labeled supernatant protein fraction obtained as described in the text. The soluble proteins were dialyzed at 4°C against several changes of 0.01 M sodium phosphate buffer (pH 6.5), containing 0.01M MgCl$_2$ and 10^{-4}M GTP to remove free ^{14}C-leucine and to alter the medium. Fifteen ml of the resulting solution containing 12-mg protein was then incubated for 1 hr at 37°C with 1 ml of the post-microsomal supernatant fraction containing the carrier microtubular protein (13.1-mg protein) and 1.8 μC of ^{3}H-colchicine (specific activity 0.5 mC/μmole). A column of DEAE-Sephadex A-50, 4.7 cm high by 1.3 cm in diameter, was equilibrated with the phosphate buffer and 16 ml of incubation mixture applied to it. The conditions for chromatography were based on those of Weisenberg et al. (1968). Step-wise elution of protein from the column was carried out with the following solutions: 25 ml of 0.1M NaCl, 40 ml of 0.3M NaCl, and 40 ml of 0.8M NaCl contained in the above buffer. Conductivity values of 2.5, 9.3, 22.8, and 47.5 mmho corresponded to 0.0, 0.1, 0.3, and 0.8M NaCl in buffer, respectively. All column eluates were collected as 2-ml fractions. Aliquots of 0.5 ml were counted in 10 ml of Aquasol under conditions described in the text. Salt gradient (——); tritium (——●——); ^{14}C (——▲——).

similar to those of Marantz, Ventilla, and Shelanski (1969) resulted in the formation of a precipitate which contained bound ^{3}H-colchicine and small amounts of ^{14}C-labeled protein, representing 3 to 4% of the total ^{14}C-labeled soluble protein. ^{14}C-Labeled soluble protein could also be precipitated with rabbit anti-serum to rat brain microtubular protein.

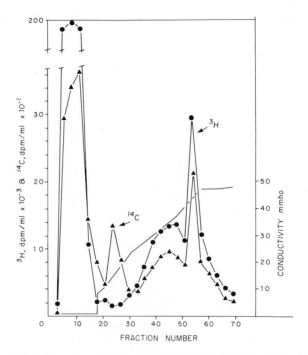

FIG. 10. Isoelectric focusing of ^{14}C-labeled supernatant protein and ^{3}H-colchicine-binding protein. The ^{14}C-labeled amino acid mixture was incubated with the cell-free system as described in the text. The resultant ^{14}C-labeled supernatant fraction, 9 ml containing 22.5 mg protein, was incubated with 1.6 ml of post-microsomal supernatant fraction, 15.4 mg of protein, and 1.8 μC of ^{3}H-colchicine (specific activity 0.5 mC/μmole), for 1 hr at 37°C. After the incubation, the mixture was dialyzed for 16 hr at 4°C against 0.01M sodium phosphate buffer (pH 6.5), containing 0.01M MgCl$_2$ and 10^{-4}M GTP, to remove free ^{3}H-colchicine and ^{14}C-labeled amino acids. During dialysis, there was significant denaturation and approximately 40% of the radioactivity was lost. After dialysis, the precipitate was removed by centrifugation, and 15 ml of the supernatant solution was electrofocused for 65 hr at 4°C in a pH gradient from pH 3 to 10, containing 1% ampholine carrier ampholytes. Following this procedure, 1-ml samples were collected and aliquots were processed for counting. pH gradient (——); ^{3}H (——●——); ^{14}C (——▲——); ^{14}C in hot trichloroacetic acid-precipitable material (○).

Further experimentation suggested that vinblastine sulfate, which is known to aggregate microtubular protein, precipitated a factor required for optimal protein synthesis. When a pH 5 supernatant fraction was added to the *in vitro* incubation system, protein-synthesizing capacity was enhanced significantly. However, pretreatment of the pH 5 supernatant fraction with 1.0 mM vinblastine sulfate (at pH 6.5 or 7.0) abolished the stimulating activity.

The nature of the factor involved in protein synthesis and precipitated by vinblastine sulfate was investigated (Raeburn and Baxter, 1972). Component reactions of protein synthesis were studied separately. Peptide synthetase (ribosome-bound peptide bond formation) and peptide chain elongation factor E.F. I (aminoacyl-tRNA binding factor) were not inhibited by vinblastine sulfate. However, amino acid activation and peptide chain elongation factor E.F. II (translocase) were inhibited. The pH 5 supernatant fraction contains large amounts of E.F. II, and it is probable therefore that vinblastine sulfate interacts either with E.F. II itself or with another protein related to E.F. II.

Since vinblastine sulfate has no absolute specificity for microtubular protein (Wilson, Bryan, Ruby, and Mazia, 1970), it is not possible at this time to assign a specific role to microtubular protein, or a subunit thereof, in the translocation reaction, but such a function is a distinct possibility.

B. The Synthesis of S-100

Early studies (McEwen and Hydén, 1966) showed the rates of S-100 synthesis and degradation to be extremely rapid, representing 15% of the total soluble protein synthesis (Rubin and Stenzel, 1965), whereas more recent work has shown that the rates of synthesis and degradation of S-100 are similar to that of other cell proteins. This problem has been reinvestigated by Lerner and Herschman (1972). A cell-free polyribosomal system from rat brain tissue was utilized, and the S-100 synthesized during a 1-hr incubation was determined by antibody precipitation and gel electrophoreses following removal of the polyribosomes by ultracentrifugation.

The S-100 obtained by this *in vitro* incubation procedure not only reacted with the antibody to S-100, but migrated at the normal position in SDS-polyacrylamide gels. This protein was found to represent 0.15% of the total soluble protein released from the ribosome. Since the S-100 protein represents 0.8% of the total soluble protein in brain tissue, this indicates that its rate of synthesis is not more rapid than that of other brain proteins.

REFERENCES

Alemà, S., Calissano, P., Rusca, G., and Giuditta, A. (1973): *Journal of Neurochemistry, (in press)*.
Arch, S. (1972*a*): *Journal of General Physiology*, 59:47.
Arch, S. (1972*b*): *Journal of General Physiology*, 60:102.
Bennett, G., and Edelman, G. (1968): Isolation of an acidic protein from rat brain. *Journal of Biological Chemistry*, 243:6234.
Berry, R. W., and Cohen, M. J. (1972): Synaptic stimulation of RNA metabolism in the giant neuron of *Aplysia californica*. *Journal of Neurobiology*, 3:209.
Bignami, A., Eng, L. F., Dahl, D., and Uyeda, C. T. (1972): Localization of the glial fibrillary acidic protein in astrocytes by immunofluorescence. *Brain Research*, 43:429.

Bock, E. (1972): Identification and characterization of water-soluble rat brain antigens. I. Brain and species specificity. *Journal of Neurochemistry,* 19:1731.

Bock, E., Mellerup, E. T., and Rafaelson, O. J. (1972): Antigen-antibody crossed electrophoresis on water-soluble rat brain antigens. *Journal of Neurochemistry,* 18:2435.

Boesch, J., Marko, P., and Cuénod, M. (1972): Effects of colchicine on axonal transport of proteins in the pigeon visual pathway. *Neurobiology,* 2:123.

Brunngraber, E., Susz, J. P., and Warecka, K. (1970): Isolation of brain-specific glycoprotein. *Journal of Neurochemistry,* 17:829.

Bryan, J., and Wilson, L. (1970): Are cytoplasmic microtubules heteropolymers? *Proceedings of the National Academy of Sciences,* 68:1762.

Busch, H. (1967): In: *Methods in Enzymology,* Vol. 12, edited by L. Grossman and K. Moldave, p. 448.

Calissano, P., Moore, B. W., and Friesen, A. (1969): Effect of calcium ion on S-100, a protein of the nervous system. *Biochemistry,* 8:4318.

Cuénod, M., Marko, P., and Niederer, E. (1973): Disappearance of particulate tectal protein during optic nerve degeneration in the pigeon. *Brain Research (in press).*

Cuénod, M., Sandri, C., and Akert, K. (1970): Enlarged synaptic vesicles as an early sign of secondary degeneration in the optic nerve terminals of the pigeon. *Journal of Cell Science,* 60:605.

Cuénod, M., Sandri, C., and Akert, K. (1972): Enlarged synaptic vesicles in optic nerve terminals induced by intraocular injection of colchicine. *Brain Research,* 39:285.

Dannies, P. S., and Levine, L. (1969): Demonstration of subunits in beef brain acidic protein (S-100). *Biochemical and Biophysical Research Communications,* 37:587.

Dannies, P. S., and Levine, L. (1971): Structural properties of bovine brain S-100 protein. *Journal of Biological Chemistry,* 246:6276.

Davies, G. E., and Stark, G. R. (1970): Use of dimethyl suberimidate, a cross-linking reagent, in studying the subunit structure of oligomeric proteins. *Proceedings of the National Academy of Sciences,* 66:651.

Delpech, B., Delpech, A., Clement, J., and Laumonier, R. (1972): *International Journal of Cancer,* 9:374.

Eng, L. F., Gerstl, B., and Vanderhaeghen, J. J. (1970): *Transactions of the American Society for Neurochemistry,* 1:42.

Eng, L. F., Vanderhaeghen, J. J., Bignami, A., and Gerstl, B. (1971): An acidic protein isolated from fibrous astrocytes. *Brain Research,* 28:351.

Frazier, W. T., Kandel, E. R., Kupfermann, I., Waziri, R., and Coggeshall, R. (1967): Morphological and functional properties of identified neurons in the abdominal ganglion of *Aplysia californica. Journal of Neurophysiology,* 30:1288.

Fulton, C., Kane, R. E., and Stephens, R. E. (1971): Serological similarity of flagellar and mitotic microtubules. *Journal of Cell Biology,* 50:762.

Giuditta, A., Moore, B. W., Prozzo, N., and Packard, A. (1971): Brain specific proteins in cephalopods. *Abstracts of the Third Congress of the International Society for Neurochemistry,* p. 18.

Gombos, G., Vincedon, G., Tardy, J., and Mandel, P. (1966): Hétérogéneité électrophorétique et préparation rapide de la fraction protéique S-100. *Comptes Rendue de l'Academie des Science (D) (Paris),* 263:1533.

Hemminki, K. (1972): Preparation of viable and morphologically intact cells from newborn rat brain. *Experimental Cell Research,* 75:379.

James, K. A. C., and Austin, L. (1970): The binding *in vitro* of colchicine to axoplasmic proteins from chicken sciatic nerve. *Biochemical Journal,* 117:773.

Kernell, D., and Peterson, R. P. (1970): The effect of spike activity versus synaptic activation on the metabolism of ribonucleic acid in a molluscan giant neurone. *Journal of Neurochemistry,* 17:1087.

Lerner, M. P., and Herschman, H. R. (1972): S-100 protein synthesis by isolated polyribosomes from rat brain. *Science,* 178:995.

Løvtrup-Rein, H., and McEwen, B. S. (1966): Isolation and fractionation of rat brain nuclei. *Journal of Cell Biology,* 30:405.

Marantz, R., Ventilla, M., and Shelanski, M. (1969): Vinblastine-induced precipitation of microtubule protein. *Science,* 165:498.

Margolis, R. K., Margolis, R. U., and Shelanski, M. L. (1972): The carbohydrate composition of brain microtubule protein. *Biochemical and Biophysical Research Communications,* 47:432.

McEwen, B. S., and Hydén, H. (1966): A study of specific brain proteins on the semi-micro scale. *Journal of Neurochemistry,* 13:823.

Moore, B. W. (1965*a*): *Biochemical and Biophysical Research Communications,* 19:739.

Moore, B. W. (1965*b*): *Proceedings of the International Conference on Neurochemistry,* Oxford, G. B. Ansell, editor.

Moore, B. W., and Perez, V. J. (1968): Specific acidic proteins of the nervous system. In: *Physiological and Biochemical Aspects of Nervous Integration,* edited by F. D. Carlson, p. 343. Prentice-Hall, Englewood Cliffs, N.J.

Raeburn, S., and Baxter, C. F. (1971): The synthesis *in vitro* of colchicine-binding protein. *Transactions of the American Society for Neurochemistry,* 2:101.

Raeburn, S., and Baxter, C. F. (1972): Vinblastine sulfate inhibition of rat brain cell-free protein synthesis. *Transactions of the American Society for Neurochemistry,* 3:115.

Roback, H. N., and Scherer, H. J. (1935): *Virchow's Archives,* 294:365.

Rosa, U., Scassellati, G. A., Pennisi, F., Riccioni, N., Giagnoni, P., and Giordani, R. (1964): Labelling of human fibrinogen with 131-I by electrolytic iodination. *Biochimica et Biophysica Acta,* 86:519.

Rubin, A. L., and Stenzel, K. H. (1965): *Proceedings of the National Academy of Sciences,* 53:963.

Steele, W. J., and Busch, H. (1963): *Cancer Research,* 23:1153.

Stewart, J. A. (1972): Tissue-specific brain S-100. A demonstration of multiple proteins. *Biochimica et Biophysica Acta,* 263:178.

Tewari, S., and Baxter, C. F. (1969): Stimulatory effect of γ-aminobutyric acid upon amino acid incorporation into protein by a ribosomal system from immature rat brain. *Journal of Neurochemistry,* 16:171.

Uyeda, C. T., Eng, L. F., and Bignami, A. (1972): Immunological study of the glial fibrillary protein. *Brain Research,* 37:81.

Uyemura, K., Vincendon, G., Gombos, G., and Mandel, P. (1971): Purification and some properties of S-100 protein fractions from sheep and pig brains. *Journal of Neurochemistry,* 18:429.

Van Nieuw Amerongen, A., Van den Eijnden, D. H., Heijlman, J., and Roukema, P. A. (1972): Isolation and characterization of a soluble glucose-containing sialoglycoprotein from the cortical gray matter of calf brain. *Journal of Neurochemistry,* 19:2195.

Vincendon, G., Waksman, A., Uyemura, K., Tardy, J., and Gombos, G. (1967): Ultracentrifugal behavior of beef brain S100 protein fraction. *Archives of Biochemistry,* 120:233.

Wang, T. Y. (1967): The isolation properties and possible functions of chromatin acidic proteins. *Journal of Biological Chemistry,* 242:1220.

Warecka, K., and Bauer, H. (1966): Studien über hirnproteine. Immunochemische untersuchungen der wasserlöslichen fractionen. *Deutsche Zeitschrift für Nervenheilkunde,* 189:53.

Warecka, K., and Bauer, H. (1967): Studies on "brain-specific" proteins in aqueous extracts of brain tissue. *Journal of Neurochemistry,* 14:783.

Warecka, K., and Müller, D. (1969): The appearance of human "brain specific" glycoprotein in ontogenesis. *Journal of Neurological Sciences,* 8:329.

Warecka, K., Müller, H. J., Vogel, H. M., and Tripatzia, J. (1972): Human brain-specific alpha$_2$-glycoprotein: Purification by affinity chromatography and detection of a new component: Localization in nervous cells. *Journal of Neurochemistry,* 19:719.

Weisenberg, R. C., Borisy, G. G., and Taylor, E. W. (1968): The colchicine-binding protein of mammalian brain and its relation to microtubules. *Biochemistry,* 7:4466.

Wilson, D. L. (1971): Molecular weight distribution of proteins synthesized in single, identified neurons of *Aplysia. Journal of General Physiology,* 57:26.

Wilson, D. L., and Berry, R. W. (1972): The effect of synaptic stimulation on RNA and protein metabolism in the R2 soma of *Aplysia*. *Journal of Neurobiology*, 3:369.

Wilson, L., Bryan, S., Ruby, A., and Mazia, D. (1970): Precipitation of proteins by vinblastine and calcium ions. *Proceedings of the National Academy of Sciences*, 66:807.

Wolff, D. J., and Siegel, F. L. (1972): Purification of a calcium-binding phosphoprotein from pig brain. *Journal of Biological Chemistry*, 247:4180.

Zomzely-Neurath, C., York, C., and Moore, B. W. (1972): Synthesis of a brain-specific protein (S-100 protein) in a homologous cell-free system programmed with cerebral polysomal messenger RNA. *Proceedings of the National Academy of Sciences*, 69:2326.

Proteins of the Nervous System
Raven Press, New York © 1973

Tissue and Cell Culture as a Tool in Neurochemistry

Harvey R. Herschman

I. INTRODUCTION

Many of the subjects discussed elsewhere in this volume have either been partially elucidated or could be approached using various tissue culture techniques. Although there are many books and reviews of cell and tissue culture which discuss either various culture techniques or various problems for which cell culture has served a specific function, no organized description of the application of alternative types of cell culture to neurochemical problems is currently available. I am presently preparing a methodological comparison of the culture systems used in neurobiology (Herschman, 1973). This review extends that format to describe neurochemical results obtained with culture techniques, as well as the possible role of cell and tissue culture in the future of neurochemistry. Despite this orientation, I would like to extend one disclaimer: tissue and cell culture should not be considered as a scientific discipline or field of research, but rather as a method or tool to be used in the analysis of specific problems. For example, my own laboratory has been interested in the appearance and regulation of macromolecules which are specific to the nervous system, and cell culture has provided us with a valuable method to analyze some aspects of these problems.

II. UNIQUE ADVANTAGES OF CULTURE SYSTEMS

The most obvious and most often exploited characteristic of culture techniques is their unique ability to isolate tissues or cells from the rest of the organism. The investigator can then maintain such isolated preparations for an extended period of time in a relatively defined and easily manipulatable environment. Consequently, one is able to study cellular interactions and biochemistry in the absence of the homeostatic effects operative *in vivo*. The *direct* effects of substances such as pharmacological agents, hormones, and growth factors can be observed when the ambiguities arising from biochemical changes produced in other tissues which mediate the neural response are removed. In addition, tissue or cell preparations can be subjected to chronic exposure to agents which would be toxic to the entire organism. Finally, environmental variables can be manipulated in either numerical or temporal combinations that are not possible *in vivo*. In this chapter I will describe the various types of culture systems currently utilized and discuss some applications of their unique properties to the resolution of problems in neurobiology. Table 1 summarizes the types of culture methods used and some of the problems to which these techniques have been applied.

Table 1.

Neural Cell and Tissue Culture

I **Primary Culture**
  1 Explant Culture
    A Myelination
    B Inborn Errors of Metabolism
    C Neurologic Mutants
    D Hormone Effects
    E Demyelinating Diseases
    F Synaptogenesis; Bioelectric Activity
    G Nerve Growth Factor
  2 Dispersed Cell Cultures
    A Growth Requirements
    B NGF Effects
    C Syaptogenesis
  3 Reggregation Culture
    A Neurologic Mutants
    B Requirements for Maturation
    C Specific Aggregation Factors
II **Continuous Cell Lines and Strains**
  1 Glia
    A S100 Protein
    B Enzyme Induction
    C Cyclic AMP
  2 Neuroblastoma
    A Morphological Maturation
    B Biochemical Differentiation
    C Electrophysiological Characteristics

III. EXPLANT CULTURES

At the close of the 19th Century the very nature of the nervous system was in doubt. One school, championed by Held and his associates, proposed that the fibrous connectives seen coursing within neural tissue were cytoplasmic bridges of a syncytial structure. The opposing school, led by Ramon y Cahal and His, maintained that these fibers grew out from individual cells and served as connectives between discrete cells comprising the nervous system. The first reported experiment using culture techniques was designed to resolve this neurobiological controversy. R. G. Harrison (1907) confirmed the neuronal theory of Cahal and His when he observed neuronal fibers growing out of a clotted lymph culture of embryonic tadpole tissue.

The great majority of culture studies of neural tissue have been performed by utilizing refinements and modifications of Harrison's method of explanting small pieces of embryonic neural tissue. Much of this work has recently been reviewed by Murray (1971), a leading contributor to this field. The most commonly utilized tissues for such studies are cerebellum, cerebrum, dorsal root ganglia, and autonomic ganglia from neonatal rodents or kittens and from chick embryos. The most commonly used procedure is the double-coverslip modification (Murray and Stout, 1942, 1947) of the Maximow assembly (Maximow, 1925). Small pieces of neonatal tissue (approximately 1 mm square) are placed on collagen-coated (Bornstein, 1958) coverslips, and the round coverslip is fixed by capillarity to a larger square coverslip. The explant is fed with a drop or two of nutrient medium containing a balanced salt solution, serum, embryo extract, and glucose (Hild, 1957, 1966; Bornstein and Murray, 1958; Peterson and Murray, 1960; Silberberg and Schutta, 1967). When the explants are firmly in place and fed properly, the assembly is completed by placing the double coverslip onto a depression slide. The chamber is then sealed with paraffin and incubated at 35°C. To feed such cultures or to change the constitution of their medium, the inner (round) coverslip is removed, washed, placed on a new square coverslip, refed with the appropriate medium, and sealed in a new depression slide. Cell migration and flattening of the explant occur as the explanted neural tissue remains in culture. Eventually, regions of the preparation can be observed which are only one cell thick, and therefore lend themselves to microscopic, histochemical, and electrophysiological analysis at the level of the defined cell. Such cultures have therefore primarily been optimized to yield histotypically organized cellular arrangements which resemble neural tissue *in vivo,* but in one dimension. However, little biochemical work has been done on such cultures because of the relatively limited amount of tissue available for analysis.

As might be imagined, the preparation and feeding of the large numbers of Maximow cultures required for biochemistry is a relatively tedious task. Since such cultures can be continuously monitored microscopically without much difficulty, however, the great majority of experiments reported describe the effects of various agents on the morphological maturation of such cultures. Most of the modifications described through the years have resulted in preparations with improved microscopic characteristics. Hild and his associates have described a similar technique in which tissue explants are grown as "flying coverslips" in roller-tubes (Hild, 1956, 1967; Hild and Tasaki, 1962). The coverslip bearing the explant is placed in a test tube and covered with medium, and the plugged tube is placed in a rotating drum in an incubator. To feed such cultures, the investigator simply aspirates the old medium every 7 to 10 days and replaces it with fresh nutrient solution. The preparation and maintenance of such cultures is clearly much simpler than in Maximow chambers. Ease of microscopic observation is sacrificed, however, since the coverslips must be removed from the tube, observed, and returned to culture under sterile conditions.

The most striking morphological event observable in explant cultures is the appearance of myelinated axons (Fig. 1). The onset and progress of myelination can be observed microscopically and continuously monitored without damage to the explant. Many of the experiments reported in the literature have dealt with the effect of various reagents, tissue fluids, hor-

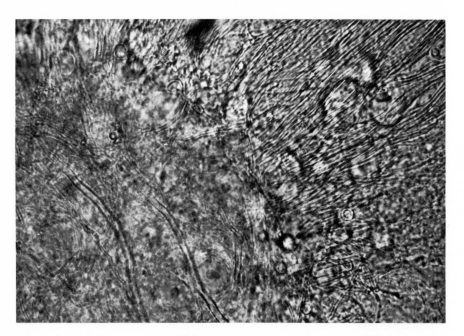

FIG. 1. Explanted culture of topographically paired mouse-brain cerebellar explants. (Photograph courtesy of Drs. Murray and C. D. Allerand.)

mones, and pharmacologically active substances on the appearance and progress of myelination in explants. Although space does not permit a detailed description of these experiments, several examples will serve to illustrate the unique contributions to neurochemistry that have been made by the analysis of explant cultures.

(1) Demyelination has been observed in several of the amino acid ureas. Silberberg (1967, 1969) cultured cerebellar explants in the presence of the various metabolites which accumulate in phenylketonurea (PKU) and maple syrup urine disease (MSUD, branched-chain ketonurea) to determine if any of these compounds are directly responsible for demyelination. Several of the indole acids and α-keto-isocaproate (metabolites which increase in PKU and MSUD, respectively) were found to cause demyelination *in vitro*.

(2) Precocious myelination of cerebellar explants in the presence of thyroxine has been demonstrated (Hamburgh, 1966), suggesting that the accelerated appearance of myelin in thyroxine-treated animals is due to the direct effect of this hormone on neural tissue.

(3) Demyelinating effects of antisera and lymphocytes from patients with multiple sclerosis and Guillain-Barré syndrome, as well as sera and lymphocytes from animals with the autoimmune diseases, experimental allergic encephalomyelitis (EAE) and experimental allergic neuritis (EAN) have been described (Bornstein and Appel, 1961; Appel and Bornstein, 1964; Berg and Kallen, 1964; Yonezawa, Ishihara, and Matsuyama, 1968; Dowling, Kim, Murray and Cook, 1968; Arnason, Winkler and Hadler, 1969; Bornstein and Iwanimi, 1971). Suppression of the complex bioelectric activity characteristic of mature neural explants (for reviews see Crain, 1966; Murray, 1971) by sera from animals suffering from EAE or patients affected with multiple sclerosis has been reported (Bornstein and Crain, 1965, 1971). The relationship of these laboratory diseases to the human afflictions, and the relative roles of cellular and humoral factors, are described elsewhere in this volume by Eylar.

(4) The work of Levi-Montalcini and her associates (1954; reviewed by Levi-Montalcini and Angeletti, 1968) has culminated in the characterization of a protein growth factor, nerve growth factor (NGF), which stimulates the proliferation and maintenance of sympathetic neurons *in vivo*. When treated with appropriate concentrations of this factor, explanted chick-embryo sensory ganglia produce a dense outgrowth of neurites (Levi-Montalcini, Meyer, and Hamburger, 1954). The explanted sensory ganglion culture system and its now classic "halo effect" have been used both for the quantitation and the elucidation of the effects of NGF. The biological and physicochemical characteristics of this remarkable protein are de-

scribed elsewhere in this volume by Angeletti, Hogue-Angeletti, and Bradshaw.

What is the potential of explant culture for additional contributions to neurochemistry and to the study of proteins specific to the nervous system? Although numerous descriptions of effects on myelination based on morphological observations have been reported, we have only recently begun to see reports of chemical measurements of myelination in culture. Sulfatide synthesis during *in vitro* myelination has recently been described by two laboratories (Silberberg, Benjamins, Hirschkowitz, and McKhann, 1972; Fry, Lehrer, and Bornstein, 1972). In addition to the limited amount of material, one of the major problems in studying myelination in explants has been the relative lack of synchronization of this process. Allerand and Murray (1968) showed that individual explants myelinated over a long time period (between 3 and 16 days), whereas paired explant cultures which came from contiguous sections of neonatal cerebellum initiated myelination in a unimodal peak at about 7 to 8 days *in vitro*. In addition to promoting synchrony of myelination, this "topographic pairing" procedure increased both the percentage of cultures which myelinated and the apparent amount of myelin in each explant. It should be possible to produce sufficient material for intensive biochemical analysis of the myelination process by culturing contiguously paired explants on flying coverslips. The isolation and characterization of several of the protein components of myelin, described elsewhere in this volume by Folch-Pi and Eylar, coupled with the sensitive analytical and immunochemical techniques now available, should permit the *in vitro* analysis of the synthesis and degradation of the myelin proteins and the effects of known demyelinating agents on their production.

Similarly, the use of such sensitive techniques as complement fixation and radioimmunoassay will permit an analysis of the regulation of the appearance of the brain-specific antigens, whose discovery, purification, isolation, and characterization are described elsewhere in this volume by Moore, Calissano, and Grasso. The unique advantages of explant culture, coupled with the ability to suppress selectively the proliferation and maturation of classes of cells with agents such as 6-hydroxydopamine or EAE sera, may help in what appears to be the formidable task of finding functions for these organ-specific proteins.

Synaptogenesis in developing explant cultures has been demonstrated by both ultrastructural (Bunge, Bunge, and Peterson, 1967) and electrophysiological (Crain, 1966) criteria. Morgan, Whittaker, and Moore have described elsewhere in this volume the isolation and characterization of synaptosomes and the subsynaptic membrane and soluble components of this organelle. Recently, two laboratories have prepared antisera to synapto-

somal membrane antigens, and these sera demonstrate serological specificity for synaptosomal plasma membrane (Herschman, Cotman, and
Matthews, 1972; Adam, *unpublished*). The interactions of these antisera
with developing neural explants may help to provide insight into the biochemical processes involved in the formation of synapses.

Explant culture techniques of neural tissue have been gradually refined
over the past 30 years. No really significant changes in the methods for
explant culture have occurred recently. Progress in neurochemistry using
this methodology will result primarily from the application of new microanalytical techniques and the use of reagents which specifically affect one
or another process of neural development or maintenance.

IV. DISSOCIATED CELL CULTURES

Dissociated cell cultures of neural tissue have been used for a funda-
mentally different purpose than explant culture. The latter technique em-
phasizes the development and activity of interacting, closely packed cells.
In contrast, when dissociated, sparsely plated cells in culture are analyzed,
the emphasis is placed on the maturation and characterization of the single
cell, either in isolation or with defined cell-to-cell interactions. This system
thus permits the experimenter to question what aspects of the biochemistry,
electrophysiology, and morphology of cells of neural origin are independent
of tissue integrity.

Most of the experiments reported employing this technique have used
spinal ganglia preparations from either chick embryo or neonatal rodents.
The extirpated ganglia are usually dissociated by treatment with trypsin
in Ca^{++}, Mg^{++}-free medium. This procedure, first described by Moscona
(1952), was applied to neural tissue about 25 years ago (Cavanaugh, 1955;
Nakai, 1956). Many laboratories have since adapted and modified this
basic procedure for dissociated spinal cord ganglion (Scott, Engelbert, and
Fisher, 1969; Varon and Raiborn, 1971) and sympathetic ganglion (Greene,
personal communication) cultures. Relatively few reports of dissociated
culture of central nervous system tissue have been published. Most of these
reports (see Sensenbrenner, Booher, and Mandel, 1971) have been concerned primarily with the nutritional requirements and supporting matrix
required for optimal morphological differentiation of chick cerebral cultures
or fractionated cells from the same tissue (Varon and Raiborn, 1969).
Only a very few biochemical analyses of dissociated brain cell cultures
have been described (Wilson, Schrier, Farber, Thompson, Rosenberg,
Blume, and Nirenberg, 1972).

Much of the emphasis on work of this nature has been devoted to determining the role of media components and exogenous growth factors such as NGF on the morphological and electrophysiological maturation of dissociated spinal ganglia (Miller, Varon, Kruger, Coates, and Orkand, 1971; Scott, 1971; Scott and Fisher, 1970, 1971). Several groups have recently described selective plating techniques which have permitted the removal of the bulk of non-neuronal cells prior to plating of the dissociated ganglia (diZerega, Johnson, Morrow, and Kasten, 1970; Okun, Ontkean, and Thomas, 1972). Recently, Fishbach (1970, 1972) used selective plating techniques and inhibitors of DNA synthesis to remove nonmyogenic and non-neuronal cells prior to the establishment of a low-density dissociated cell culture system in which neuromuscular synaptogenesis by isolated motor neurons on individual muscle fibers can be detected by electrophysiological techniques. A representative neuromuscular culture is shown in Fig. 2.

Neurochemical studies of dissociated cell culture will obviously depend on extremely sensitive microanalytical methods. Single-cell chemistry at this level of complexity is practiced by only a very few laboratories. Analysis of dissociated cell cultures will probably be confined primarily to morphological, ultrastructural, and electrophysiological investigations of single cells and specific pairs or groups of cells within such cultures. The effects

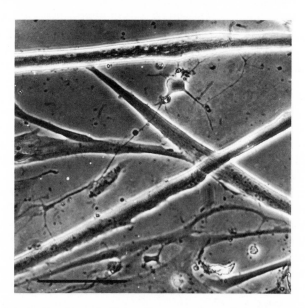

FIG. 2. Dissociated cell culture of chick embryo spinal ganglion neurons and embryonic myoblasts. (Photograph courtesy of Dr. Gerald Fishbach.)

of a variety of hormones, growth factors, pharmacological reagents, etc., on morphology, ultrastructure, and synaptogenesis will certainly be heavily investigated in the future. Thus many of the phenomena previously examined in explant cultures (e.g., effects of EAE and EAN sera, glucose concentration) will be reinvestigated at a single-cell level.

V. REAGGREGATION CULTURE

Dissociated cells in culture (particularly growing in suspension) often tend to aggregate into clumps. This interaction, which is affected by the cell type, the culture vessel, and the culture media, often results in cell aggregates which histotypically resemble the tissue of origin. The self-aggregating property of dissociated tissue has been developed into a controlled quantitative methodology by Moscona (1961) and his associates (reviewed by Moscona, 1965). Problems of cell sorting and relative adhesiveness have been studied by observing the aggregates formed in rotation cultures derived from mixed-cell populations of trypsin-dissociated embryonic organs. The effects of nutritional factors, age, and tissue-specific extracts have been observed on aggregating cultures of dissociated cells from single organs, from co-mingled cells from different organs of the same species, or from cells of the same organ from differing species (Garber, 1967; Orr, 1968; Lilien, 1968).

Reaggregation culture techniques have only recently been applied to neural tissue. The earliest reports utilizing this procedure describe sorting out of neural retina cells from cerebellar cells (Ishii, 1966) and the characterization by electron microscopy of structures which morphologically resemble synapses (Stefanelli, Zacchei, Caravita, Cataldi, and Ieradi, 1967). More complex reaggregation and sorting out of dissociated cells from a defined brain region have recently been described by DeLong (1970). In these studies, dissociated fetal isocortex and hippocampal tissue reaggregated into defined cell layers which resemble the *in vivo* cellular organization (Fig. 3).

Neurochemical studies of reaggregation cultures, still in their infancy, have proceeded along two different tracks. The first of these has been concerned with the ability of neural aggregates to develop properties characteristic of nervous system tissue. Seeds (1971) has measured the increase in several enzymes (acetylcholinesterase, choline acetyltransferase, and glutamate decarboxylase) and shown that these increase during culture of whole-brain aggregates. Similar biochemical studies on myelination, myelin components, brain-specific protein antigens, synaptic membrane components, hormonal effects, etc., are obviously waiting to be analyzed by

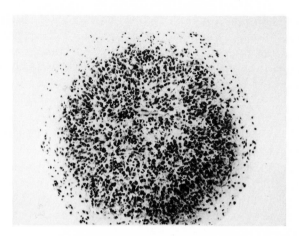

FIG. 3. Reaggregation culture of fetal mouse isocortex. (Photograph courtesy of Drs. George DeLong and Richard Sidman.)

neurochemists in this promising system. The reaggregation culture, coupled with cell-separation techniques, offers an excellent system to analyze both the role of various cell types in the formation of histotypic structures and the relationship between histotypic association and expression of specific neural chemistry.

Previous studies on non-neural tissues have shown that tissue-specific surface components which promote the reaggregation of dissociated homologous tissue, but not of cells derived from a different organ, can be extracted from monolayer cell cultures. Garber and Moscona (1972*a,b*) have recently analyzed neural tissue for similar factors. In their initial paper on this subject, they reported the age-dependence profiles for the reaggregation of various brain regions from chick and mouse embryo cells and the results obtained with co-mingled cultures of various brain regions from homologous and heterologous species. Once these parameters had been characterized, they sought factors which could promote the reaggregation of specific brain regions. Supernatants from monolayer cultures of 14-day-old fetal mouse cerebrum could promote the aggregation of cells of the same source and age, but did not enhance the aggregation of cells derived from other brain regions or from other tissues of mouse embryos. However, these supernatants are active on reaggregating cells derived from the homologous brain region of chick embryo. Maximal effect of the soluble factor derived from monolayer cultures of 14-day fetal cerebrum was observed on reaggregating cerebral cells derived from 14-day mouse embryos; cells from either older or younger fetuses were affected to varying degrees. The 14-day fetal cerebral aggregates were increased in volume approximately 350-fold at optimal concentrations of the factor. These results suggest the presence of region-specific factors which promote the mutual recognition and interaction of neural cells during development. Purification and characterization of these macromolecules and the use of antisera to them—both *in vivo* and *in vitro*—coupled with the analysis of specific proteins of the nervous system suggest a potentially exciting approach to the study of the cellular interactions required for the expression of neurochemical uniqueness during development.

VI. CELL CULTURE OF DIFFERENTIATED NEURAL TUMORS

A. Introduction

Explant culture, culture of dissociated neural tissue, and reaggregation culture are all variations of *primary culture* techniques, in which tissue is (1) removed from the embryo, (2) placed in culture, and (3) analyzed *without subculture*. Consequently, even with the use of extensive cell-fractionation procedures, these cultures consist of mixtures of heterogeneous cells. Measurement of a biochemical parameter thus yields an average determination for a mixed population of tissue. Such results are subject to the same criticisms and restrictions that apply to measurements made directly on neural tissue taken from developing animals. The difficulty of extrapolating from an analysis of a heterogeneous collection of developing cells to the events occurring in a single cell are familiar to all neurochemists, and have been discussed in many contexts.

The ideal experimental system to overcome the disadvantage of cellular heterogeneity would be a homogeneous population of continuously dividing cells which express the biochemical function of interest to the investigator. Cells could be propagated indefinitely, analyzed, and the results extrapolated to events occurring in a single cell. Populations of *clonal* (i.e., stemming from a single cell) lines which maintain organ-specific biochemical functions apparently indefinitely have been derived from differentiated *tumors* of tissues as diverse as pituitary (Yasamura, Tashjian, and Sato, 1966), liver (Richardson, Tashjian, and Levine, (1969), and adrenal (Buonassisi, Sato, and Cohen, 1962). The methodology and application of culture, cloning, and maintenance of differentiated cell lines has been reviewed on several occasions (see Yasamura, 1968; Herschman, 1973).

The interactions of differing cells is obviously one of the most vital aspects of neural tissue. However, the study of clonal cell lines expressing biochemical functions unique to the nervous system provides some obvious advantages to the neurochemist. Several reports have appeared describing the adaptation to cell culture of naturally occurring human tumors of the sympathetic nervous system (Lyon, 1970; Tumilowicz, Nichols, Cholon, and Greene, 1970), as well as central nervous system gliomas (Manuelidis, 1965; Pontén and Macintyre, 1968). Nervous system-specific biochemical parameters in these human tumors have not been described until recently (Herschman and Lerner, 1973). Two tumor-cell systems, a naturally occurring transplantable mouse neuroblastoma (Klebe and Ruddle, 1969; Schubert, Humphreys, Baroni, and Cohen, 1969; Augusti-Tocco and Sato, 1969) and a chemically induced rat astrocytoma (Benda, Lightbody, Sato, Levine, and Sweet, 1968), have been adapted to clonal cell culture and analyzed extensively. In the following sections I will review briefly some of the biochemical studies reported with clonal neural cell lines.

B. Neuroblastoma Cell Lines

Clonal cell lines derived from the mouse C1300 neuroblastoma tumor exhibit a number of biochemical functions that are unique to neural tissue. The initial reports describing the culture of this tumor demonstrated the presence of tyrosine hydroxylase (Augusti-Tocco and Sato, 1969; Schubert et al., 1969). Clones were subsequently isolated from this tumor which were classified either as adrenergic or cholinergic. The adrenergic clones produce high levels of tyrosine hydroxylase and low levels of choline acetyltransferase, whereas the reverse is found in the cholinergic clones (Amano, Richelson, and Nirenberg, 1972). Electrophysiological studies of C1300 clones have confirmed their neuronal characteristics. The cultured cells have electrically excitable membranes (Nelson, Ruffner, and Nirenberg, 1969; Nelson, Peacock, Amano, and Minna, 1971) and are electrically responsive to iontophoretically applied acetylcholine (Harris and Dennis, 1970; Nelson, Peacock, and Amano, 1971). Although these cells are uniquely sensitive to 6-hydroxydopamine (Angeletti and Levi-Montalcini, 1970), reflecting a property of adrenergic neurons, they are not responsive to NGF and are not affected by anti-NGF antisera (Herschman and Stahn, *unpublished*). However, extension of neurites in response to NGF application has recently been described in two human neuroblastoma culture systems (Goldstein, *personal communication*).

We have examined several clonal cell lines derived from the C1300 tumor, the uncloned culture-adapted cells, and the tumor tissue itself for the brain-specific antigens S-100 and 14–3–2. We have not been able to demonstrate the presence of either of these proteins, although we have characterized the production of 14–3–2 in the human neuroblastoma strain

14-3-2
in IMR strain.

IMR (Herschman and Lerner, 1973). In contrast, Kolber, Goldstein, and Moore *(personal communication)* have found the 14–3–2 protein in a C1300 clone, as well as in two human neuroblastoma strains.

Neurite extension of C1300 mouse neuroblastoma clones (Fig. 4) has been reported in response to a variety of experimental manipulations, including serum withdrawal (Seeds, Gilman, Amano, and Nirenberg, 1970), X-irradiation (Prasad, 1971), or the application of 5-bromodeoxyuridine (Schubert and Jacob, 1970), dibutyryl cyclic AMP (Prasad and Hsie, 1971) or prostaglandins (Gilman and Nirenberg, 1971*a*). This morphological alteration has been interpreted by some as an indication of a more differentiated state. Several parameters have been monitored in an attempt to discover biochemical correlates of this morphological phenomenon. These include acetylcholinesterase levels (Blume, Gilbert, Wilson, Farber, Rosenberg, and Nirenberg, 1970; Kates, Winterton, and Schlessinger, 1971; Schubert, Tarikas, Harris, and Heinemann, 1971), tyrosine hydroxylase, choline acetyltransferase, microtubule protein (Kates et al., 1971), surface glycopeptides (Brown, 1971), and glycosphingolipids (Dawson, Kemp, Stoolmiller, and Dorfman, 1972). The results of these and other reports suggest that, although cholinesterase levels increase under these conditions (Blume et al., 1970), this change is in part nonspecific (Schubert et al., 1971) and can be induced in a manner which does not cause concomitant neurite extension (Prasad and Vernadakis, 1972). Although surface glycopeptide changes do occur in cells extending neurites (Brown, 1972), significantly increased levels of presumably neuron-specific biochemical parameters have not yet been demonstrated, with the exception of acetylcholinesterase.

Synapse formation using clonal cell lines has not been reported, although a trophic interaction resulting in localized sensitivity to iontophoretically

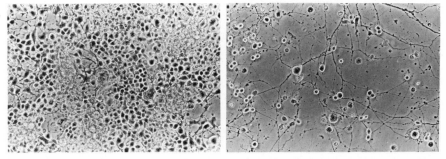

FIG. 4. Neuroblastoma clone 18 cells (derived from the C1300 tumor) grown in *(left)* Dulbecco's modified Eagle's medium containing 10% fetal calf serum and *(right)* on serum-free medium.

applied acetylcholine does occur in a C1300 neuroblastoma and clonal muscle-cell culture system (Harris, Heinemann, Schubert, and Tarikas, 1971). The obvious advantages of clonal cells capable of forming synapses under defined culture conditions for the study of the unique biochemical and electrophysiological events occurring in synaptogenesis need no elaboration. Several laboratories are currently attempting to induce additional neuronal tumors, in the hope of ultimately developing such experimental systems.

C. Differentiated Glial Cell Lines

In 1968, Benda et al. described the adaptation to culture of cells derived from a chemically induced rat astrocytoma. This line, C-6 (Fig. 5), produces the brain-specific S-100 protein. More recently, another glial cell line (Lightbody, Pfeiffer, Kornblith, and Herschman, 1970) and a cell line derived from a Schwann cell tumor (Pfeiffer and Wechsler, 1972) which produce this protein have been characterized. The latter cell line also produces myelin basic protein. These cloned glial cells have been used to study the regulation of several brain-specific biochemical characteristics.

Low-density growing cultures of C-6 cells do not accumulate S-100 protein. Accumulation of this protein (Fig. 6) occurs only after cell-to-cell contact is achieved and cell division is reduced (Pfeiffer, Herschman, Lightbody, and Sato, 1970). This accumulation is apparently related to changes in the membrane antigenicity of C-6 cells (Pfeiffer, Herschman, Lightbody, Sato, and Levine, 1971; Herschman, Breeding, and Nedrud,

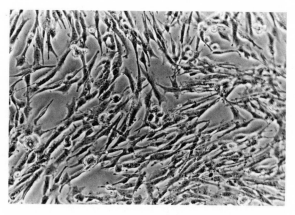

FIG. 5. Astrocytoma clone C-6 cells growing in cell culture.

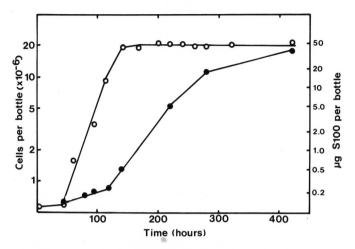

FIG. 6. Accumulation of S-100 protein during growth of C-6 cells. Open circles, cell number; filled circles, amount of S-100. Data are redrawn from Pfeiffer et al. (1970).

1972). To determine if this accumulation is due to an induction of S-100 protein synthesis in confluent cultures, an immunochemical-electrophoretic method of isolating S-100 protein from pulse-labeled cultured cells has been developed (Herschman, 1971) and applied to exponentially growing and stationary C-6 cultures. These results (Herschman, Grauling, and Lerner, 1973) suggest that the observed increase of S-100 protein in stationary C-6 cultures is due to a density-dependent contact-mediated induction of synthesis.

Hormonal regulation of enzymes and cyclic AMP has also been studied in clonal C-6 cells. The level of glycerol phosphate dehydrogenase in C-6 cells is elevated almost 20-fold after the administration of cortisol (de Vellis, Inglish, and Galey, 1971) (Fig. 7), which is similar to the regulation by cortisol of glycerol phosphate dehydrogenase in brain (de Vellis and Inglish, 1968). Studies with inhibitors of RNA and protein synthesis suggest that the induction is due to *de novo* protein synthesis (de Vellis et al., 1971). Norepinephrine increases the levels of lactic dehydrogenase (de Vellis et al., 1971) and cyclic AMP (Shimizu, Creveling, and Daly, 1970; Gilman and Nirenberg, 1971*b;* de Vellis and Brooker, 1972), as well as adenyl cyclase activity (Schimmer, 1971), in C-6 cells. A similar cyclic AMP response to norepinephrine and also to histamine has been reported in a human glial-cell culture line (Clark and Perkins, 1971). The physiological significance of the regulation of these enzyme levels and cyclic AMP by

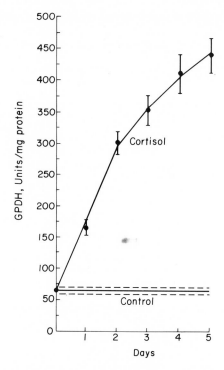

FIG. 7. Induction of glycerolphosphate dehydrogenase in C-6 cells in response to cortisol. Cortisol concentration was 5×10^{-7} M. Culture medium was changed daily. (Illustration provided by Dr. J. de Vellis.)

hormones and neurotransmitters in glial cells is open to question. Such questions probably reflect far more our current ignorance of the role of glial cells in neurobiology than a lack of functional significance.

REFERENCES

Allerand, C. D., and Murray, M. R. (1968): Myelin formation *in vitro*. Endogenous influences on cultures of newborn mouse cerebellum. *Archives of Neurology,* 19:292.

Amano, T., Richelson, E., and Nirenberg, M. (1972): Neurotransmitter synthesis by neuroblastoma clones. *Proceedings of the National Academy of Sciences,* 69:258.

Angeletti, P. U., and Levi-Montalcini, R. (1970): Cytolytic effect of 6-hydroxydopamine on neuroblastoma cells. *Cancer Research,* 30:2863.

Appel, S. H., and Bornstein, M. B. (1964): The application of tissue culture to the study of experimental allergic encephalomyelitis. II. Serum factors responsible for demyelination. *Journal of Experimental Medicine,* 119:303.

Arnason, B. G. W., Winkler, G. F., and Handler, N. M. (1969): Cell-mediated demyelination of peripheral nerve in tissue culture. *Laboratory Investigation,* 21:1.

Augusti-Tocco, G., and Sato, G. (1969): Establishment of functional clonal lines of neurons from mouse neuroblastoma. *Proceedings of the National Academy of Sciences*, 64:311.

Benda, P. J., Lightbody, J., Sato, G. H., Levine, L., and Sweet, W. (1968): Differentiated rat glial cell strain in tissue culture. *Science*, 161:370.

Berg, O., and Kallen, B. (1964): Effect of mononuclear blood cells from multiple sclerosis patients on neuroglia in tissue culture. *Journal of Neuropathology and Experimental Neurology*, 23:550.

Blume, A., Gilbert, F., Wilson, S., Farber, J., Rosenberg, R., and Nirenberg, M. (1970): Regulation of acetylcholinesterase in neuroblastoma cells. *Proceedings of the National Academy of Sciences*, 67:786.

Bornstein, M. B. (1958): Reconstituted rat-tail collagen used as substrate for tissue cultures on coverslips in Maximow slides and roller tubes. *Laboratory Investigation*, 7:134.

Bornstein, M. B., and Appel, S. H. (1961): The application of tissue culture to the study of experimental "allergic" encephalomyelitis. I. Patterns of demyelination. *Journal of Neuropathology and Experimental Neurology*, 20:141.

Bornstein, M. B., and Crain, S. M. (1965): Functional studies of cultured brain tissues as related to "demyelinative disorders." *Science*, 148:1242.

Bornstein, M. B., and Crain, S. M. (1971): Lack of correlation between changes in bioelectric functions and myelin in cultured CNS tissues chronically exposed to sera from animals with EAE. *Journal of Neuropathology and Experimental Neurology*, 30:129.

Bornstein, M. B., and Iwanami, H. (1971): Experimental allergic encephalomyelitis: Demyelinating activity of serum and sensitized lymph node cells on cultured nerve tissues. *Journal of Neuropathology and Experimental Neurology*, 30:240.

Bornstein, M. B., and Murray, M. R. (1958): Serial observations on patterns of growth, myelin formation, maintenance and degeneration in cultures of new-born rat and kitten cerebellum. *Journal of Biophysical and Biochemical Cytology*, 4:499.

Brown, J. C. (1971): Surface glycoprotein characteristic of the differentiated state of neuroblastoma cells. *Experimental Cell Research*, 69:440.

Bunge, M. B., Bunge, R. P., and Peterson, E. R. (1967): A light and electron microscope study of long-term organized cultures of rat dorsal root ganglia. *Brain Research*, 6:728.

Buonassisi, V., Sato, G., and Cohen, A. I. (1962): Hormone-producing cultures of adrenal and pituitary tumor origin. *Proceedings of the National Academy of Sciences*, 48:1184.

Cavanaugh, M. W. (1955): Neuron development from trypsin-dissociated cells of differentiated spinal cord of the chick embryo. *Experimental Cell Research*, 9:42.

Clark, R. B., and Perkins, J. P. (1971): Regulation of adenosine $3',5'$-cyclic monophosphate concentration in cultured human astrocytoma cells by catecholamine and histamine. *Proceedings of the National Academy of Sciences*, 68:2757.

Crain, S. M. (1966): Development of "organotypic" bioelectric activities in central nervous tissues during maturation in culture. *International Review of Neurobiology*, 9:1.

Dawson, G., Kemp, S. F., Stoolmiller, A., and Dorfman, A. (1972): Biosynthesis of glycosphingolipids by mouse neuroblastoma. *Biochemical and Biophysical Research Communications*, 44:687.

DeLong, G. R. (1970): Histogenesis of fetal mouse isocortex and hippocampus in reaggregating cell cultures. *Developmental Biology*, 22:563.

de Vellis, J., and Brooker, G. (1972): Effect of catecholamines on cultured glial cells: Correlation between cyclic AMP levels and lactic dehydrogenase induction. *Federation Proceedings*, 31:513a.

de Vellis, J., and Inglish, D. (1968): Hormonal control of glycerolphosphate dehydrogenase in the rat brain. *Journal of Neurochemistry*, 15:1061.

de Vellis, J., Inglish, D., and Galey, F. (1971): Effects of cortisol and epinephrine on glial cells in culture. In: *Cellular Aspects of Neural Growth and Differentiation*, edited by D. Pease, p. 23. University of California Press, Berkeley.

diZerega, G., Johnson, L., Morrow, J., and Kasten, F. H. (1970): Isolation of viable neurons from embryonic spinal ganglia by centrifugation through albumin gradients. *Experimental Cell Research*, 63:189.

Dówling, P. C., Kim, S. U., Murray, M. R., and Cook, S. D. (1968): Serum 19S and 7S demyelinating antibodies in multiple sclerosis. *Journal of Immunology,* 101:1101.

Fischbach, G. D. (1970): Synaptic potentials recorded in cell cultures of nerve and muscle. *Science,* 169:1331.

Fischbach, G. D. (1972): Synapse formation between dissociated nerve and muscle cells in low density cell cultures. *Developmental Biology,* 28:407.

Fry, J. M., Lehrer, G. M., and Bornstein, M. B. (1972): Sulfatide synthesis: Inhibition by experimental allergic encephalomyelitis serum. *Science,* 175:192.

Garber, B. (1967): Aggregation *in vivo* of dissociated cells. II. Role of developmental age in tissue reconstruction. *Journal of Experimental Zoology,* 164:339.

Garber, B. B., and Moscona, A. A. (1972*a*): Reconstruction of brain tissue from cell suspensions. I. Aggregation patterns of cells dissociated from different regions of the developing brain. *Developmental Biology,* 27:217.

Garber, B. B., and Moscona, A. A. (1972*b*): Reconstruction of brain tissue from cell suspensions. II. Specific enhancement of aggregation of embryonic cerebral cells by supernatant from homologous cell cultures. *Developmental Biology,* 27:235.

Gilman, A. G., and Nirenberg, M. (1971*a*): Regulation of adenosine 3',5'-cyclic monophosphate metabolism in cultured mouse neuroblastoma cells. *Nature,* 234:356.

Gilman, A. G., and Nirenberg, M. (1971*b*): Effect of catecholamines on the adenosine 3',5'-cyclic monophosphate concentrations of clonal satellite cells of neurons. *Proceedings of the National Academy of Sciences,* 68:2165.

Hamburgh, M. (1966): Evidence for a direct effect of temperature and thyroid hormone on myelinogenesis *in vitro. Developmental Biology,* 13:15.

Harris, A. J., and Dennis, M. J. (1970): Acetylcholine sensitivity and distribution on mouse neuroblastoma cells. *Science,* 167:1253.

Harris, A. J., Heinemann, S., Schubert, D., and Tarakis, H. (1971): Trophic interaction between cloned tissue culture lines of nerve and muscle. *Nature,* 231:296.

Harrison, R. G. (1907): Observation on the living developing nerve fiber. *Proceedings of the Society for Experimental Biology and Medicine,* 4:140.

Herschman, H. R. (1971): Synthesis and degradation of a brain specific protein (S-100 by clonal cultured human glial cells. *Journal of Biological Chemistry,* 246:7569.

Herschman, H. R. (1973): Culture of neural tissue and cells. In: *Research Methods in Neurochemistry,* Vol. II, edited by N. Marks and R. Rodnight. Plenum Press, New York *(in press).*

Herschman, H. R., Breeding, J., and Nedrud, J. (1972): Sialic acid masked membrane antigens of clonal functional glial cells. *Journal of Cellular Physiology,* 79:249.

Herschman, H. R., Cotman, C., and Matthews, D. (1972): Serologic specificities of brain subcellular organelles. I. Antisera to synaptosomal fractions. *Journal of Immunology,* 108:1362.

Herschman, H., Grauling, B., and Lerner, M. (1973): Nervous system specific proteins in cultured neural cells. In: *Tissue Culture of the Nervous System,* edited by G. Sato. Plenum Press, New York *(in press).*

Herschman, H., and Lerner, M. P. (1973): Production of a nervous system specific protein (14–3–2) by human neuroblastoma cells in culture. *Nature (in press).*

Hild, W. (1957): Myelinogenesis in cultures of mammalian central nervous tissue. *Zeitschrift für Zellforschung und Mikroskopische Anatomie,* 46:71.

Hild, W. (1966): Cell types and neuronal connections in cultures of mammalian central nervous tissue. *Zeitschrift für Zellforschung and Mikroskopische Anatomie,* 69:155.

Hild, W., and Tasaki, I. (1962): Morphological and physiological properties of neurons and glial cells in tissue cultures. *Journal of Neurophysiology,* 25:277.

Ishii, K. (1966): Reconstruction of dissociated chick brain cells in rotation-mediated culture. *Cytologica,* 31:89.

Kates, J., Winterton, R., and Schlessinger, K. (1971): Induction of acetylcholinesterase activity in mouse neuroblastoma tissue culture lines. *Nature,* 229:345.

Klebe, R., and Ruddle, F. (1969): Neuroblastoma: Cell culture analysis of a differentiating stem cell system. *Journal of Cell Biology,* 43:69a.

Levi-Montalcini, R., and Angeletti, P. U. (1968): Nerve growth factor. *Physiological Reviews,* 48:534.

Levi-Montalcini, R., Meyer, H., and Hamburger, V. (1954): *In vitro* experiments on the effects of mouse sarcoma 180 and 37 on the spinal and sympathetic ganglia of the chick embryo. *Cancer Research,* 14:49.

Lightbody, J., Pfeiffer, S. E., Kornblith, P. L., and Herschman, H. R. (1970): Biochemically differentiated human glial cells in tissue culture. *Journal of Neurobiology,* 1:411.

Lilien, J. E. (1968): Specific enhancement of cell aggregation *in vitro. Developmental Biology,* 17:657.

Lyon, G. M., Jr. (1970): Growth stimulation of tissue culture cells derived from patients with neuroblastoma. *Cancer Research,* 30:2521.

Manuelidis, E. E. (1965): Long-term lives of tissue cultures of intracranial tumors. *Journal of Neurosurgery,* 22:368.

Maximow, A. (1925): Tissue cultures of young mammalian embryos. *Contributions to Embryology (Carnegie Institute),* 16:47.

Miller, R., Varon, S., Kruger, L., Coates, P. W., and Orkand, P. M. (1970): Formation of synaptic contacts on dissociated chick embryo ganglion cells *in vitro. Brain Research,* 24:356.

Moscona, A. A. (1952): Cell suspensions from organ rudiments of chick embryo. *Experimental Cell Research,* 3:535.

Moscona, A. A. (1961): Rotation mediated histogenic aggregation of dissociated cells. A quantifiable approach to cell interactions *in vitro. Experimental Cell Research,* 22:455.

Moscona, A. A. (1965): Recombination of dissociated cells and the development of cell aggregates. In: *Cells and Tissues in Culture,* Vol. I, edited by E. N. Willmer, p. 489. Academic Press, London.

Murray, M. R. (1971): Nervous tissues isolated in culture. In: *Handbook of Neurochemistry,* Vol. 5a, edited by A. Lajtha, p. 373. Plenum Press, London.

Murray, M. R., and Stout, A. P. (1942): Characteristics of human Schwann cells *in vitro. Anatomical Record,* 84:275.

Murray, M. R., and Stout, A. P. (1947): Distinctive characteristics of the sympatheticoblastoma cultivated *in vitro.* A method for prompt diagnosis. *American Journal of Pathology,* 23:429.

Nakai, J. (1956): Dissociated dorsal root ganglia in tissue culture. *American Journal of Anatomy,* 99:81.

Nelson, P. G., Peacock, J. H., and Amano, T. (1971): Responses of neuroblastoma cells to iontophoretically applied acetylcholine. *Journal of Cell Physiology,* 77:353.

Nelson, P., Peacock, J. H., Amano, T., and Minna, J. (1971): Electrogenesis in mouse neuroblastoma cells *in vitro. Journal of Cell Physiology,* 77:337.

Nelson, P., Ruffner, W., and Nirenberg, M. (1969): Neuronal tumor cells with excitable membranes grown *in vitro. Proceedings of the National Academy of Sciences,* 64:1004.

Okun, L. M., Ontkean, F. K., and Thomas, C. A. (1972): Removal of non-neuronal cells from suspensions of dissociated embryonic dorsal root ganglia. *Experimental Cell Research,* 73:226.

Orr, M. F. (1968): Histogenesis of sensory epithelium in reaggregates of dissociated embryonic chick otocysts. *Developmental Biology,* 17:39.

Peterson, E. R., and Murray, M. R. (1960): Modification of development in isolated dorsal root ganglia by nutritional and physical factors. *Developmental Biology,* 2:461.

Pfeiffer, S. E., Herschman, H. R., Lightbody, J., and Sato, G. (1970): Synthesis by a clonal line of rat glial cells of a protein unique to the nervous system. *Journal of Cellular Physiology* 75:329.

Pfeiffer, S. E., Herschman, H. R., Lightbody, J., Sato, G., and Levine, L. (1971): Modification of cell surface antigenicity as a function of culture conditions. *Journal of Cellular Physiology,* 78:145.

Pfeiffer, S. E., and Wechsler, W. (1972): Biochemically differentiated neoplastic clone of Schwann cells. *Proceedings of the National Academy of Sciences,* 69:2885.

Pontén, J., and Macintyre, E. H. (1968): Interaction between normal and transformed bovine fibroblasts in culture. *Acta Pathologica et Microbiologica Scandinavica; Section A: Pathology,* 74:465.

Prasad, K. N. (1971): X-Ray induced morphological differentiation of mouse neuroblastoma cells *in vitro. Nature,* 234:471.

Prasad, K. N., and Hsie, A. W. (1971): Morphologic differentiation of mouse neuroblastoma cells induced *in vitro* by dibutyryl adenosine 3′,5′-cyclic monophosphate. *Nature New Biology,* 233:141.

Prasad, K. N., and Vernadakis, A. (1972): Morphological and biochemical study in X-ray and dibutyryl cyclic AMP induced differentiated neuroblastoma cells. *Experimental Cell Research,* 70:27.

Richardson, U. I., Tashjian, A. H., Jr., and Levine, L. (1969): Establishment of a clonal strain of hepatoma cells which secrete albumin. *Journal of Cell Biology,* 40:236.

Schimmer, B. P. (1971): Effects of catecholamines and monovalent cations on adenylate cyclase activity in cultured glial tumor cells. *Biochimica et Biophysica Acta,* 252:567.

Schubert, D., Humphreys, S., Baroni, C., and Cohen, M. (1969): *In vitro* differentiation of a mouse neuroblastoma. *Proceedings of the National Academy of Sciences,* 64:316.

Schubert, D., and Jacob, F. (1970): 5-Bromodeoxyuridine-induced differentiation of a neuroblastoma. *Proceedings of the National Academy of Sciences,* 67:247.

Schubert, D., Tarikas, H., Harris, A. J., and Heinemann, S. (1971): Induction of acetylcholine esterase activity in a mouse neuroblastoma. *Nature New Biology,* 233:79.

Scott, B. S. (1971): Effect of potassium on neuron survival in cultures of dissociated human nervous tissue. *Experimental Neurology,* 30:297.

Scott, B. S., Englebert, V. E., and Fisher, K. C. (1969): Morphological and electrophysiological characteristics of dissociated chick embryonic spinal ganglion cells in culture. *Experimental Neurology,* 23:230.

Scott, B. S., and Fisher, K. C. (1970): Potassium concentration and number of neurons in cultures of dissociated ganglia. *Experimental Neurology,* 27:16.

Scott, B. S., and Fisher, K. C. (1971): Effect of choline, high potassium and low sodium on the number of neurons in cultures of dissociated chick ganglia. *Experimental Neurology,* 31:183.

Seeds, N. W. (1971): Biochemical differentiation in reaggregating brain cell culture. *Proceedings of the National Academy of Sciences,* 68:1858.

Seeds, N. W., Gilman, A. G., Amano, T., and Nirenberg, M. W. (1970): Regulation of axon formation by clonal lines of a neural tumor. *Proceedings of the National Academy of Sciences,* 66:160.

Sensenbrenner, M., Booher, J., and Mandel, P. (1971): Cultivation and growth of dissociated neurons from chick embryo cerebral cortex in the presence of different substrates. *Zeitschrift für Zellforschung und Mikroskopische Anatomie,* 117:559.

Shimizu, H., Creveling, C. R., and Daly, J. (1970): Stimulated formation of adenosine 3′-5′-cyclic phosphate in cerebral cortex: Synergism between electrical activity and biogenic amines. *Proceedings of the National Academy of Sciences,* 65:1033.

Silberberg, D. H. (1967): Phenylketonurea metabolites in cerebellum culture morphology. *Archives of Neurology,* 17:524.

Silberberg, D. H. (1969): Maple syrup urine disease metabolites; studies in cerebellum cultures. *Journal of Neurochemistry,* 16:1141.

Silberberg, D., Benjamins, J., Herschkowitz, N., and McKhann, G. M. (1972): Incorporation of radioactive sulphate into sulfatide during myelination in cultures of rat cerebellum. *Journal of Neurochemistry,* 19:11.

Silberberg, D., and Schutta, H. (1967): The effects of unconjugated bilirubin and related pigments on cultures of rat cerebellum. *Journal of Neuropathology and Experimental Neurology,* 26:572.

Stefanelli, A., Zacchei, A. M., Caravita, S., Cataldi, A., and Ieradi, L. A. (1967): New-forming retinal synapses *in vitro. Experientia,* 23:199.

Tumilowicz, J. J., Nichols, W. W., Cholon, J. J., and Greene, A. E. (1970): Definition of a continuous human cell line derived from neuroblastoma. *Cancer Research,* 30:2110.

Varon, S., and Raiborn, C. W., Jr. (1969): Dissociation, fractionation and culture of embryonic brain cells. *Brain Research,* 12:180.

Varon, S., and Raiborn, C., Jr. (1971): Excitability and conduction in neurons of dissociated ganglionic cell cultures. *Brain Research,* 30:83.

Wilson, S. H., Schrier, B. K., Farber, J. L., Thompson, E. J., Rosenberg, R. N., Blume, A. J., and Nirenberg, M. W. (1972): Markers for gene expression in cultured cells from the nervous system. *Journal of Biological Chemistry,* 247:3159.

Yasumura, Y. (1968): Retention of differentiated function in clonal animal cell lines, particularly hormone-secreting cultures. *American Zoologist,* 8:285.

Yasumura, Y., Tashjian, A. H., Jr., and Sato, G. (1966): Establishment of four functional clonal strains of animal cells in culture. *Science,* 154:1186.

Yonezawa, T., Ishihara, Y., and Matsuyama, H. (1968): Studies on experimental allergic peripheral neuritis. Demyelinating patterns studies *in vitro. Journal of Neuropathology and Experimental Neurology,* 27:453.

Proteins of the Nervous System
Raven Press, New York © 1973

The Recognition of Proteins by Hormone-Binding Properties

Bruce S. McEwen

I. INTRODUCTION

There are four basic strategies that can be used to study or recognize proteins of the central nervous system. The most obvious approach is on the basis of the enzymatic or other functional activity of the protein in question. A second approach is the separation of a protein mixture by electrophoretic or other physical methods, and immunological identification of a brain-specific protein such as S-100 and 14–3–2. As described elsewhere in this volume by Dr. Barondes, proteins can be labeled in the cell soma and their transport to presynaptic endings studied by following the movement of the radioactive label. A fourth approach is to study the ability of proteins to bind specific ligands, such as hormones or neurotransmitters; our work has involved the study of the presumptive receptors for steroid hormones in the brain.

In order to study the binding of hormones by such "receptor" proteins, it is necessary to first identify the responsive target tissues containing the receptor, and to determine the cellular site of action of the hormone. After the target tissues and site of action have been identified, the binding reaction can be analyzed using various agonists and antagonists, in the way that the α-bungarotoxin has been used to characterize the acetylcholine receptor (Berg, Kelly, Sargent, Williamson, and Hall, 1972; Clark, Wolcott, and Raftery, 1972; de Plazas and de Robertis, 1972; Fulpius, Cha, Klett, and Reich, 1972).

There are several criteria which must be fulfilled before a binding protein is recognized as a hormone receptor. First, target or sensitive tissues should contain binding sites, and insensitive tissues or cells should not. Studies on nonneural target tissues for steroid hormones have established the existence of binding proteins in both the cytosol and nucleus, which appear to mediate and therefore be receptors for steroid hormones. In certain cases where there is a lack of hormone responsiveness, the target tissue can be shown to lack the binding protein. A good example of this is the androgen insensitivity mutation that results in the testicular feminizing syndrome, in which a genetic male produces relatively normal amounts of androgen but cannot show the proper response to the hormone, and in which the androgen target tissues either lack or are grossly deficient in androgen-binding protein (Bullock, Bardin, and Ohno, 1971). An additional criterion is that the cellular location of the binding protein should be reasonable in view of what is known about the cellular mechanism of action of the hormone. Lastly, agonists and antagonists of the hormone action should bind to the receptor protein, and inactive hormones should not bind. Many of these criteria are being used not only for steroid hormones but also for protein hormones, the hypothalamic-releasing factors, and neurotransmitters (Cuatrecasas, 1971; de Kretser, Catt, and Paulsen, 1971; Lefkowitz and Haber, 1971; Grant, Vale and Guillemin, 1972; Means and Vaitukaitis, 1972).

II. MECHANISMS OF STEROID HORMONE ACTION

Steroid hormones enter the target cell and are bound to proteins in the cytoplasm, after which they are transported to the nucleus where they exert their action at the level of regulation of the genome (Jensen and DeSombre, 1972; Liao and Fang, 1969; O'Malley, Spelsburg, Schrader, Chytil, and Steggles, 1972; Swaneck, Highland, and Edelman, 1969; Williams-Ashman and Reddi, 1972). There does not appear to be any transformation of the estrogenic or glucocorticoid hormones prior to or during binding. In contrast, testosterone is converted to 5α-dihydrotestosterone in many target tissues prior to its binding by cytoplasmic receptors and entrance into the nucleus. Thus, the mechanism of steroid hormone action differs markedly from that of the protein and peptide hormones such as ACTH, glucagon, or norepinephrine, in which the hormone interacts with a receptor at the cell surface, which in turn stimulates the formation of cyclic AMP, the "second messenger" (Robison, Butcher, and Sutherland, 1971).

The best evidence that cyclic AMP is not an obligatory mediator of steroid hormone action has been obtained by de Vellis and co-workers (de Vellis, Inglish, Cole, and Molson, 1971), using cultured glial tumor material. These tumor cells are responsive to both glucocorticoids and epinephrine, which induce the synthesis of glycerol phosphate dehydrogenase (GDPH) and lactic dehydrogenase (LDH), respectively. The specificity of the enzyme inductions in response to the two hormones indicates that they utilize two completely separate mechanisms. If the glucocorticoid induction involved cyclic AMP, as is known to be the case for the norepinephrine induction, such a clear separation could not occur.

Table 1 summarizes the methodology used to study the binding of steroid

TABLE 1. *Methodology for the study of steroid "receptors"*

Autoradiography
Cell fractionation: nucleus, cytosol
Physical separation of soluble proteins
    Density gradient centrifugation in sucrose or glycerol
    Gel electrophoresis
    Column chromatography

hormones. Autoradiography is of particular importance for the study of brain tissue, due to its extensive heterogeneity and anatomical complexity. Cell fractionation studies are utilized for the determination of the subcellular location of the binding protein. The binding of steroid hormones tends to occur both in the cell nucleus and in the cytosol, or soluble cytoplasmic supernatant. The binding proteins can be further characterized by subjecting the cytosol or nuclear extract to various types of fractionation.

III. THE EFFECTS OF ESTROGEN ON BRAIN TISSUE

The important effects of estrogens on the CNS include both the regulation of pituitary function and of certain components of mating behavior (Table 2). For example, the lordosis reflex which is characteristic of the estrous state in the female rat is abolished by gonadectomy and can be restored by systemic administration of estradiol. The ability of estradiol to restore this reflex is dependent on the presence of an intact hypothalamus and preoptic region (Fig. 1*A*). Lesions in this area also abolish other estrogen-dependent functions. Conversely, local implants of estradiol in the anterior hypothalamus or preoptic area can duplicate the effects of systemically administered estradiol to restore estrous behavior in ovariectomized female rats. Implants in other brain areas are generally ineffective.

This type of study thus established that the brain is a target tissue for estrogenic hormones for the production of both behavioral and neuro-

TABLE 2. *Estrogen effects on neurally mediated effects in rats*

Function	Region of brain	Reference
Female lordosis reflex	anterior hypothalamus, preoptic area	Lisk, 1967
Food intake	hypothalamus	Wade and Zucker, 1970
Gonadotrophin secretion	pituitary, hypothalamus amygdala	Lisk, 1967; Tindal, Knaggs, and Turvey, 1967

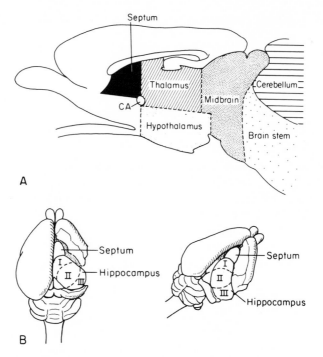

FIG. 1. *(A)* Sagital section of the rat brain; *(B)* corticosterone-binding areas (from McEwen, Weiss, and Schwartz, 1969).

endocrine effects, and further localized the target tissue to be the hypothalamus and preoptic area. These regions were therefore reasonable tissues in which to search for estrogen receptors. As was predicted on the basis of these observations, the injection of radioactive estradiol to ovariectomized rats does result in a selective accumulation of estradiol in the hypothalamus and preoptic area (Eisenfeld and Axelrod, 1965; Kato and Villee, 1967; McEwen and Pfaff, 1970). An analysis of subcellular fractions showed that there is a time-dependent accumulation of radioactivity in the nuclear fraction, to levels much higher than that of the total homogenate (Zigmond and McEwen, 1970; Kato, Atsumi, and Muramatsu, 1970; Notides, 1970; Chader and Villee, 1970). This accumulation is highest in nuclei from the hypothalamus and preoptic area, in agreement with functional observations and tissue uptake studies (Fig. 2*B*).

We have also studied the soluble cytosol-binding protein in hypothalamus, pituitary, and uterus. Sucrose density gradient separation reveals a similar peak of estradiol-binding protein in all three tissues, having a sedimentation

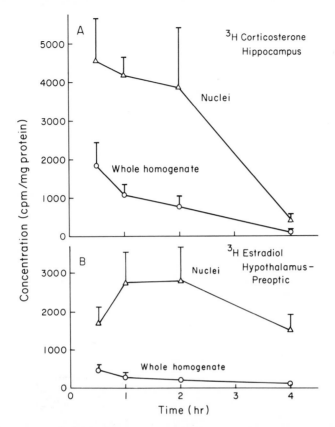

FIG. 2. The selective uptake of labeled steroids by cell nuclei. Uptake of ^{3}H-corticosterone by hippocampal cell nuclei as compared to whole homogenate *(A)*. Uptake of ^{3}H-estradiol by cell nuclei of the hypothalamic-preoptic area *(B)*. Labeled steroid was administered intraperitoneally to adrenalectomized and ovariectomized animals, respectively (from McEwen, Zigmond, and Gerlach, 1972).

value of 8S, with the smallest amount present in the hypothalamus. The cytosol-binding protein shows the same kind of regional specificity as the nuclear binding, with activity in the hypothalamus and preoptic area and an absence of binding activity in regions such as the cerebral cortex. Similar observations have been made by other investigators (Kahwanago, Heinrichs, and Herrmann, 1969; Eisenfeld, 1970; Kato, Atsumi, and Inaba, 1970).

An important aspect of hormone binding is that of the chemical specificity of the binding reaction, which must agree with the known specificity of action of the various estrogens. Figure 3 shows a competition experiment

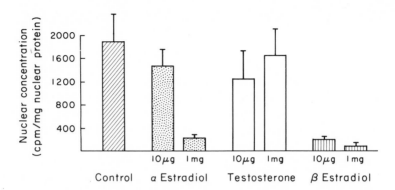

FIG. 3. The competition of unlabeled steroids for labeled 17β-estradiol. Competing steroid was administered simultaneously with the ³H-estrogen 17β at dose indicated (from McEwen, Zigmond, and Gerlach, 1972).

in which we attempted to block the binding of labeled estradiol by the simultaneous administration of a large amount of unlabeled steroid. The most significant competition of ³H-17β-estradiol binding was shown by the unlabeled natural estrogen, whereas the inactive optical isomer 17α-estradiol was effective only in high concentration, probably as the result of contamination with the 17β form, and no competition was demonstrated by testosterone. The synthetic highly potent estrogen diethylstilbestrol was found to compete as well as 17β-estradiol (Zigmond, *unpublished*). There is thus a strong correlation between potency in the induction of the behavioral and neuroendocrine effects of estrogens and extent of binding. A similar specificity has been observed for the cytosol binding protein.

The appearance of estrogen-binding capacity in the hypothalamus and preoptic area was found to appear approximately 10 days prior to the onset of puberty, which normally occurs at 35 to 40 days of age, whereas other areas show little change with age (Kato, Atsumi, and Inaba, 1971; Plapinger and McEwen, *unpublished*). It is not yet known whether the appearance of the estrogen-binding protein is a response to secretion of the hormone, to other factors such as pituitary hormones, or whether it is a spontaneous event unrelated to any of the factors which later regulate reproductive function. There is a binding protein for estradiol which is present extracellularly in the cerebrospinal fluid and blood prior to 21 days of age, which may act to protect the brain from the effects of maternal estrogen and other adverse influences which may be present *in utero* (Plapinger and McEwen, *unpublished;* Raynaud, Mercier-Bodard, and Baulier, 1972).

IV. THE INTERACTION OF ADRENAL STEROIDS WITH BRAIN TISSUE

The interaction between the adrenal cortex and the brain is much less well understood than that involving the gonadal steroids. The natural glucocorticoid in the rat is corticosterone, and the predominant human glucocorticoid is hydrocortisone. In contrast to the binding of labeled estrogen by brain tissue, the region most heavily labeled with ^{3}H-corticosterone was the hippocampus (McEwen, Weiss, and Schwartz, 1969). This structure is related to the cerebral cortex and is part of the limbic system, which is concerned with the mediation of vegetative and emotional events (Fig. 1*B*).

Autoradiographic examination of the hippocampus revealed that the greatest binding of corticosterone was localized to the pyramidal neurons of the CA1 and CA2 regions of the hippocampus, with much less binding by CA3 and CA4 (Gerlach and McEwen, 1972). There is also some accumulation of corticosterone in the small neurons of the dentate gyrus, but to a much smaller extent than in the pyramidal neurons of CA1 and CA2. This pattern of uptake has thus far not been interpreted in terms of hippocampal function.

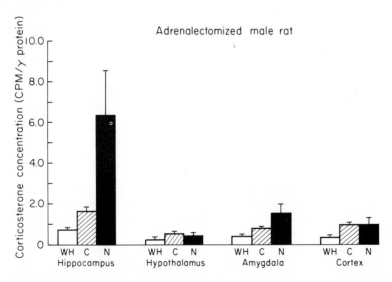

FIG. 4. The binding of ^{3}H-corticosterone to cytosol macromolecules and cell nuclei. Note binding in hippocampus. The amygdala also shows a small but significant nuclear binding (from McEwen, Magnus, and Wallach, 1971).

We then proceeded to investigate the binding of corticosterone as we did for estradiol, by determining the subcellular distribution of binding. We again found that there was a selective nuclear accumulation, in this case with the most extensive binding in the hippocampus (Figs. 2*A* and 4; McEwen, Weiss, and Schwartz, 1970). We have also been able to demonstrate the same regional pattern of cell nuclear uptake of corticosterone using brain tissue slices, thus proving that the binding selectivity is an intrinsic property of the binding sites rather than a result of factors such as blood flow (McEwen and Wallach, 1973).

We have also examined the uptake of labeled corticosterone by autoradiographic methods (Fig. 5), which has confirmed the nuclear accumulation of the labeled steroid. If we compete for the corticosterone-binding sites with unlabeled steroid and prepare similar autoradiograms, the specific uptake over the cell nucleus is abolished, and the level of radiographic

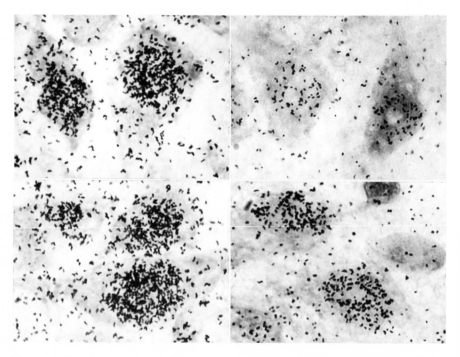

FIG. 5. Radioautogram of pyramidal neurons in the cornu ammonis of the rat brain hippocampus, illustrating the concentration of ³H-corticosterone in the nuclear region. The duration of exposure was 248 days *(left)* or 178 days *(right)*. The autoradiograms on the left were stained with methyl green-pyronin Y, and on the right with Darrow red and light green (1,481 ×). For details, see Gerlach and McEwen, 1972.

labeling is similar for all regions of the tissue. This provides histologic confirmation of our observations with cell fractionation that the binding of corticosterone in the hippocampal pyramidal neurons involves a saturable mechanism. Cultured glial cells have also been shown to contain nuclear binding sites for corticosteroids (de Vellis and McEwen, *unpublished*), and we must consider that there may be a certain amount of nuclear accumulation by glial cells. However, it is clear that the greatest proportion of uptake occurs in neurons.

An acidic nuclear protein that binds corticosterone can be extracted with strong salt solutions and separated on Sephadex G-200 (Fig. 6). Digestion with proteolytic enzymes indicates that the binding factor is indeed a protein, as has been shown in other tissues (McEwen and Plapinger, 1970). We have also been able to identify a soluble brain protein that binds corticosterone (McEwen, Magnus, and Wallach, 1972; McEwen, 1973), and another laboratory has made similar observations (Grosser, Stevens, Bruenger, and Reed, 1971). The cytosol-binding proteins are stereospecific and bind both active and antagonistic steroids. They have a limited capacity and a high affinity for the steroid, with a dissociation constant in the range of 10^{-8} to 10^{-9} M. Nuclear-binding sites are generally thought to be a part of the acidic protein fraction, and can be extracted with moderate salt concentrations (Fig. 6). Our present view is that these nuclear-binding sites

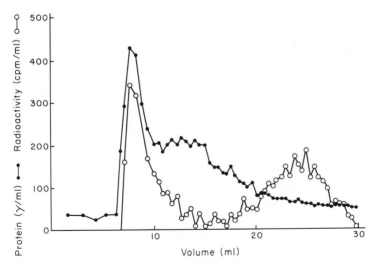

FIG. 6. Separation on Sephadex G-200 of a nuclear-binding protein extracted from isolated brain cell nuclei with 0.4 M NaCl, after *in vivo* labeling with ^{3}H-corticosterone. For details, see McEwen and Plapinger, 1970.

are probably derived from the cytoplasm through transport of the hormone, and possibly the binding proteins as well.

In order to demonstrate that the cellular corticosterone-binding protein was a distinct entity unrelated to the corticosterone-binding protein found in the blood, referred to as CBG or transcortin (Westphal, 1971), we compared the two proteins by a number of different parameters (Table 3). The two proteins show markedly different sedimentation patterns on poly-acrylamide gel electrophoresis, and the rates of exchange with unlabeled corticosterone are markedly different. A slow rate of exchange appears to be characteristic of tissue receptors, whereas a serum transport protein would be expected to show a rapid dissociation. Only the tissue protein could be precipitated with protamine sulfate, demonstrated dexamethasone binding, and could be inhibited with sulfhydryl reagents. The two binding factors are thus distinctly different.

TABLE 3. *Comparison of brain and serum corticoid-binding proteins**

Protein	Brain	Serum
Protamine sulfate	precipitated	not precipitated
Dexamethasone	binds	does not bind
—SH group antagonists	blocks	does not block
Polyacrylamide gels	slow migration	fast migration
Exchange rate	slow	fast

* Based on data from McEwen, Magnus, and Wallach, 1972, and McEwen, 1973.

V. *IN VITRO* STUDIES OF CORTICOSTERONE BINDING

There are a number of advantages in the use of *in vitro* methods for studies of the cellular mechanism of hormone uptake, since it is possible to manipulate factors such as hormone concentration and incubation conditions. Table 4 summarizes some of the basic characteristics of the *in vitro* uptake of ^{3}H-corticosterone.

These *in vitro* studies have confirmed our *in vivo* demonstration of the regional specificity of nuclear uptake to the hippocampus. We were also able to demonstrate competition with unlabeled corticosterone, and found a temperature dependence of uptake, with maximum results obtained at 25°C rather than 37°C. Uptake by the nuclear fraction is much more temperature dependent than uptake by the whole homogenate, with a much greater percentage reduction in response to lower temperature. This may be relevant to the mechanism of binding.

When uptake in the whole homogenate of hippocampal tissue is com-

TABLE 4. *Corticosterone uptake by 300μ brain tissue slices*[a]

Brain region	Conditions[b]	Nuclear radioactivity DPM/mg protein
Hippocampus	Control	15,800
	Competition[c]	1,350
	0°C	3,800
Hypothalamus-preoptic area	Control	5,500
	Competition[c]	400

[a] Based on data presented by McEwen, 1973.
[b] 25°C unless indicated.
[c] 30 min incubation at 5×10^{-9} M ^{3}H-corticosterone + 2.5×10^{-7} M unlabeled corticosterone.

pared with uptake by the nuclear fraction, a saturation point is reached at 2×10^{-8} M corticosterone in the medium. Uptake of cortisol or hydrocortisone is much lower, in agreement with corticosterone being the natural glucocorticoid in the rat (McEwen and Wallach, 1973).

When we compared the hippocampal nuclear uptake of corticosterone and cortisol with that of progesterone and estradiol, we found the relative uptake of these steroids by the whole homogenate to follow a polarity rule, with the least polar steroid showing the greatest uptake, i.e., progesterone > estradiol > corticosterone cortisol. The nuclear uptake did not show this pattern, but showed a specificity for the glucocorticoids over the gonadal steroids.

VI. GLUCOCORTICOID EFFECTS ON NEURAL FUNCTION

The general approach used in our work was to initially demonstrate that an area of the brain that responded to a hormone, specifically estradiol, contained binding sites for that hormone. We turned to the glucocorticoid system, which was not as clearly understood either in terms of precise functions or of precise localization of functions within the brain. Recent advances in this area have led us to recognize a number of neurally mediated events which are in some way dependent on glucocorticoids.

Bohus (1970, 1971) and de Wied (1967) have found effects of glucocorticoids both on the formation of a discrimination and on the extinction of a conditioned avoidance response, which is consistent with the concept that the glucocorticoids facilitate adaptation of the animal to a particular situation. Improvement of the formation of a conditioned response or the performance of that response is of obvious adaptive advantage. Facilitation of the extinction of a conditioned response, such as an avoidance response, is also of adaptive significance, because by definition the retention of such behavior is unnecessary when the situation responded to is absent.

ACTH secretion occurs episodically, with peak amounts during the later phase of the sleep cycle in both the rat and human. Secretion occurs during the period of REM or paradoxical sleep in the human, and glucocorticoids have been shown to selectively suppress the appearance of paradoxical sleep. Johnson and Sawyer (1971) showed that adrenalectomy results in the disappearance of the diurnal rhythmicity of paradoxical sleep in the rat, whereas administration of a synthetic glucocorticoid results in the specific suppression of REM sleep in the human, without altering the amount of slow wave sleep. Gillin, Jacobs, Fram, and Snyder (1972) found that a synthetic glucocorticoid suppressed the occurrence of paradoxical sleep in human subjects and did not affect slow wave sleep.

Henkin (1970) has demonstrated a clear relationship between glucocorticoids and the sensory thresholds for both the detection and recognition of various sensory stimuli. These effects are observed for a number of sensory modalities in the human. Patients with adrenal insufficiency have decreased thresholds for detecting particular odors, tastes, and sounds, but the threshold for recognition is increased. They are thus able to detect stimuli at very low intensities, but are less able than normal individuals to recognize what they are.

Only in the case of ACTH secretion and REM sleep is it possible thus far to suggest some involvement of the hippocampus. This region is the site of the theta rhythm which is very prominent during REM sleep, and disruption of the diurnal rhythmicity of ACTH secretion follows section of the fornix (Moberg, Scapagnini, DeGroot, and Ganong, 1971), the main pathway from the hippocampus, or implantation of corticosteroid in the hippocampus (Slusher, 1966). It is possible that the binding of corticosterone can be utilized to elucidate some of the functional effects of the hormone on the brain, as in the extensive binding in the CA1 and CA2 regions of the hippocampus in contrast to the much lower binding in CA3 and CA4.

VII. CONCLUSIONS

If we examine to what extent our studies of the binding of steroid hormones by brain tissue have met the criteria for receptors which I outlined earlier, it will be clear that we have not yet proved unequivocally that these binding sites are actually receptors. Our strongest argument comes from the analogy with other systems. We have found that the cellular site of binding agrees with that found in nonneural target tissues, where the hormones have been shown to have direct effects on the genome.

We have also demonstrated a correlation between the regions which bind hormone and those which respond to the hormone. This is particularly clear for the estrogenic steroids, although it has not yet been carried from the regional to the cellular level of correlation. Finally, there is very good agreement between the binding of various hormones and their analogues to these binding sites and the ability of these substances to induce lordosis behavior or to regulate gonadotrophin secretion.

It will be of great interest in the future to find out whether the binding proteins from different target tissues, such as the estrogen-binding proteins from the uterus, pituitary, and brain, are identical or whether there are major or minor differences in their structure. This is critical for the understanding of the cellular mechanism of action of the hormone, because if they are identical we will have to look elsewhere within the cell to explain their differential effects on different tissues.

REFERENCES

Berg, D. K., Kelly, R. B., Sargent, P. B., Williamson, P., and Hall, Z. W. (1972): Binding of α-bungarotoxin to acetylcholine receptors in mammalian muscle. *Proceedings of the National Academy of Sciences,* 69:147–151.

Bohus, B. (1970): Central nervous structures and the effect of ACTH and corticosteroids on avoidance behavior: A study with intra cerebral implantation of corticosteroids in the rat. In: *Pituitary, Adrenal and the Brain,* edited by D. de Wied and J. A. W. M. Weijnen, pp. 171–183. Elsevier, Amsterdam.

Bohus, B. (1971): Adrenocortical hormones and central nervous function: The site and mode of their behavioural action in the rat. In: *Proceedings of the Third International Congress on Hormonal Steroids, Hamburg 1970,* edited by V. H. T. James and L. Martini, pp. 752–758. Excerpta Medica, Series 219, Basel.

Bullock, L. P., Bardin, C. W., and Ohno, S. (1971): The androgen insensitive mouse: Absence of intranuclear androgen retention in the kidney. *Biochemical and Biophysical Research Communications,* 44:1537–1543.

Chader, G. J., and Villee, C. A. (1970): Uptake of oestradiol by the rabbit hypothalamus. *Biochemical Journal,* 118:93–97.

Clark, D. G., Wolcott, R. G., and Raftery, M. A. (1972): Partial characterization of an α-bungarotoxin-binding component of electroplax membranes. *Biochemical and Biophysical Research Communications,* 48:1061–1067.

Cuatrecasas, P. (1971): Insulin-receptor interactions in adipose tissue cells: Direct measurement and properties. *Proceedings of the National Academy of Sciences,* 68:1264–1268.

de Kretser, D. M., Catt, K. J., and Paulsen, C. A. (1971): Studies on the *in vitro* testicular binding of iodinated luteinizing hormone in rats. *Endocrinology,* 80:332.

de Plazas, S. F., and de Robertis, E. (1972): Binding of α-bungarotoxin to the cholinergic receptor proteolipid from *Electrophorus* electroplax. *Biochimica et Biophysica Acta,* 274:258–265.

de Vellis, J., Inglish, D., Cole, R., and Molson, J. (1971): Effects of hormones on the differentiation of cloned lines of neurons and glial cells. In: *Influence of Hormones on the Nervous System, Proceedings of the First International Society of Psychoneuroendocrinology, Brooklyn, 1970,* pp. 25–39. Karger, Basel.

De Wied, D. (1967): Opposite effects of ACTH and glucocorticosteroids on extinction of conditioned avoidance behavior. In: *Proceedings of the Second International Congress on Hormonal Steroids, Milan,* pp. 945–951. Excerpta Medica International Congress Series, No. 132.

Eisenfeld, A. J. (1970): ³H-Estradiol: *In vitro* binding to macromolecules from the rat hypothalamus, anterior pituitary and uterus. *Endocrinology,* 86:1313–1318.

Eisenfeld, A. J., and Axelrod, J. (1965): Selectivity of estrogen distribution in tissues. *Journal of Pharmacology and Experimental Therapeutics,* 150:469–475.

Fulpius, B., Cha, S., Klett, R., and Reich, E. (1972): Properties of the nicotinic acetylcholine receptor macromolecule of *Electrophorus electricus. Federation of European Biochemical Societies. Letters,* 24:323–326.

Gerlach, J. L., and McEwen, B. S. (1972): Rat brain binds adrenal steroid hormone: Radioautography of hippocampus with corticosterone. *Science,* 175:1133–1136.

Gillin, J. C., Jacobs, L. S., Fram, D. H., and Snyder, F. (1972): Acute effect of a glucocorticoid on normal human sleep. *Nature,* 237:398–399.

Grant, G., Vale, W., and Guillemin, R. (1972): Interaction of thyrotoxin releasing factor with membrane receptors of pituitary cells. *Biochemical and Biophysical Research Communications,* 46:28.

Grosser, B. I., Stevens, W., Bruenger, F. W., and Reed, D. J. (1971): Corticosterone binding by rat brain cytosol. *Journal of Neurochemistry,* 18:1725–1732.

Henkin, R. I. (1970): The effects of corticosteroids and ACTH on sensory systems. *Progress in Brain Research,* 32:270–293.

Jensen, E. V., and DeSombre, E. R. (1972): Estrogens and progestins. In: *Biochemical Actions of Hormones,* Vol. 2, edited by G. Litwack, pp. 215–255. Academic Press, New York and London.

Johnson, J. H., and Sawyer, C. H. (1971): Adrenal steroids and the maintenance of a circadian distribution of paradoxical sleep in rats. *Endocrinology,* 89:507–512.

Kahwanago, I., Heinrichs, W. L., and Herrmann, W. L. (1969): Isolation of oestradiol "receptors" from bovine hypothalamus and anterior pituitary gland. *Nature,* 223:313–314.

Kato, J., Atsumi, Y., and Inaba, M. (1970): A soluble receptor for estradiol in rat anterior hypophysis. *Journal of Biochemistry,* 68:759–761.

Kato, J., Atsumi, Y., and Inaba, M. (1971): Development of estrogen receptors in the rat hypothalamus. *Journal of Biochemistry,* 70:1051–1053.

Kato, J., Atsumi, Y., and Muramatsu, M. (1970): Nuclear estradiol receptor in rat anterior hypophysis. *Journal of Biochemistry,* 67:871–872.

Kato, J., and Villee, C. A. (1967): Preferential uptake of estradiol by the anterior hypothalamus of the rat. *Endocrinology,* 80:567–575.

Lefkowitz, R. J., and Haber, E. (1971): A fraction of the ventricular myocardium that has the specificity of the cardia beta-adrenergic receptor. *Proceedings of the National Academy of Sciences,* 68:1773–1777.

Liao, S., and Fang, S. (1969): Receptor proteins for androgens and the mode of action of androgens on gene transcription in ventral prostate. *Vitamins and Hormones,* 27:17–90.

Lisk, R. D. (1967): Sexual behavior: Hormonal control. In: *Neuroendocrinology,* Vol. 2, edited by L. Martini and W. F. Ganong, pp. 197–239. Academic Press, New York.

McEwen, B. S. (1973): Glucocorticoid binding sites in rat brains: Subcellular and anatomical localizations. *Progress in Brain Research, in press.*

McEwen, B. S., Magnus, C., and Wallach, G. (1971): Biochemical studies of corticosterone binding to cell nuclei and cytoplasmic macromolecules in specific regions of the rat brain. In: *Steroid Hormones and Brain Function,* edited by C. H. Sawyer and R. A. Gorski, pp. 247–258. University of California Press, Berkeley.

McEwen, B. S., Magnus, C., and Wallach, G. (1972): Soluble corticosterone-binding macromolecules extracted from rat brain. *Endocrinology,* 90:217–226.

McEwen, B. S., and Pfaff, D. W. (1970): Factors influencing sex hormones uptake by rat brain regions: I. Effects of neonatal treatment, hypophysectomy, and competing steroid on estradiol uptake. *Brain Research,* 21:1–16.

McEwen, B. S., and Plapinger, L. (1970): Association of corticosterone-1,2-H³ with macromolecules extracted from brain cell nuclei. *Nature,* 226:263–264.

McEwen, B. S., and Wallach, G. (1973): Corticosterone binding to brain: *In vitro* studies of cytosol and nuclear binding. *Brain Research,* 57:373–386.

McEwen, B. S., Weiss, J. M., and Schwartz, L. S. (1969): Uptake of corticosterone by rat brain and its concentration by certain limbic structures. *Brain Research,* 16:227–241.

McEwen, B. S., Weiss, J. M., and Schwartz, L. S. (1970): Retention of corticosterone by cell nuclei from brain regions of adrenalectomized rats. *Brain Research,* 17:471–482.

McEwen, B. S., Zigmond, R. E., and Gerlach, J. L. (1972): Sites of steroid binding and action in the brain. In: *Structure and Function of the Nervous System,* edited by G. H. Bourne, pp. 205–291. Academic Press, New York.

Means, A. R., and Vaitukaitis, J. (1972): Peptide hormone "receptors": Specific binding of ^{3}H-FSH to testis. *Endocrinology,* 90:39–46.

Moberg, G. P., Scapagnini, U., DeGroot, J., and Ganong, W. F. (1971): Effect of sectioning the fornix on diurnal fluctuation in plasma corticosterone levels in the rat. *Neuroendocrinology,* 7:11–15.

Notides, A. C. (1970): Binding affinity and specificity of the estrogen receptor of the rat uterus and anterior pituitary. *Endocrinology,* 87:987–992.

O'Malley, B. W., Spelsburg, T. C., Schrader, W. T., Chytil, F., and Steggles, A. W. (1972): Mechanisms of interaction of a hormone-receptor complex with the genome of a eukaryotic target cell. *Nature,* 235:141–144.

Raynaud, J. P., Mercier-Bodard, C., and Baulieu, E. E. (1972): Rat estradiol binding plasma protein (EBP). *Steroids,* 18:767–788.

Robison, G. A., Butcher, R. W., and Sutherland, E. W. (1971): *Cyclic AMP.* Academic Press, New York.

Slusher, M. A. (1966): Effects of cortisol implants in the brainstem and ventral hippocampus on diurnal corticosterone levels. *Experimental Brain Research,* 1:184–194.

Swaneck, G. E., Highland, E., and Edelman, I. S. (1969): Stereospecific nuclear and cytosol aldosterone-binding proteins of various tissues. *Nephron,* 6:297–316.

Tindal, J. S., Knaggs, G. S., and Turvey, A. (1967): Central nervous control of prolactin secretion in the rabbit: Effect of local oestrogen implants in the amygdaloid complex. *Journal of Endocrinology,* 37:279–287.

Wade, G., and Zucker, I. (1970): Modulation of food intake and locomotor activity in female rats by diencephalic hormone implants. *Journal of Comparative and Physiological Psychology,* 72:328–336.

Westphal, U. (1971): *Steroid-Protein Interactions.* Springer-Verlag, New York.

Williams-Ashman, H. G., and Reddi, A. H. (1972): Androgenic regulation of tissue growth and function. In: *Biochemical Actions of Hormones,* Vol. 2, edited by G. Litwack, pp. 257–294. Academic Press, New York and London.

Zigmond, R. E., and McEwen B. S. (1970): Selective retention of oestradiol by cell nuclei in specific brain regions of the ovariectomized rat. *Journal of Neurochemistry,* 17:889–899.

Proteins of the Nervous System
Raven Press, New York © 1973

Nerve Growth Factor

Pietro U. Angeletti, Ruth Hogue Angeletti,
William A. Frazier, and Ralph A. Bradshaw

I. INTRODUCTION

During the course of studies on the effect of peripheral tissue on the developing nervous system, Bueker (1948) observed a marked hypertrophy of chick embryonic sensory and sympathetic ganglia following the transplantation of mouse sarcoma tissue. Levi-Montalcini (1952) and Levi-Montalcini and Hamburger (1953) subsequently found that this hypertrophy was due to the release of a humoral factor by the tumor explants, and designated this substance *nerve growth factor* (NGF). When tissue extracts containing NGF were added to explanted sensory ganglia from chick embryo that had been maintained *in vitro* in plasma clots for 12 to 14 hr, a dramatic nerve fiber outgrowth from the ganglia was observed (Fig. 1). The introduction of such outgrowth from cultured ganglionic tissue became the basis of a semiquantitative assay of NGF that has only recently been supplemented by immunological and radiochemical methods (Hendry, 1972).

After purification of NGF from mouse submaxillary glands (Cohen, 1959), *in vivo* experiments with the purified protein established that NGF selectively stimulated the growth of the sympathetic system of para- and prevertebral ganglia (Fig. 2). This selectivity of the NGF effect on the sympathetic system has occasionally been questioned. There have been several reports that NGF also stimulates other cell types in addition to sympathetic neurons. However, the magnitude of such effects is minor, supporting the view that its principal physiological action is centered on the sympathetic nervous system.

Additional evidence for this specificity is provided by studies with antiserum to the NGF molecule. It has been known for many years that injection of NGF antiserum produces a rapid and complete destruction of all para- and prevertebral ganglia (Levi-Montalcini and Booker, 1960; Levi-Montalcini and Angeletti, 1966), an effect referred to as immunosympathectomy. The morphological effects of the antiserum are quite different from the destructive process following treatment with other cytotoxic agents (Fig. 3). The initial morphological changes seen following treatment

133

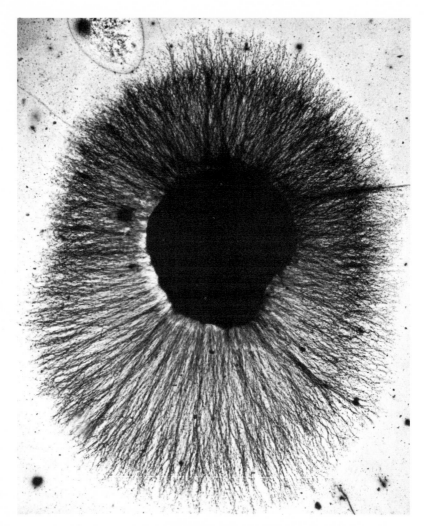

FIG. 1. Induction by NGF of fiber outgrowth from the dorsal root ganglion of chick embryo (NGF, 0.01 µg/ml).

with a cytotoxic agent such as 6-hydroxydopamine are found in the cytoplasm, with a gradual spreading to the nucleus followed by cell death (Fig. 3). In contrast, the early lesions following administration of NGF antiserum are nuclear, with nucleolar segregation and condensation of the chromatin (Fig. 4). Cytoplasmic lesions appear only secondarily (P. U. Angeletti, Levi-Montalcini, and Caramia, 1971).

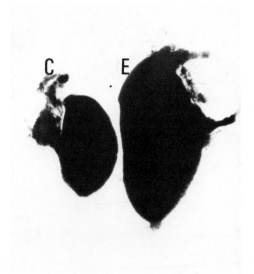

FIG. 2. *In vivo* stimulation of mouse superior cervical ganglion by NGF. The experimental (E) animal was treated with 10 μg NGF per g body weight daily for 10 days, starting at birth.

The specific interaction with sympathetic neurons of antibodies directed against the NGF molecule implies that the NGF present in these ganglia is available to a large molecule located on or near the cell surface. It has been shown with radioimmunoassay and uptake studies of ^{125}I-labeled NGF that NGF is specifically concentrated in sympathetic ganglia, its concentration there being 40- to 50-fold that of plasma (Hendry, 1972). These data, in addition to the observed structural similarities between NGF and insulin (see below), suggest the presence of specific NGF receptors on the surface of sympathetic neurons. Experiments to localize, isolate, and characterize such receptors employing ferritin-labeled antibodies, insolubilized NGF, and affinity chromatography are currently in progress.

It is also noteworthy that Sjöstrand and Angeletti have obtained evidence that NGF may be taken up from the nerve endings and be transported to the cell soma via a retrograde transport system. Sjöstrand found that NGF treatment induced an increase in axonal density and the fluorescence intensity of norepinephrine terminals in the iris of the 1-week-old rat (Fig. 5). Injection of the NGF into the vitreous humor produced a three- to fourfold increase in growth, followed by a decrease. No changes were observed at the cell body, and the initial effect appears to occur on the growth cones.

The hypertrophy of sympathetic ganglia in response to NGF is the result

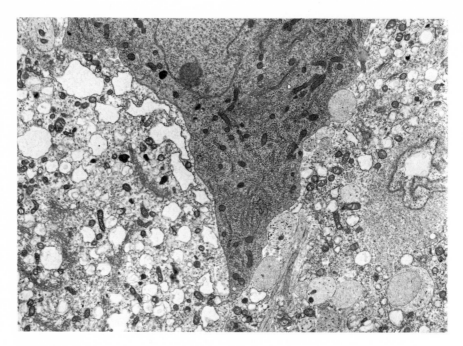

FIG. 3. Ultrastructural lesion produced in a sympathetic neuron by injection of 6-hydroxy-dopamine (100 μg/g in newborn mice.

of increases both in cell number and size. Electron microscopic studies showed that treatment with NGF produced significant changes in cellular ultrastructure (Levi-Montalcini, Caramia, and Angeletti, 1969; P. U. Angeletti et al., 1971), with an enrichment of membranous constituents such as the endoplasmic reticulum and Golgi apparatus. The most characteristic feature of these cells was the appearance of large bundles of microtubules and microfilaments (Fig. 6). These morphological observations are still the most well-defined response of ganglia to NGF, but it is now possible to describe, albeit in less rigorous terms, the metabolic responses underlying these changes in cellular ultrastructure.

II. METABOLIC EFFECTS OF NGF

Initial experiments on measuring the effect of NGF on cellular metabolism demonstrated that NGF increased all synthetic and oxidative processes within the sympathetic ganglia. NGF treatment increased glucose oxidation,

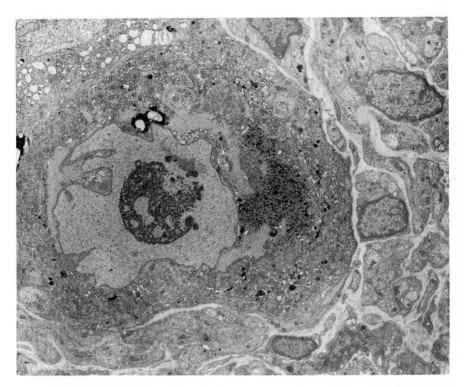

FIG. 4. Electron micrograph of the superior cervical ganglion of the mouse following the administration of NGF antiserum.

primarily via the direct oxidative pathway (P. U. Angeletti, Liuzzi, Levi-Montalcini, and Gandini-Attardi, 1964*b*), and increased the incorporation of acetate into lipid (P. U. Angeletti, Liuzzi, and Levi-Montalcini, 1964*a*), amino acid into protein (P. U. Angeletti, Gandini-Attardi, Toschi, Salvi, and Levi-Montalcini, 1965), and uridine into RNA (P. U. Angeletti et al., 1965). The increase in RNA synthesis was particularly marked, and, on the basis of this observation, it was hypothesized that NGF might act via stimulation of the synthesis of a new messenger RNA. However, Larrabee (1972) has found that nerve fiber outgrowth in response to NGF is independent of new RNA synthesis. It has since been demonstrated that other protein hormones, such as insulin, are able to stimulate RNA synthesis in sympathetic ganglia without stimulating neurite outgrowth (Levi-Montalcini, 1966), a fact of interest since NGF has now been shown to be structurally related to insulin (see below).

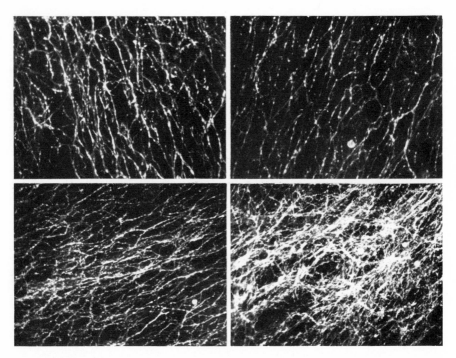

FIG. 5. Effect of NGF on the outgrowth of sympathetic axon terminals.

More recently, several laboratories have been concerned with the question of whether cyclic adenosine monophosphate (cyclic AMP) is a mediator of the NGF response. Roisen, Murphy, Pichichero, and Braden (1972) have noted stimulation of neurite outgrowth from 8-day-old chick sensory ganglia explanted on collagen-coated coverslips after the addition of 1 to 5 mM dibutyryl cyclic AMP. A similar result has been obtained employing the plasma-clot culture system routinely used for NGF bioassay (Frazier, Ohlendorf, Boyd, Johnson, Ferrendelli, and Bradshaw, *in preparation*). However, attempts to demonstrate an effect of NGF on intracellular cyclic AMP levels in sensitive neurons have produced the apparently contradictory result that there is no significant variation in cyclic AMP levels in sensory ganglia between 10 min and 24 hr after the addition of NGF *in vitro*, and NGF does not affect the activity of adenyl cyclase from this tissue. Furthermore, no effect of cyclic AMP or its dibutyryl derivative on sympathetic neurons has been detected. It is perhaps significant that the positive effect of dibutyryl cyclic AMP is pH dependent; it is manifested

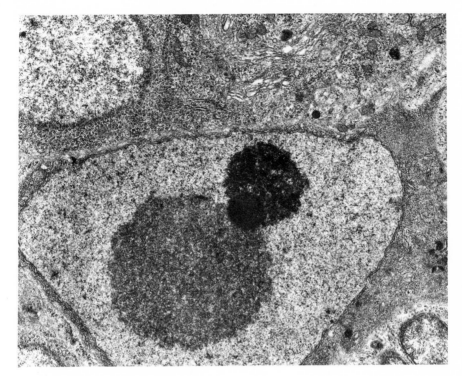

FIG. 6. Electron micrograph of mouse superior cervical ganglion tissue obtained from an animal treated with 10 μg NGF per g body weight for 7 days. Note the abundance of microfilaments and microtubules.

at pH 8.0 but not at pH 7.0. These observations suggest that the response to dibutyryl cyclic AMP is not related to the NGF response and that NGF does not mediate its effect via this "second messenger." Hier, Arnason, and Young (1972) have reached a similar conclusion from measurements of microtubule levels in sensitive ganglia. L. Frati *(personal communication)* has also been unable to demonstrate cyclic AMP involvement in the epidermal growth factor (EGF)-induced outgrowth of epidermis, and the purified EGF-receptor complex appears to be without adenyl cyclase activity.

Studies have also been focused on the effects of NGF on biochemical processes that are unique to the sympathetic neuron. It has been found that NGF induces a striking 15- to 20-fold increase in the activities of two enzymes in the biosynthetic pathway for the synthesis of the adrenergic transmitter norepinephrine; these enzymes are tyrosine hydroxylase and dopamine-β-hydroxylase, which catalyze the conversions of tyrosine to DOPA and of dopamine to norepinephrine, respectively (Thoenen, Angeletti, Levi-Montalcini, and Kettler, 1971). An increase in catecholamine biosynthesis is also indicated by a large increase of histofluorescence in cells treated *in vivo* with NGF, suggesting that there is a functional stimulation of these neurons by the NGF.

The specificity of this effect was demonstrated by a comparison of the effects of NGF on these enzymes in sympathetic ganglia and adrenal medullary cells, which contain an almost identical composition of enzymes and utilize the same metabolic pathway for the production of epinephrine. NGF had virtually no effect on the activities of either tyrosine hydroxylase or dopamine-β-hydroxylase in adrenal medullary tissue (Fig. 7).

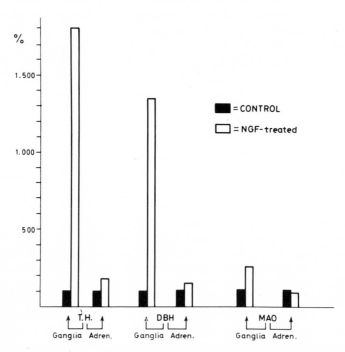

FIG. 7. A comparison of the effects of NGF on the levels of tyrosine hydroxylase and dopamine-β-hydroxylase in sympathetic ganglia and adrenal medullary tissue. (From P. U. Angeletti, Levi-Montalcini, Kettler, and Thoenen, 1972.)

III. DISTRIBUTION AND STRUCTURE OF NGF

In a strict sense, NGF is not a protein of the nervous system. It is not brain specific, or even tissue or species specific. The availability of pure NGF and of radioimmunoassay methods for the detection of proteins has made it possible to compare NGF levels in many tissues. The NGF level in the submaxillary gland is approximately 1,000-fold higher than in other tissues, with the lowest concentration in the brain. In mice, there are no sex differences in NGF for any tissue except the submaxillary gland, where the level in male animals is always higher. Plasma concentrations are also higher in male animals.

Since NGF acts specifically on the sympathetic nervous system, it might be associated with the adrenergic nerve terminals which are present in the microsomal pellet following centrifugation at $100,000 \times g$. However, there is no difference in the NGF content of this fraction in tissue from control animals and in tissue obtained from animals treated with 6-hydroxydopamine, which selectively destroys adrenergic terminals. Thus, NGF is present in peripheral tissue even in the absence of the sympathetic system on which it has a selective effect.

Similar values of NGF concentration in peripheral tissues from different animal species have been obtained by microcomplement fixation (P. U. Angeletti, Levi-Montalcini, and Vigneti, 1972). After subcellular fractionation, most of the NGF is recovered with the microsomal fraction, indicating that it is present within the cell in a membrane-bound form. The concentration of NGF in the microsomal fraction is 0.1 to 0.2 mg% of the total protein in this fraction (Fig. 8). Considerable immunological cross-reactivity among different species can be observed with microcomplement fixation. The immunological similarity is very high among different mammalian species, and some cross-reactivity can be demonstrated between mammalian and snake venom NGF (R. H. Angeletti, 1971).

Since the most abundant source of NGF is the male mouse submaxillary gland, the structure of NGF isolated from this tissue has been most well defined. NGF is found in the tubules of the gland and is secreted with the saliva. The significance of the high levels and the function, if any, of the NGF within the gland are completely unknown. NGF has not yet been identified with any of the enzymes or biologically active proteins known to be present in the salivary gland (Levi-Montalcini and Angeletti, 1968).

NGF was partially purified from submaxillary gland extracts by Cohen (1959), who found it to be a basic protein with a molecular weight of 44,000. However, this preparation was contaminated with trace amounts of various

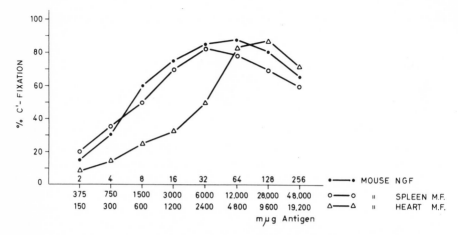

FIG. 8. Microcomplement fixation of purified mouse NGF versus the microsomal fraction of mouse spleen and heart. The concentration of protein in a tissue is calculated from the amount of protein required to give 50% complement fixation.

hydrolytic activities. The later development of more refined techniques of column chromatography and the use of Sephadex gel filtration permitted the purification of NGF by two different methods to a state of homogeneity sufficient for use in physiochemical studies.

Varon, Nomura, and Shooter (1967a,b) have isolated NGF as a large aggregate with a sedimentation coefficient of 7S, which corresponds to a molecular weight in excess of 100,000. This aggregate has been further purified to homogeneity and shown to contain three classes of subunits, α, β, and γ. Although the function of the α subunit is not yet certain, the γ subunit has been found to be an arginine esterase. The β subunit is the only one possessing NGF activity. Although the stoichiometry of this complex is not fully established, Perez-Polo, DeJong, Strauss, and Shooter (1972) have obtained evidence suggesting that the interaction of the α and γ subunits with the β subunit is specific, since the high molecular weight complex appears to form even in the presence of crude submaxillary gland extracts. However, the increase of NGF activity accompanying aggregation may be a protective effect at the low concentrations of protein employed in the bioassay.

The NGF used for more detailed structural analysis was purified according to a modification (Bocchini and Angeletti, 1969) of the procedure of Cohen (1959), which yields an active unit and appears to be slightly larger than the β subunit as measured by gel-filtration techniques. Zanini, Angeletti, and Levi-Montalcini (1968) later found this preparation to contain a smaller, 14,000 molecular weight species. Experiments were thus begun to determine the minimum molecular weight of the NGF protein. The amino acid composition of NGF revealed the presence of 12 half-cystinyl residues (R. H. Angeletti, Bradshaw, and Wade, 1970), which must all participate in disulfide linkages, since there are no free sulfhydryl groups in the native protein (Bocchini, 1970). As measured by sedimentation equilibrium methods, denaturation of the native NGF in guanidine HCl at pH 3.3 caused the molecular weight to decrease to 16,200 from 29,000, demonstrating that the larger protein isolated is indeed a dimer. Moreover, the molecular weight of NGF did not decrease significantly further when the disulfide linkages were reduced and alkylated with iodoacetate prior to treatment with guanidine HCl. Thus, native NGF is not only a dimer of two subunits, but these units are associated noncovalently, with the disulfide bridges internal to each. Column tryptic fingerprint analysis of ^{14}C-S-carboxymethyl NGF unequivocally established this hypothesis and further demonstrated that the two components of the dimer are very similar or identical in amino acid sequence.

The combined data from the tryptic digests of NGF and analyses of the peptides purified from chymotryptic, peptic, and thermolytic digests permitted the construction of an internally consistent, primary and secondary structure for mouse NGF (Figs. 9 and 10; R. H. Angeletti and Bradshaw, 1971). The single polypeptide chain of 118 amino acid residues yields a monomeric molecular weight of 13,259 and a dimeric molecular weight of 26,518. Structural studies of β NGF indicate a close similarity of the two preparations (E. M. Shooter, *personal communication*). The molecule possesses several interesting and unusual features. The isoelectric point of 9.3 (Bocchini, 1970) is in agreement with the content of eight lysines, seven arginines, and eight (of 19) amidated acidic residues. The more acidic and hydrophobic residues are clustered near the amino terminus, whereas the carboxy terminal end has a high concentration of basic residues. By use of the protein sequencer, it was found that the NGF preparations were not always homogeneous and that the first eight amino terminal residues were sometimes removed. Most preparations analyzed contained an approximately equal mixture of the 110 and 118 residue chains. In contrast, the β subunit prepared by Shooter consists almost entirely of the 118 residue chain (E. M. Shooter, *personal communication*), indicating that the 110-residue polypeptide may actually be an artifact of preparation. It is interesting that the amino terminal octapeptide sequence has about 50% sequence homology with angiotensin. Studies attempting to determine if the cleavage of this peptide from the amino terminus of the NGF molecule has physiological significance are currently in progress.

The carboxy terminus of NGF as prepared by the method of Bocchini and Angeletti (1969) has been found to be arginine. However, the fact that this amino acid is not always present in the purified molecule points to a heterogeneity at the carboxy terminus as well as at the amino terminus (W. A. Frazier. *personal communication;* J. Bamburg and E. M. Shooter, *personal communication*). Taylor, Cohen, and Mitchell (1967) have found that the EGF is extracted from submaxillary gland in association with an arginine esterase, as is NGF. They have proposed that EGF, which also possesses a carboxy terminal arginine, is cleaved from another large molecule by the esterase, and that these two proteins are actually part of a biosynthetic complex. Attempts are being made to determine if a similar mechanism exists for the genesis of the NGF molecule. J. Bamburg and E. M. Shooter *(personal communication)* have, in fact, reported that purification under acidic conditions results in an NGF molecule that has a carboxy terminal arginine, whereas preparation under basic conditions results in a loss of this arginine. The terminal arginine appears to be necessary for binding of the α and γ subunits to the β subunit in the 7S NGF complex.

The placement of the three disulfide bridges (Fig. 12) restricts the NGF molecule to a fairly tight and compact structure consisting of a series of loops, the smallest being a 14-residue ring. Crystals of NGF have recently been prepared, and structural analysis using X-ray techniques should yield more precise information concerning the tertiary and quarternary structure (C. E. Ohlendorf, R. A. Bradshaw, and F. S. Matthews, *personal communication*). Correlation of the conformation of NGF in solution with that in the crystalline state will be possible using data from studies of the rates and effects of specific chemical modification (R. H. Angeletti, Frazier, and Bradshaw, 1972b; Frazier, Angeletti, Sherman, and Bradshaw, *in preparation*).

IV. NGF AND INSULIN

Many of the effects of NGF resemble those of insulin in sensitive tissues. As noted above, neurons sensitive to NGF also respond to high levels of insulin with an increased uridine incorporation (Partlow, 1969; P. U. Angeletti et al., 1965), enhanced protein synthesis (Partlow, 1969; P. U. Angeletti et al., 1965; P. U. Angeletti, Liuzzi and Levi-Montalcini, 1966), and an increased energy metabolism (Liuzzi, Pocchiari, and Angeletti, 1968). Structural homologies which might explain these common effects were therefore sought.

Significant structural similarities were observed between NGF and both guinea pig insulin and human proinsulin (Fig. 9). When activated to insulin, the proinsulin molecule produces three chains, A, B, and C, with the A and B chains remaining covalently linked by two disulfide bonds (Oyer, Cho, Peterson, and Steiner, 1971; Nolan, Margoliash, Peterson, and Steiner, 1971). The regions of highest homology are located in the segments of the NGF sequence which correspond to the A and B chains. In the NGF sequence, these segments are separated by 35 residues, the exact spacing required to allow the alignment of the C peptide of proinsulin with no deletions. This alignment (Fig. 9) can be obtained by the introduction of only five deletions into the NGF molecule. Although the NGF subunit contains 32 more residues than human proinsulin, a repetition of the proinsulin molecule allows the incorporation of a second complete B chain, designated as B'. The rationale for this duplication is considered below.

These similarities in structure suggest that proinsulin and NGF are related to a common ancestral gene. Although many types of statistical analyses have been used to calculate similarities between protein sequences, the relatedness-odds relationship (Dayhoff, 1969) seems to be the most appropriate for distantly related proteins. This type of analysis showed a similarity among identical residues that is higher than random for the A, B and B' segments with NGF (Frazier, Angeletti, and Bradshaw, 1972). Corresponding values for nonidentical residues were essentially random, as may be expected for proteins at an evolutionary distance corresponding to only 15 to 20% identity. Thus, structural relationships that reflect evolution from a common precursor in the case of distantly related proteins can be inferred only in regions of identity.

In addition to the regions of homology, the conservation of three of the six half-cystinyl residues present in both NGF and proinsulin suggest that at least some regions of the two proteins may also have similar three-dimensional structures. As depicted schematically in Fig. 10, two of the three conserved half-cystinyl residues retain pairing identical to that of the corresponding residues in insulin, and this disulfide bond connects the two regions of the NGF sequence which are most identical to insulin. The third half-cystinyl residue, conserved in the NGF structure, is linked to a half-cystinyl residue found in the B' segment. The presence of this B' segment imparts added structural constraints to the NGF molecule, and the overall changes in structure resulting from the incorporation of the B' region may be reflected in those properties which distinguish it from insulin. The extent to which the similarity in three-dimensional structures exists, as indicated by the conserved disulfide bridge, will best be established by X-ray crystallographic analysis of NGF followed by comparison to the known structure of insulin (Blundell, Cutfield, Cutfield, Dodson, Dodson, Hodgkin, Mercola, and Vijayan, 1971).

In lieu of a defined three-dimensional model for NGF, chemical modi-

Mouse NGF   1   5   10   15

Mouse NGF: Ser- - -[Ser]-Thr-His-Pro- - -Val-Phe-His-Met-Gly-Glu- - - - Phe-Ser-Val-Cys-Asp-Ser
Human PI: Phe-Val-Asn-Gln-His-Leu-Cys-Gly-Ser-His-Leu-Val-Glu-Ala-Leu-Tyr-Leu-Val-Cys-Gly-Glu
Gn.Pig Ins.: Phe-Val-Ser-Arg-His-Leu-Cys-Gly-Ser-Asn-Leu-Val-Glu-Thr-Leu-Tyr-Ser-Val-Cys-Gln-Asp
   B-1   B-5   B-10   B-15   B-20

   20   25   30   35

Mouse NGF: Val-Ser-Val-Trp-Val-Gly-Asp-Lys-Thr-Thr-Ala-Thr-Asn-Ile-Lys-Gly-Lys-Glu-Val-Thr-Val
Human PI: Arg-Gly-Phe-Phe-Tyr-Thr-Pro-Lys-Thr-Arg-Arg-Glu-Ala-Glu-Asp-Leu-Gln-Val-Gly-Gln-Val
Gn.Pig Ins.: Asp-Gly-Phe-Phe-Tyr-Ile-Pro-Lys-Asp-[
   B-25   B-30   C-1   C-5   C-10
   *   *   *

   40   45   50   55

Mouse NGF: Leu-Ala-Glu-Val-Asn-Ile-Asn-Asn-Ser-Val-Phe-Arg-Gln-Tyr-Phe-Phe-Glu-Thr-Lys-Cys-Arg
Human PI: Glu-Leu-Gly-Gly-Gly-Pro-Gly-Ala-Gly-Ser-Leu-Gln-Pro-Leu-Ala-Leu-Glu-Gly-Ser-Leu-Gln
Gn.Pig Ins.:
   C-15   C-20   C-25   C-30

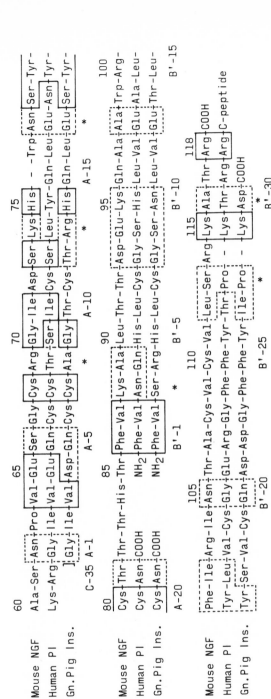

FIG. 9. The alignment of the amino acid sequence of the primary subunit of mouse NGF (R. H. Angeletti et al., 1972b) with those of human proinsulin (Oyer et al., 1971) and guinea pig insulin (Smith, 1966). Numbers above the lines are those of the NGF residue positions, and numbers below the lines indicate the positions of the proinsulin or insulin residues. Solid lines enclose sets of identical residues, and dotted lines enclose sets of residues considered to be favored amino acid substitutions, defined as those pairs of residues with an R_{ij} value (relatedness odds) greater than the random value of 10 (Dayhoff, 1969). B' denotes the repeated B chain of insulin (see text). Asterisks indicate positions at which residues from other insulins and proinsulins increase the number of observed similarities (Frazier et al., 1972). Copyright 1972 by the American Association for the Advancement of Science.

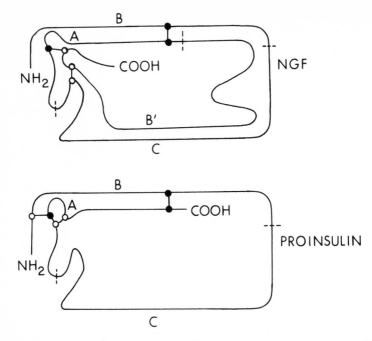

FIG. 10. A schematic representation of the alignment of disulfide bonds in the NGF and proinsulin molecules. Circles represent half-cystinyl residues; those indicated as filled circles have been conserved in the NGF sequence whereas open circles have not. Dotted bars divide the schematic peptide chains into the regions of the proinsulin molecule corresponding to the B chain, C peptide, A chain, repeated B chain, and B' (Frazier et al., 1972). Copyright 1972 by the American Association for the Advancement of Science.

fication experiments to map the topography of the molecule have been initiated. These studies serve a dual purpose in that derivatives synthesized for such studies can provide information about structures in the protein required for biological activity as well. Modification of tyrosine with tetranitromethane results in a dinitrotyrosyl derivative that is fully active. Thus both residues are relatively available to solvent. A similar derivative, in which tyrosyl residues A 14 and A 19 have been nitrated, has been prepared for insulin (Morris, Mercola, and Arquilla, 1970). It possesses at least 75% of the biological activity of the native hormone. Modification of the tryptophan residues of NGF by N-bromosuccinimide or 2-hydroxy-5-nitrobenzyl sulfonium bromide indicates that one tryptophan residue (Trp 21) is fully available and unnecessary for biological activity, one (Trp 99) is partially buried, and one (Trp 76) is unavailable for reaction, presumably because it is located in the interior of the protein. The contribution of the last two residues is obscured by the fact that oxidation of these amino acids leads to changes in the state of polymerization and the conformation of the molecule. It is probable that they are not required for direct interaction with a receptor. The assignment of these three residues permits a comparison with the residues occupying the corresponding positions in the known structure of insulin. Both residues 21 and 76 possess corresponding environments in insulin. The environment of Trp 99 cannot be assessed in this manner because it occurs in the repeated B′ segment. The sum of these studies indicates that the location of the tyrosyl and tryptophyl residues in NGF is consistent with the concept that the two proteins have at least partially similar three-dimensional structures and that neither residue class contains members directly required for biological activity (R. H. Angeletti et al., 1972*b*).

The relationship of NGF and proinsulin, detailed in Fig. 9, is of the type displayed by proteins that have evolved independently from a common ancestral gene. A plausible scheme detailing possible major events that are consistent with the present relationship is depicted in Fig. 11. This scheme

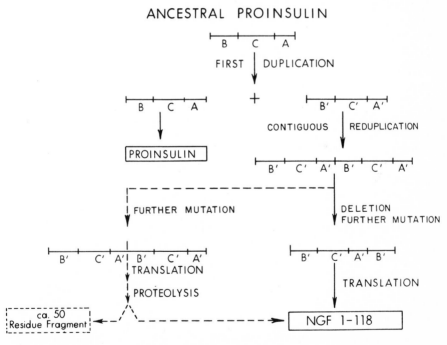

FIG. 11. A hypothetical scheme depicting the evolution of a gene coding for NGF from an ancestral proinsulin gene by way of accepted genetic mechanisms. Genes are shown as lines with bars indicating segments corresponding to those of the gene products. Gene products (proteins) are enclosed in boxes: the dashed box indicates a hypothetical protein (Frazier et al., 1972). Copyright 1972 by the American Association for the Advancement of Science.

proposes that a complete duplication of the ancestral gene was followed by a contiguous reduplication which resulted in the formation of a structural gene with sufficient genetic information to code for a polypeptide twice as long as proinsulin. An analogous situation has been described for the human haptoglobins (Dixon, 1966) and the immunoglobins (Hill, Delaney, Fellows, and Lebovitz, 1966).

There are two possible subsequent routes for the production of the 118-residue NGF molecule. A deletion event (or sum of events) could have removed the genetic material coding for the carboxyl terminal A chain and C peptide region, leaving a structural gene with sufficient information for a polypeptide chain of 118 amino acids. Alternatively, synthesis of the product of the longer gene followed by subsequent proteolysis to remove about 50 residues from the carboxyl terminal end could occur.

There are several lines of evidence in favor of the latter hypothesis. Taylor et al. (1967) have suggested that EGF may be formed by proteolytic cleavage of a larger protein. Furthermore, the carboxyl terminal arginine of NGF corresponds to one of the sites at which proinsulin is cleaved to release the C peptide (Nolan et al., 1971), and could therefore be located in a region of the molecule which retains the features necessary for the limited proteolysis required in zymogen activation (Fig. 12). In addition, NGF is isolated from the submaxillary gland as part of a multisubunit complex that includes a potent arginine esterase (Varon et al., 1967*b*). The proximity of an enzyme capable of such a cleavage is therefore assumed. Further studies will be required to differentiate between these possibilities.

The observations, detailed above, indicating a structural relationship between NGF and insulin, provide a new experimental approach to the question of how NGF exerts its multifaceted effects on the nervous system. Although it seems likely that the common structural features shared by NGF and insulin account for the limited cross-reactivity seen, it is unlikely that this phenomenon is either extensive or physiologically significant. Rather, it suggests that there are common features in the mechanism of action, as each acts in its own responsive tissue, as well as the structural and physiological differences that clearly distinguish the two. Thus, the demonstrations that NGF is biologically active in an insolubilized form (Bradshaw, Frazier, and Angeletti, 1972), that it is bound specifically to responsive cells and not to unresponsive ones (Frazier, Boyd, and Bradshaw, *unpublished experiments*), and that it can be visualized at the surface membrane under the electron microscope by means of ferritin-labeled antibodies (M. N. Goldstein, *unpublished experiments*) all point to a mechanism of action requiring a membrane-bound receptor, completely analogous to the behavior already demonstrated for insulin (Cuatrecasas,

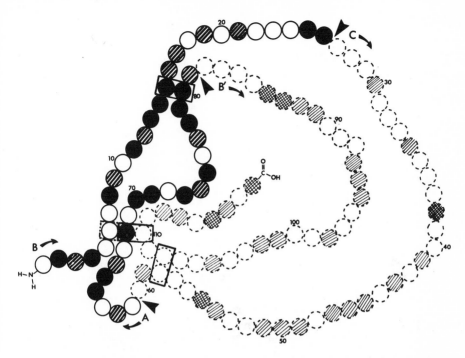

FIG. 12. Schematic representation of the comparison of the covalent structure of human proinsulin and mouse 2.5S NGF (Bradshaw et al., 1972). Solid circles indicate the portions of the NGF sequence which correspond to the functional B and A chains of insulin as indicated. (NGF 1-26 and NGF 61–81). Broken circles represent the segments of NGF which correspond to the insulin C-peptide and the repeated B chain, B'. Filled or cross-hatched circles indicate residues identical in both sequences. Diagonally shaded circles indicate favored amino acid replacements. The deletions introduced into the NGF sequence (Fig. 9) are not considered. The solid boxes enclose pairs of half-cystinyl residues which form disulfide bonds in NGF. The dotted extension of the box enclosing residues 68 and 110 in NGF indicates the corresponding disulfide bridge in human proinsulin. Arrowheads mark the peptide bonds for NGF which correspond to the cleavage points for the activation of proinsulin.

1969, 1971, 1972). How far the parallel between these two trophic factors extends remains to be established. Its elucidation should provide considerable insight not only into the chemistry and biology of NGF but also into the development and stabilization of its neuronal target tissues.

ACKNOWLEDGMENTS

R. A. B. is a U.S. Public Health Service Research Career Development Awardee (AM-23968). Portions of this work were supported by U.S. Public Health Service Grants AM-13362 and NS-10229.

REFERENCES

Angeletti, P. U., Gandini-Attardi, D., Toschi, G., Salvi, M. L., and Levi-Montalcini, R. (1965): Metabolic aspects of nerve growth factor on sympathetic and sensory ganglia: Protein and ribonucleic acid synthesis. *Biochimica et Biophysica Acta,* 95:111–120.

Angeletti, P. U., Levi-Montalcini, R., and Caramia, F. (1971): Analysis of the effects of the antiserum to the nerve growth factor in adult mice. *Brain Research,* 27:343–355.

Angeletti, P. U., Levi-Montalcini, R., Kettler, R., and Thoenen, H. (1972): Comparative studies on the effects of the nerve growth factor on sympathetic ganglia and adrenal medulla in newborn rats. *Brain Research,* 44:197–206.

Angeletti, P. U., Levi-Montalcini, R., and Vigneti, I. (1972): Localization of the nerve growth factor in subcellular fractions of peripheral tissues. In: *Nerve Growth Factor and Its Antiserum,* edited by E. Zaimis, pp. 39–45. Athlone Press, London.

Angeletti, P. U., Liuzzi, A., and Levi-Montalcini, R. (1964a): Stimulation of lipid biosynthesis in sympathetic and sensory ganglia by a specific nerve growth factor. *Biochimica et Biophysica Acta,* 84:778–781.

Angeletti, P. U., Liuzzi, A., and Levi-Montalcini, R. (1966): Effetti dell'insulina sulla sintesi di RNA e di lipidi nei gangli sensitivi embrionali. *Annales di Instituto Superiore de Sanità,* 2:420–422.

Angeletti, P. U., Liuzzi, A., Levi-Montalcini, R., and Gandini-Attardi, D. (1964b): Effects of a nerve growth factor on glucose metabolism by sympathetic and sensory nerve cells. *Biochimica et Biophysica Acta,* 90:445–450.

Angeletti, R. H. (1971): Immunological relatedness of nerve growth factors. *Brain Research,* 25:424–427.

Angeletti, R. H., Angeletti, P. U., and Levi-Montalcini, R. (1972a): Selective accumulation of 125-I labelled nerve growth factor in sympathetic ganglia. *Brain Research,* 46:421–425.

Angeletti, R. H., and Bradshaw, R. A. (1971): The amino acid sequence of 2.5 S mouse submaxillary gland nerve growth factor. *Proceedings of the National Academy of Sciences,* 68:2417–2420.

Angeletti, R. H., Bradshaw, R. A., and Wade, R. D. (1970): The subunit structure and amino acid composition of mouse submaxillary gland nerve growth factor. *Biochemistry,* 10:463–469.

Angeletti, R. H., Frazier, W. A., and Bradshaw, R. A. (1972b): Topography of nerve growth factor: Reactivity of tyrosine and tryptophan. *Abstracts of the Eighth Meeting of the Federation of European Biological Societies,* North-Holland, Amsterdam, p. 462.

Blundell, T. L., Cutfield, J. F., Cutfield, S. M., Dodson, E. J., Dodson, G. G., Hodgkin, D. C., Mercola, D. A., and Vijayan, M. (1971): Atomic positions in rhombohedral 2-zinc insulin crystals. *Nature,* 231:508–511.

Bocchini, V. (1970): The nerve growth factor: Amino acid composition and physico-chemical properties. *European Journal of Biochemistry,* 15:127–131.

Bocchini, V., and Angeletti, P. U. (1969): The nerve growth factor: Purification as a 30,000 molecular weight protein. *Proceedings of the National Academy of Sciences,* 64:787–794.

Bradshaw, R. A., Frazier, W. A., and Angeletti, R. H. (1972): A comparison of the structural and functional properties of nerve growth factor and insulin. In: *The Chemistry and Biology of Peptides,* edited by J. Meienhofer, pp. 423–439. Ann Arbor Science Publishers, Ann Arbor, Mich.

Bueker, E. D. (1948): Implantation of tumors in the hind-limb field of the embryonic chick and developmental response of the lumbosacral nervous system. *Anatomical Record,* 102:369–390.

Cohen, S. (1959): Purification and metabolic effects of a nerve-growth-promoting protein from snake venom. *Journal of Biological Chemistry,* 234:1129–1137.

Cuatrecasas, P. (1969): Interaction of insulin with the cell membrane: The primary action of insulin. *Proceedings of the National Academy of Sciences,* 63:450–457.

Cuatrecasas, P. (1971): Insulin-receptor interactions in adipose tissue cells: Direct measurement and properties. *Proceedings of the National Academy of Sciences,* 68:1264–1268.

Cuatrecasas, P. (1972): Affinity chromatography and purification of the insulin receptor from liver cell membranes. *Proceedings of the National Academy of Sciences,* 69:1277–1281.

Dayhoff, M. O., editor (1969): *Atlas of Protein Sequence and Structure,* Vol. 4, Chapter 9. National Biomedical Research Foundation, Silver Spring, Md.

Dixon, G. H. (1966): Mechanisms of protein evolution. In: *Essays in Biochemistry,* Vol. 2, pp. 147–204. Academic Press, New York.

Frazier, W. A., Angeletti, R. H., and Bradshaw, R. A. (1972): Nerve growth factor and insulin. *Science,* 176:482–488.

Hendry, I. A. (1972): Developmental changes in tissue and plasma concentrations of the biologically active species of nerve growth factor, by using a two-site radioimmunoassay. *Biochemical Journal,* 128:1265–1272.

Hier, D. D., Arnason, B. G., and Young, M. (1972): Studies on the mechanism of action of nerve growth factor. *Proceedings of the National Academy of Sciences,* 69:2268–2272.

Hill, R. L., Delaney, R., Fellows, R. E., Jr., and Lebovitz, H. E. (1966): The evolutionary origin of the immunoglobulins. *Proceedings of the National Academy of Sciences,* 56:1762–1769.

Larrabee, M. G. (1972): Metabolism during development in sympathetic ganglia of chickens: Effects of age, nerve growth factor and metabolic inhibitors. In: *Nerve Growth Factor and Its Antiserum,* edited by E. Zaimus, pp. 71–88. Athlone Press, London.

Levi-Montalcini, R. (1952): Effects of mouse tumor transplantation on the nervous system. *Annals of the New York Academy of Sciences,* 55:330–343.

Levi-Montalcini, R. (1966): The nerve growth factor: Its mode of action on sensory and sympathetic nerve cells. *Harvey Lectures,* Series 60:217–259.

Levi-Montalcini, R., and Angeletti, P. U. (1966): Immunosympathectomy. *Pharmacological Reviews,* 18:619–628.

Levi-Montalcini, R., and Angeletti, P. U. (1968): Nerve growth factor. *Physiological Reviews,* 48:534–569.

Levi-Montalcini, R., and Booker, B. (1960): Destruction of the sympathetic ganglia in mammals by an antiserum to the nerve growth promoting factor. *Proceedings of the National Academy of Sciences,* 42:384–391.

Levi-Montalcini, R., Caramia, F., and Angeletti, P. U. (1969): Alterations in the fine structure of nucleoli in sympathetic neurons following nerve growth factor antiserum treatment. *Brain Research,* 12:54–73.

Levi-Montalcini, R., and Hamburger, V. (1953): A diffusible agent of mouse sarcoma producing hyperplasia of sympathetic ganglia and hyperinnervation of the chick embryo. *Journal of Experimental Zoology,* 123:233–388.

Liuzzi, A., Pocchiari, F., and Angeletti, P. U. (1968): Glucose metabolism in embryonic ganglia: Effect of nerve growth factor (NGF) and insulin. *Brain Research,* 7:452–454.

Morris, J. W. S., Mercola, D. A., and Arquilla, E. R. (1970): Preparation and properties of 3-nitrotyrosine insulins. *Biochemistry,* 9:3930–3937.

Nolan, C., Margoliash, E., Peterson, J. D., and Steiner, D. F. (1971): The structure of bovine proinsulin. *Journal of Biological Chemistry,* 246:2780–2795.

Oyer, P. E., Cho. S., Peterson, J. D., and Steiner, D. F. (1971): Studies on human proinsulin: Isolation and amino acid sequence of the human pancreatic C peptide. *Journal of Biological Chemistry,* 246:1375–1386.

Partlow, L. M. (1969): Metabolic effects of nerve growth factor on the sympathetic nervous system of the chick embryo. Ph.D. Thesis, Johns Hopkins University.

Perez-Polo, J. R., DeJong, W. W. W., Straus, D., and Shooter, E. M. (1972): The physical and biological properties of β and 7S nerve growth factor from the mouse submaxillary gland. In: *Functional and Structural Proteins of the Nervous System, Advances in Experimental Medicine and Biology,* Vol. 32, edited by A. N. Davison, P. Mandel, and I. G. Morgan, pp. 91–98. Plenum Press, New York.

Roisen, F. J., Murphy, R. A., Pichichero, M. E., and Braden, W. G. (1972): Cyclic adenosine monophosphate stimulation of axonal elongation. *Science,* 175:73–74.

Smith, L. F. (1966): Species variation in the amino acid sequence of insulin. *American Journal of Medicine,* 40:662–666.

Taylor, J. M., Cohen, S., and Mitchell, W. M. (1967): Epidermal growth factor: High and low molecular weight forms. *Proceedings of the National Academy of Sciences,* 67:164–171.

Thoenen, H., Angeletti, P. U., Levi-Montalcini, R., and Kettler, R. (1971): Selective induction by nerve growth factor of tyrosine hydroxylase and dopamine β hydroxylase in the rat superior cervical ganglion. *Proceedings of the National Academy of Sciences,* 68:1598–1602.

Varon, S., Nomura, J., and Shooter, E. M. (1967a): The isolation of the mouse nerve growth factor protein in a high molecular weight form. *Biochemistry,* 6:2202–2209.

Varon, S., Nomura, J., and Shooter, E. M. (1967b): Subunit structure of a high molecular weight form of the nerve growth factor from mouse submaxillary gland. *Proceedings of the National Academy of Sciences,* 57:1782–1789.

Zanini, A., Angeletti, P. U., and Levi-Montalcini, R. (1968): Immunochemical properties of the nerve growth factor. *Proceedings of the National Academy of Sciences,* 61:835–842.

Proteins of the Nervous System
Raven Press, New York © 1973

The Structural and Chemical Properties of Synaptic Vesicles

Victor P. Whittaker*

I. THE ELECTRIC ORGAN OF *TORPEDO* AS A SOURCE OF CHOLINERGIC SYNAPSES

A. Introduction

Highly homogeneous preparations of synaptic vesicles can be obtained from mammalian cerebral cortical tissue by the methods described by Whittaker, Michaelson, and Kirkland (1964) and Whittaker and Sheridan (1965). They suffer from the disadvantage that they are derived from many different types of nerve endings utilizing different transmitters. There is increasing evidence that vesicles storing particular transmitters have specific proteins associated with them (for a review see Bloom, Iversen, and Schmitt, 1970); a preparation derived from such a complex region of the nervous system would thus be expected to contain a rather complex pattern of proteins. In addition, the yield of vesicle protein is low, only a few micrograms per gram of cortex.

We therefore began to look for a tissue that was richly innervated with nerve terminals utilizing a single transmitter, and we found the electric organ of *Torpedo,* which has a purely cholinergic innervation and an acetylcholine content 10 to 30 times higher than that of mammalian cortex. The electric organ is a large lobe of tissue on each side of the head formed from closely packed stacks of electroplaques, flattened cells derived embryologically from muscle cells. Each cell is profusely innervated on its underside only. The release of acetylcholine generates small potentials in these cells, analogous to end-plate potentials. The geometrical arrangement of innervation ensures that the potentials of individual electroplaques sum in series following a synchronous discharge, resulting in a polarization of the stacks of cells. This polarization may amount to 50 V in large specimens of *Torpedo marmorata,* or even 400 V in the big *Torpedo nobiliana* of the North Atlantic.

---

* Present address: Abteilung für Neurochemie, Max-Planck Institut für Biophysikalische Chemie, D-3400 Göttingen-Nikolausberg, Postfach 968, Germany.

Synaptic transmission in this tissue appears to be quite similar to that found in muscle. It is possible to record miniature potentials in the organ, but no direct estimate has yet been made of the number of acetylcholine molecules per quantum. It is therefore not yet possible to decide whether the calculated number of acetylcholine molecules per isolated vesicle (70,000; Whittaker, Essman and Dowe, 1972*b*) is equal to that required to produce the observed miniature potentials.

B. Isolation of the Cholinergic Receptor

Besides serving as a source of cholinergic synaptic vesicles, the electric organ is also rich in cholinergic receptors. Following the discovery that certain snake venoms are powerful postsynaptic cholinergic-blocking agents (e.g., Lee, 1970), several groups have used purified neurotoxins derived from these venoms as biochemical labels in attempts to isolate receptors (Changeux, 1972; Miledi, Molinoff, and Potter, 1971; Schmidt and Raftery, 1972). One of the most recent studies is that of Heilbronn, Karlsson, and Widlund (1972). The tissue is extracted with a phosphate buffer containing 1% Triton X-100, as described by Miledi et al. (1971), and the supernatant obtained after centrifugation is passed through a column of ECD-Sepharose 4B to which a purified neurotoxin derived from the venom of *Naja naja siamensis* has been conjugated. The Sepharose is washed with 1 M NaCl in phosphate buffer, pH 7.5, followed by carbachol in phosphate buffer containing 0.1% Triton X-100.

A small proportion of the protein (~ 2%) present in the original extract is bound by the gel. Only traces of acetylcholinesterase are bound and these are removed by elution with 1 M NaCl. Elution with carbachol, whose pharmacological activity resembles that of acetylcholine, removes two protein fractions that have strong affinities both for the reversible cholinergic blocking agent D-tubocurarine and for the neurotoxin, as measured by equilibrium dialysis or gel filtration experiments. The final product (representing 0.14% of the original protein) is about 25 times more effective in this respect per milligram protein than the original extract. The apparent molecular weight of these purified proteins is 400,000 to 450,000, and they contain considerable amounts of acidic and hydroxy amino acid residues but rather small amounts of basic residues.

In further experiments using higher ionic strengths during the original elution of the organ and 1% Triton X-100 when eluting the column, material with an apparent molecular weight of about 140,000 and having one or two neurotoxin-binding sites was eluted (Karlsson, Heilbronn, and Widlund, 1972). The main part of the receptor protein (~ 0.3% of total protein) was, however, eluted from the column only in an acidic carbachol medium (Heilbronn and Mattson, *unpublished*), and this protein binds approximately 35 times as much tubocurarine as the original extract.

C. Isolation of Synaptic Vesicles

Synaptic vesicles were first prepared from electric tissue by Sheridan, Whittaker, and Israël (1966), and the method used was subsequently improved by Israël, Gautron, and Lesbats (1970), using low-viscosity sucrose-NaCl gradients isoosmotic with elasmobranch plasma. The tissue is difficult to homogenize with conventional techniques, and in our latest procedure (Whittaker et al., 1972*b*) it is comminuted by pounding after rendering it brittle by freezing it in liquid Freon 12 or liquid nitrogen. Electron microscopic examination of the fragments demonstrated that tissue organization

[handwritten margin note: Comminute ↓ shattered, crunched up...]

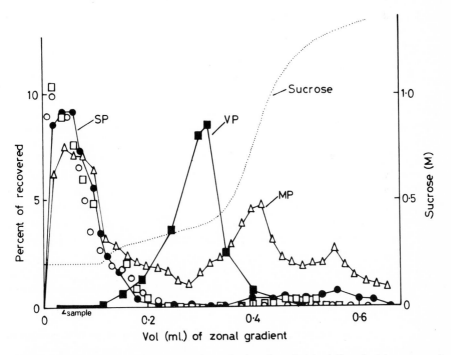

FIG. 1. Distribution of components of a cytoplasmic extract of the electric organ of *Torpedo* after separation on a sucrose-NaCl density gradient in a Ti-14 zonal rotor at 48,000 rpm for 3 hr. Key: ●, protein; ○, lactate dehydrogenase; □, choline acetyltransferase; ■, bound acetylcholine; △, acetylcholinesterase; SP, soluble protein peak; VP, synaptic vesicle peak; MP, membrane peak (from Whittaker, Dowdall, and Boyne, 1972*a*).

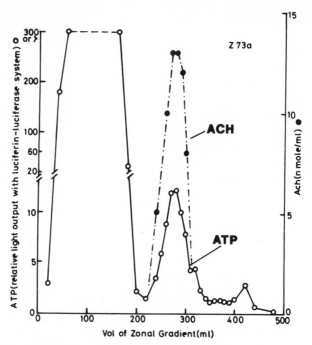

FIG. 2. Distribution of ATP in the gradient. Note the presence of large amounts in the SP peak and smaller amounts in the VP peak. Abbreviation: ACh, acetylcholine (from Whittaker, Dowdall, and Boyne, 1972a).

is well preserved at the ultrastructural level but that the external membranes of the presynaptic nerve terminals are extensively damaged, thus exposing the terminal cytoplasm. Extraction of the tissue fragments with ice-cold 0.2 M sucrose in 0.3 M NaCl followed by centrifugation to remove coarse particles yields a preparation of synaptic vesicles suspended in cytoplasmic protein having only a small amount of contamination by larger membrane fragments.

This cytoplasmic extract is then fractionated by sucrose density gradient centrifugation using a zonal rotor (Fig. 1). Soluble cytoplasmic proteins, including cytoplasmic enzymes such as lactate dehydrogenase and choline acetyltransferase, form a peak (SP) which occupies the volume originally taken up by the sample, with little diffusion into the gradient. Synaptic vesicles are recovered as a sharp peak (VP) with an equilibrium density equivalent to 0.38 M sucrose–0.21 M NaCl. This peak has a very high acetylcholine content (600 to 1,300 nmoles of acetylcholine/mg of protein) and we have recently shown (Fig. 2) that it is also rich in ATP (Whittaker, Dowdall, and Boyne, 1972a). Both the acetylcholine and the ATP of this fraction are immune to the action of hydrolytic enzymes (i.e., in a "bound"

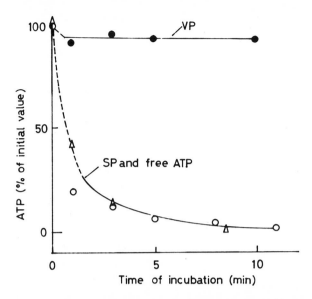

FIG. 3. Hydrolysis of ATP by an apyrase-myokinase-adenylate deaminase mixture. The material present (Fig. 2) in SP (○) is rapidly hydrolyzed at the same rate as an equivalent amount of free ATP (△); vesicular ATP (●) is resistant to hydrolysis (from Whittaker, Dowdall, and Boyne, 1972a).

state; Fig. 3) unless first released by any one of a variety of disruptive treatments (Fig. 4): treatment with detergents (including lysolecithin), phospholipase A_2 (Heilbronn, Boyne, and Edwards, 1972), osmotic shock, freezing and thawing, or storage for a few hours or days. The acetylcholine tends to be released more readily than the ATP. The molar ratio of acetylcholine to ATP varies from one experiment to another, but is usually approximately two to four.

The vesicular (VP) peak is followed by a peak of larger membrane fragments (MP, Fig. 1) having a density equivalent to that of 0.8 M sucrose or more. Many of these fragments appear to be derived from pinched-off infoldings of postsynaptic membranes which are rich in acetylcholinesterase. This peak often contains a few synaptosome-like structures, which probably accounts for the small amounts of bound acetylcholine and ATP usually found in this region of the gradient; unlike brain tissue, synaptosomes are not formed in large numbers when the electric organ is comminuted.

II. PROTEIN CONSTITUENTS OF VESICLES

As shown in Fig. 4d, the synaptic vesicles are osmotically sensitive, and can easily be disrupted by dialysing the VP fraction against distilled water. Subsequent freeze-drying produces a fraction called the FDVP fraction,

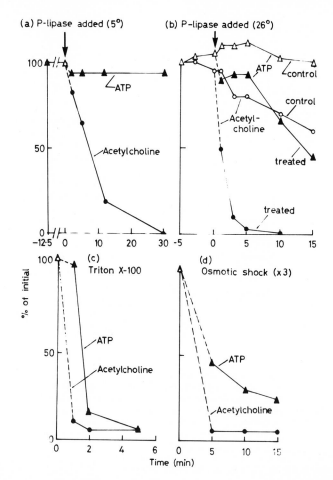

FIG. 4. Release of acetylcholine (○,●) and ATP (△,▲) from synaptic vesicles as a result of cobra venom phospholipase A$_2$ action at *(a)* 5°C and *(b)* 26°C, or treatment by *(c)* detergent or *(d)* osmotic shock (dilution 1:2 with water). Control measurements are represented by open symbols. Note that in each case, acetylcholine is liberated faster than ATP. In *(a)* very little morphological disruption occurred, whereas in *(b)* vesicle membranes had been very largely broken up.

and releases a low-molecular weight soluble protein, vesiculin. Figure 5 shows the result of submitting fraction FDVP to gel filtration on Sephadex G-200. The void volume peak (1) contains protein and phospholipids and consists mainly of the vesicle membrane. Disc gel electrophoresis of this material (Fig. 5, insert *a*) reveals three main protein components. The second main protein peak (2) contains vesiculin, a single component with

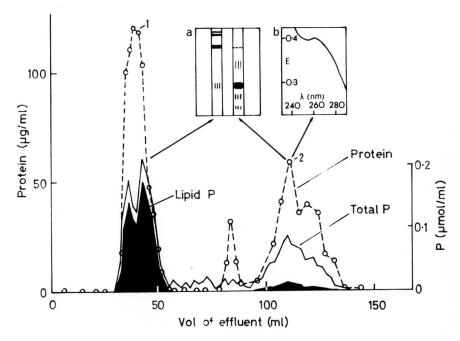

FIG. 5. Separation of membrane-bound and soluble protein from dialyzed and freeze-dried vesicle preparation. Key: (○) protein; continuous line, phosphorus; black profiles, proportion of total P in each peak that was chloroform-methanol soluble. Inserts: *(a)* disc gel electrophoresis in sodium dodecylsulfate of peaks 1 and 2; *(b)* ultraviolet absorption of peak 2. The small intermediate peak of protein is soluble protein that had diffused from SP.

a molecular weight of approximately 10,000 as shown by disc gel electrophoresis (Fig. 5, insert *a*) and by calibration of the Sephadex gel column with proteins of known molecular weight in the usual way.

The vesiculin peak contains nonlipid phosphorus, which probably represents nucleotide phosphorus, since the ultraviolet spectrum of vesiculin prepared in this way has a prominent peak or shoulder at 260 to 265 nm (Fig. 5, insert *b*). We believe that this nucleotide is a mixture of AMP and IMP, formed by the breakdown of vesicular ATP during dialysis, freeze-drying, and subsequent chromatography. This nucleotide can be largely removed by gel filtration through Sephadex G-50, whereupon vesiculin appears to dimerize. In control runs on Sephadex G-200 and similar materials with intact vesicles, all the vesicle protein and lipid and the associated acetylcholine and ATP pass through in the void volume.

Vesiculin behaves as an acidic protein with an isoelectric point at ap-

IMP - *inosine monophosphate*

TABLE 1. *Amino acid content of hydrolysates of vesiculin*

	Amino acid content		
Amino acid	mole %	moles/mole of Tyr	Assumed no. of vesicles/mole
Alanine	9.3 ± 0.24	7.7	8
Arginine	2.4 ± 0.40	2.0	2
Aspartic acid	8.9 ± 0.54	1.4	7
Glutamic acid	18.8 ± 0.54	15.7	16
Glycine	13.3 ± 1.50	11.1	11
Histidine	2.0 ± 0.17	1.7	2
Isoleucine	2.5 ± 0.02	2.1	2
Leucine	4.5 ± 0.55	3.7	4
Lysine	3.4 ± 0.66	2.8	3
Ornithine	2.8 ± 0.67	2.3	2
Phenylalanine	2.0 ± 0.32	1.7	2
Proline	4.8 ± 0.50	4.0	4
Serine	13.7 ± 1.69	11.4	11
Threonine	5.2 ± 0.39	4.3	4
Tyrosine (Tyr)	1.2 ± 0.20	1.0	1
Valine	4.1 ± 0.49	3.4	3
		Molecular weight (1 Tyr/molecule)	9,891

Samples containing approximately 200 μg of Lowry-positive protein were hydrolyzed for 17 to 24 hr in 6 M HCl in an atmosphere of N_2. Values are means ± SEM of three determinations. The component here listed as ornithine was cochromatographed with authentic ornithine (from Whittaker, Dowdall, and Boyne, 1972a).

proximately pH 3.5. Analysis of hydrolysates in 6 M HCl (Table 1) showed it to be rich in acidic and hydroxy amino acid residues. The function of vesiculin is not known, but it may well serve as a polyanion to neutralize the charge on the vesicular acetylcholine cations. The protein moiety of vesiculin may be conjugated with ATP *in vivo*, which would serve to increase the negative charge on the macromolecule.

III. CHANGES IN VESICLE MORPHOLOGY AND COMPOSITION AS A RESULT OF STIMULATION

A. Physiological Effects of Stimulation

The identification of ATP and vesiculin as vesicular components in addition to acetylcholine prompts the questions: "Is acetylcholine alone released on stimulation or are the other vesicular components released also?" and "Can vesicles depleted in acetylcholine be isolated from stimulated organs?" Dr. H. Zimmermann and I have recently been trying to answer these questions.

Anesthetized electric organs were stimulated by placing a stimulating electrode on the lobe in the brainstem containing the cells of origin of the cholinergic innervation; stimuli were usually either single square-wave shocks with a strength of 10 V and a duration of 1.5 msec or trains of such shocks with a frequency of 5/sec. The nerves to one organ were sectioned before stimulation in order to provide an unstimulated control. The response of the organ was recorded by electrodes placed on the dorsal and ventral skin above and below the organ. Repetitive stimulation was usually inter-

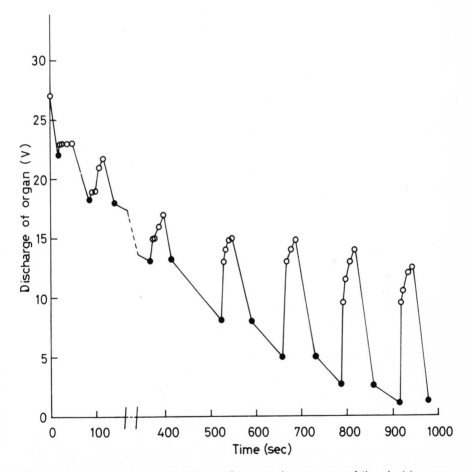

FIG. 6. Effect of repetitive stimulation at 5 sec on the response of the electric organ (●). Note the recovery of the response during rest periods in which recovery was tested by single shocks (○) at 5, 10, 20, and 30 sec. Stimuli were square-wave pulses of amplitude 10 V and duration 1.2 msec.

rupted at intervals and the ability of the summed postsynaptic potentials to recover tested by means of single shocks (Fig. 6). The effect of long continued repetitive stimulation is to reduce the postsynaptic response to negligible proportions (<1 V); however, even when "exhausted," the organ has considerable powers of recuperation. The response of the organ recovers to approximately 50% of its initial value within 30 sec (Table 2). The postsynaptic potential again declines upon resumption of repetitive stimulation after a 30-sec rest period; this is a slow process initially, but it declines rapidly after stimulation to exhaustion. Complete recovery is a slow process and takes many hours.

TABLE 2. *Effects of stimulation on the electric organ*

Parameter	Stimulated tissue (as % of unstimulated)
Whole tissue	
Organ response[a] (V) after reduction	
of response to 1 V and 30-sec recovery	35 ± 8 (3)
No. of vesicle profiles/μm^2	49 ± 7 (2)
Fraction VP[b]	
Membrane protein[c]	45 ± 3 (2)
Vesiculin[c]	94 ± 14 (2)
ATP[d]	16 ± 3 (4)
Acetylcholine[d]	12 ± 3 (4)

[a] Expressed as % of initial value.

[b] Isolated from tissue excised while stimulus was continued.

[c] Isolated on Sephadex G-200 after freeing fraction VP from traces of soluble protein by filtration through porous glass beads.

[d] Peak VP tubes.

Measurements relate to observations made with intact tissue or on fraction VP isolated at the end of the experiment. Values are means ± range (2) or SEM (more than two experiments; No. of experiments in parentheses) and are for tissue stimulated repetitively to exhaustion expressed (unless otherwise stated) as a percentage of the corresponding value for the unstimulated, denervated organ.

B. Morphological Observations

Very clear morphological changes occur as the result of stimulation: the terminal cytoplasm is depleted of vesicles and the mean diameter of the vesicles falls. Depletion is observed after as little as 600 stimuli and reaches a limiting value of approximately 50% (Table 2, Fig. 7) on prolonged

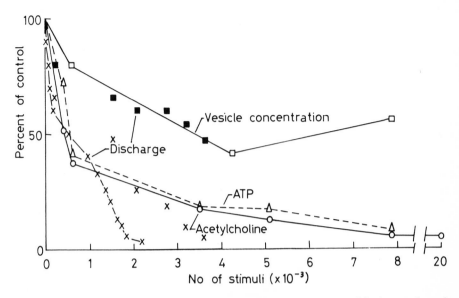

FIG. 7. Effect of stimulation on the electrical response of the organ (x), the number of vesicles/μm^2 ($\square$), and the composition of fraction VP ($\bigcirc$,$\triangle$). Values are expressed as a percentage of controls. The black squares show the ability of organ response to recover in a separate experiment in which organ response to repetitive stimulation is indicated by x's unconnected by lines.

stimulation, and mean vesicle size diminishes simultaneously (Fig. 8). The distribution of vesicle diameters is bimodal; stimulation has the effect of increasing the proportion of the population of small diameter vesicles while concomitantly reducing total vesicle number.

In addition to reducing the number and size of vesicles, prolonged stimulation also alters the appearance of the terminals. More, smaller terminals are seen in sections, and there is a marked increase in infoldings and blebs, suggesting an increase in the area of the external presynaptic membrane. The morphological changes resemble those seen by Korneliusson (1972) in muscle, but are apparently produced much more readily.

C. Biochemical and Morphological Changes in Isolated Vesicles

The VP fraction was prepared from stimulated and unstimulated tissue in two successive zonal runs by our standard method, and membrane protein and vesiculin were separated and measured as in Fig. 5. Results are given in Table 2 and Fig. 8.

Vesicle membrane protein declined on stimulation *pari passu* with

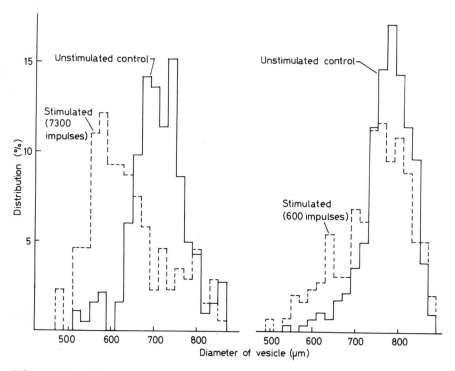

FIG. 8. Effect of stimulation on vesicle size. The abscissas are measurements of electron micrographs at 18,500 magnification uncorrected for fixation and instrumentation errors.

vesicle counts in whole tissue sections. However, vesiculin did not decline, possibly because it was more easily extractable from vesicles of stimulated organs. Both ATP and acetylcholine declined to low levels; thus, the conclusion could be drawn that the vesicles that remained after stimulation were, on the average, less effective at retaining ATP and acetylcholine than vesicles in unstimulated tissue. This was partly, but by no means entirely, accounted for by a decrease in vesicle size, since the observed 20% reduction in vesicle diameter would correspond to a 60% reduction in the volume of the surviving vesicle population or an 80% reduction in total vesicle volume compared with unstimulated tissue, whereas the reduction in vesicular ATP and acetylcholine concentrations was up to 95%. Some depletion of ATP and acetylcholine (Fig. 7) and some change in vesicle morphology (Fig. 8) were observed after only 600 stimuli, showing that synaptic vesicles are involved even during short periods of synaptic activity.

D. Conclusions

Our results were obtained with electric organs *in situ* and not on excised pieces as studied by Dunant, Gautron, Israël, Lesbats, and Manaranche (1972), and they differ in some respects from those of the Paris group. Interpretation is complicated by our ignorance of the extent to which the reduced response of the organ on repetitive stimulation is due to a failure in transmitter release or to a failure of the postsynaptic membrane to respond to transmitter release. Furthermore, comparisons of the composition of vesicle fractions isolated from stimulated and unstimulated organs depend on the assumption that the yield of vesicles from both is identical. Evidence that the efficiency of extraction is not affected by stimulation is provided by the constancy of composition of the cytoplasmic extract and of fraction SP with respect to soluble protein and soluble cytoplasmic enzymes.

Our results certainly suggest that prolonged stimulation of the cholinergic synapses of electric tissue promotes the release of the small molecular constituents of synaptic vesicles (ATP and acetylcholine), loss of vesicles, perhaps by fusion with external membranes, and reduction in size of the surviving population. Total exocytosis of vesicles apparently did not occur, since vesiculin did not decline *pari passu* with ATP and acetylcholine nor with vesicle numbers or vesicle membrane protein. The reason for this is not understood, but it may be that vesiculin is normally in an aggregated or lipid-bound form in the vesicle core and is more readily extractable by dialysis and freeze-drying from vesicles from stimulated endings than from those from nonstimulated endings. Since excision of the organ for the purpose of fractionation probably itself involves stimulation, we are inclined to think that the very low vesicular ATP and acetylcholine in tissue stimulated to exhaustion corresponds to the state of exhaustion observed electrophysiologically during prolonged repetitive stimulation and not to the partially recovered state observed after a 30-sec rest, but that the number of vesicles found in the tissue at this time is an index of its ability to recover. If this is so, then vesicles are clearly capable of being reutilized, perhaps through a limited number of cycles, before being discarded or losing their identity.

The role of ATP in the vesicle remains obscure. Is its only function to provide negative charges to neutralize the acetylcholine ion? Or is it an auxiliary transmitter, a trophic factor, or an energy source concerned with transmitter uptake, vesicle translocation, or fusion?

ACKNOWLEDGMENTS

The original work on synaptic vesicles described in this chapter was carried out by A. F. Boyne, M. J. Dowdall, W. Edwards, E. Heilbronn, S. J. Morris, V. P. Whittaker, and H. Zimmermann with funds provided by the U.K. Medical and Science Research Councils, the Leverhulme trust, and the Deutsche Forschungsgemeinschaft. P. Bystricky, C. Denston, G. H. C. Dowe, F. Henderson, G. Rowe, and B. Thurley rendered valuable technical assistance. We are most grateful to Professor C. Cazaux for arranging the supply of *Torpedos*.

REFERENCES

Bloom, F. E., Iversen, L. L., and Schmitt, F. O. (1970): Macromolecules in synaptic function. *Neurosciences Research Bulletin,* 8.

Changeux, J-P. (1972): Études sur le mécanism moléculaire de la réponse d'une membrane excitable aux agents cholinergiques. In: *Le Système Cholinergique en Anesthésiologie et Réanimation,* edited by G.-G. Nahas, J.-C. Salamagne, P. Viars, and G. Vourc'h, pp. 99–112. Librairie Arnette, Paris.

Dunant, Y., Gautron, J., Israël, M., Lesbats, B., and Manaranche, R. (1972): Les compartiments d'acétylcholine de l'organe électrique de la torpille et leur modification par la stimulation. Acetylcholine compartments in stimulated electric organ of *Torpedo marmorata. Journal of Neurochemistry,* 19:1987.

Heilbronn, E., Boyne, A. F., and Edwards, W. (1973): The effect of phospholipase A_2 on isolated cholinergic synaptic vesicles. *To be published.*

Heilbronn, E., Karlsson, E., and Widlund, L. (1972): Purification of constituents of the synaptic membranes by affinity chromatography. *Proceedings Symposium Internationale de l'INSERM,* Paris, *in press.*

Israël, M., Gautron, J., and Lesbats, B. (1970): Fractionnement de l'organe électrique de la torpille: Localisation subcellulaire de l'acétylcholine. Subcellular fractionation of the electric organ of *Torpedo marmorata. Journal of Neurochemistry,* 17:1441.

Karlsson, E., Heilbronn, E., and Widlund, L. (1972): Isolation of the nicotinic acetylcholine receptor by biospecific chromatography on insolubilized *Naja Naja* neurotoxin. *Federation of European Biochemical Societies. Letters,* 28:107.

Korneliusson, H. (1972): Ultrastructure of normal and stimulated motor end plates. *Zeitschrift für Zellforschung und Mikroskopische Anatomie,* 130:28.

Lee, C. Y. (1970): Elapid neurotoxins and their mode of action. *Clinical Toxicology,* 3:457.

Miledi, R., Molinoff, P., and Potter, L. T. (1971): Isolation of the cholinergic receptor protein of *Torpedo* electric tissue. *Nature,* 229:554.

Schmidt, J., and Raftery, M. A. (1972): Use of affinity chromatography for acetylcholine receptor purification. *Biochemical and Biophysical Research Communications,* 49:572.

Sheridan, M. N., Whittaker, V. P., and Israël, M. (1966): The subcellular fractionation of the electric organ of *Torpedo. Zeitschrift für Zellforschung und Mikroskopische Anatomie,* 74:291.

Whittaker, V. P., Dowdall, M. J., and Boyne, A. F. (1972a): The storage and release of acetylcholine by cholinergic nerve terminals: recent results with non-mammalian preparations. *Biochemical Society Symposia,* 36:49.

Whittaker, V. P., Essman, W. B., and Dowe, G. H. C. (1972b): The isolation of pure cholinergic synaptic vesicles from the electric organs of elasmobranch fish of the family *Torpedinidae*. *Biochemical Journal*, 128:833.

Whittaker, V. P., Michaelson, I. A., and Kirkland, R. J. A. (1964): The separation of synaptic vesicles from nerve-ending particles ("synaptosomes"). *Biochemical Journal*, 90:293.

Whittaker, V. P., and Sheridan, M. N. (1965): The morphology and acetylcholine content of isolated cerebral cortical synaptic vesicles. *Journal of Neurochemistry*, 12:363.

Proteins of the Nervous System
Raven Press, New York © 1973

The Proteins of Nerve-Ending Membranes

Ian G. Morgan, W. C. Breckenridge, G. Vincendon, and G. Gombos

I. INTRODUCTION

Synaptosomes consist of three major membrane systems: synaptic vesicles, the synaptosomal plasma membrane, and synaptic mitochondria. In addition, they contain more complex, but quantitatively minor, constituents such as coated vesicles and vacuoles. Although these minor constituents may be of great functional importance, it is clear that with present techniques the major problem is the characterization of synaptic vesicles and the synaptosomal plasma membrane.

II. ISOLATION AND CHARACTERIZATION OF FRACTIONS

A. Isolation of Synaptosomes

Synaptosomes were first prepared by fractionation of brain mitochondrial fractions on discontinuous sucrose density gradients (De Robertis, Pellegrino de Iraldi, Rodriguez de Lores Arnaiz, and Salganicoff, 1962; Gray and Whittaker, 1962). This approach has since been progressively modified and improved, primarily by the introduction of continuous sucrose gradients, which appear to give the purest synaptosomes (Whittaker, 1968). However, it is difficult to adapt the fine continuous gradient fractionations to the large-scale preparations needed for compositional studies.

As methodology has improved, it has become clear that synaptosomal fractions are only enriched in synaptosomes, but are by no means pure. These fractions are contaminated with glial fragments and axonal processes (Lemkey-Johnston and Larramendi, 1968), which can be quantitatively important components (Lemkey-Johnston and Dekirmenjian, 1970). In addition, they can be contaminated with varying amounts of myelin, mitochondria, and microsomes.

Partially successful attempts to eliminate contaminants have been made by replacing the initial sucrose gradients with isotonic Ficoll-sucrose

171

(Tanaka and Abood, 1963; Kurokawa, Sakamoto, and Kato, 1965; Abdel-Latif, 1966; Autilio, Appel, Pettis, and Gambetti, 1968) or cesium chloride (Kornguth, Anderson, and Scott, 1969; Kornguth, Flangas, Siegel, Geison, O'Brien, Lamar, and Scott, 1971; Kornguth, Flangas, Perrin, Geison, and Scott, 1972). Cesium chloride gradients appear to eliminate the ribosome-containing particles which have interfered with studies of synaptosomal protein synthesis (Levitan, Mushynski, and Ramirez, 1972; Ramirez, Levitan, and Mushynski, 1972), but in other respects the cesium chloride fractions seem to be less satisfactory.

Isotonic Ficoll-sucrose gradients do not completely eliminate contamination, but they do resolve the glial fragments which cosediment with synaptosomes on sucrose gradients (Cotman, Herschman and Taylor, 1971a). In general, synaptosomes prepared on Ficoll-sucrose gradients are less contaminated with membrane fragments (Morgan, Wolfe, Mandel, and Gombos, 1971), which suggests that this separation is not due to any specific density properties of glial membranes. Rather, in gradients which are not spun to equilibrium, membrane fragments may simply sediment less in the viscous Ficoll-sucrose solutions. Other advantages of Ficoll-sucrose gradients include better preservation of morphology and greater susceptibility of the synaptosomes to osmotic shock.

Despite these advantages of Ficoll-sucrose gradients, the choice of a gradient depends upon the aim of the experiment. Synaptosomes can be prepared relatively free of mitochondrial or membrane contamination by taking fractions of lower or higher density, but there is correspondingly greater contamination with membranes or mitochondria, respectively. For the preparation of synaptic vesicles and the synaptosomal plasma membrane, we have taken relatively high-density fractions from Ficoll-sucrose gradients to minimize contamination with membrane fragments.

B. Isolation of synaptosomal plasma membranes

The details of the isolation of synaptosomal plasma membranes are shown in Fig. 1. The crude mitochondrial fractions were prepared at moderate centrifugal forces (Cotman, Brown, Harrell, and Anderson, 1970) and then extensively washed (Morgan et al., 1971), in order to limit contamination with microsomal elements. Crude membrane fractions were prepared on sucrose density gradients after isolation of synaptosomes and osmotic shock (Whittaker, Michaelson, and Kirkland, 1964). All material whose sedimentation properties had not been changed by the osmotic shock was then eliminated from the crude fractions by centrifugation under approximately the same conditions used to prepare the crude mitochondrial

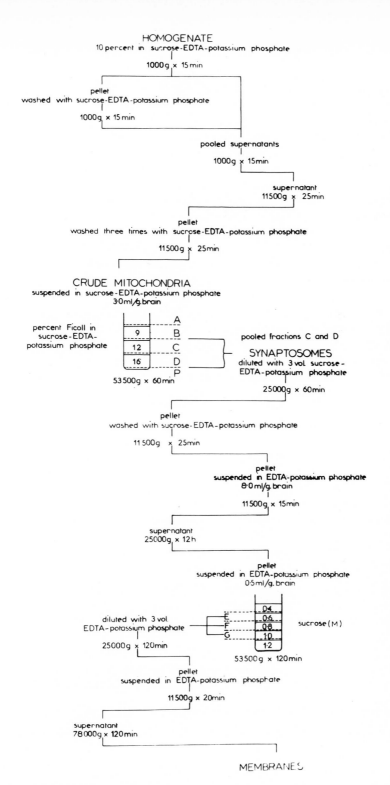

FIG. 1. The preparation of synaptosomes and synaptosomal membranes from rat brain (Morgan, Wolfe, Mandel, and Gombos, 1971).

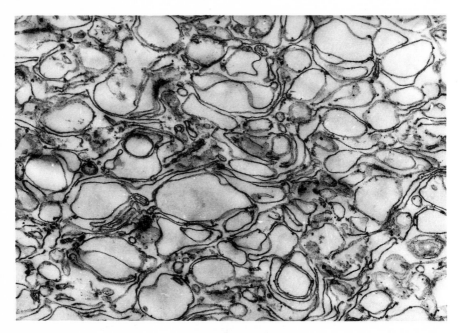

FIG. 2. Electron micrograph of synaptosomal plasma membranes from rat brain, prepared by the method described in Fig. 1. Relatively little synaptic junctional material is observed in this preparation or in the initial synaptosomal fraction (Morgan, Wolfe, Mandel, and Gombos, 1971).

fraction; otherwise, the fractions were heavily contaminated with myelin (Morgan et al., 1971; Morgan, Reith, Marinari, Breckenridge, and Gombos, 1972). Such purification may not always be necessary, since there should theoretically be little myelin contamination (Doyle and Cotman, 1972), but in practice the Ficoll-sucrose gradients are grossly overloaded and un- stable (Garey, Harper, Best, and Goodman, 1972). The use of high-capacity zonal rotors may render this step unnecessary.

The final preparations consist primarily of large membranous sacs of synaptosomal dimensions (Fig. 2). There was no microscopic evidence of mitochondrial, lysosomal, or myelin contamination. It should be noted that synaptic junctions were only rarely seen, even at the synaptosome stage.

C. Demonstration of Plasma Membrane Origin

Two contaminants were detected by following a series of negative enzymatic and chemical markers (Table 1). Several markers of the endo-

TABLE 1. *Contamination of synaptosomal plasma membranes*

Contaminant	Marker	% Contamination
Soluble proteins	Lactate dehydrogenase	<1
Lysosomes	β-Galactosidase β-Glucosidase	<1
Rough endoplasmic reticulum	RNA	<1
Smooth endoplasmic reticulum	NADPH: Cytochrome c reductase PAPS: Cerebroside sulfotransferase UDP-glucose: Ceramide glucosyl transferase CDP-choline: Diglyceride phosphocholine transferase	<5
Golgi apparatus	UDP-galactose: N-Acetylglucosamine Galactosyl transferase	<5
Inner mitochondrial membrane	Succinate dehydrogenase Cytochrome c oxidase	<1
Outer mitochondrial membrane	Monoamine oxidase NADH: Cytochrome c reductase	<5
Myelin	Cerebrosides and sulfatides Myelin-specific proteins	<1

plasmic reticulum set a limit of 5% to the contamination from this source, and a similar amount of contamination with external mitochondrial membranes was detected from the monoamine oxidase activity. The membranes were free of contamination with soluble proteins, myelin, inner mitochondrial membranes, and lysosomes.

It must be stressed that most of the markers used are not well established in brain, but are assumed by analogy with liver, an analogy which is not always valid. It is also difficult to evaluate the significance of low activities. For example, assuming that all the galactosyl transferase activity detected in the membrane fractions is due to Golgi apparatus contamination, the preparations need only be 5% contaminated to account for the activity detected. However, it has been suggested that synaptosomes and the synaptosomal plasma membrane have intrinsic glycosyl transferases (Den, Kaufman, and Roseman, 1970; Broquet and Louisot, 1971; Festoff, Appel, and Day, 1971; Bosmann, 1972), and there is no way at the present time to distinguish between the two possibilities. In the case of the monoamine oxidase activity, it has been possible to show that the observed kinetic properties are identical to those of the mitochondrial enzyme, thus strongly suggesting that the enzyme is due to contamination.

Taken together, these data suggest that the membranes are 85 to 90% pure as plasma membrane, with limited contamination from the endoplasmic reticulum, Golgi apparatus, and external mitochondrial membranes.

D. Demonstration of Neuronal Origin

One approach to determining the contamination with glial material depends upon the content of soluble glial markers detected in the synaptosomal fractions. There was a marked decrease in the levels of butyryl cholinesterase and the S-100 protein fraction in synaptosomes compared to total brain (Table 2). There was a corresponding enrichment of a soluble neuronal marker (glutamate decarboxylase). From these data it was possible to calculate a glial contamination of 10 to 20% *at the synaptosome stage.*

TABLE 2. *Contamination of synaptosomal fractions with soluble glial and neuronal markers*

Marker	Specific activity ratio
Butyryl cholinesterase	0.13
S-100 protein fraction	0.22
Glutamate decarboxylase	1.50

However, it is obviously more satisfactory to estimate glial contamination at the membrane stage, since the soluble contamination is not necessarily representative of the real membrane contamination. Although no myelin was detected (Fig. 2, Table 1), 2',3'-cyclic AMP 3'-phosphohydrolase activity was detected in the membrane preparations. This enzyme was earlier believed to be a myelin marker (Kurihara and Tsukada, 1967, 1968), but has now been shown to be associated with glial cells as well (Pfeiffer and Wechsler, 1972; Poduslo and Norton, 1972; Zanetta, Benda, Gombos, and Morgan, 1972). From these data, it would appear that the glial contamination is approximately 5%.

Another parameter which can be used to estimate glial contamination is the presence of long-chain fatty acids in the membrane sphingomyelins (Table 3). The synaptosomal plasma membrane sphingomyelins are almost devoid of long-chain fatty acids (Kishimoto, Agranoff, Radin, and Burton, 1969; Breckenridge, Gombos, and Morgan, 1972*b,c*), in contrast to the

TABLE 3. *Long-chain fatty acids of membrane sphingomyelin*

Source	Percent of sphingomyelin fatty acid	
	24:0	24:1
Neuronal plasma membrane	1.3	0.9
Myelin[1]	8.0	40.0
Oligodendrocytes[2]	11.6	23.1
Astrocytes[3]	1.3	2.8
Astrocytes[4]	9.2	13.8

[1] O'Brien and Sampson, 1965.
[2] Fewster and Mead, 1968.
[3] Pomazanskaya et al., 1969.
[4] Clone C6 astrocytes.

sphingomyelins of myelin (O'Brien and Sampson, 1965) and oligodendrocytes (Fewster and Mead, 1968). Our data indicate that C6 clone astrocytes in tissue culture contain a significant quantity of 24:0 and 24:1 in their sphingomyelins *(unpublished results),* but other data on rat brain astrocyte sphingomyelins are in conflict with these observations (Pomanzanskaya, Freysz, and Mandel, 1969). It may be significant that most nonneural sphingomyelins are rich in long-chain fatty acids (Svennerholm, Ställberg-Stenhagen, and Svennerholm, 1966). On the assumption that the long-chain fatty acids detected are due to contamination, the contamination on a sphingomyelin basis is less than 10%. Since the synaptosomal plasma membrane is poorer in sphingomyelin than most plasma membranes (Cotman, Blank, Moehl, and Snyder, 1969; Breckenridge et al., 1972b,c), the contamination on a protein basis is probably less than 5%.

These three independent estimates set the glial contamination at less than 20%, with the most likely figure being less than 10%. However, it should be noted that these tests may all be more reliable for oligodendrocytes than for astrocytes. Attempts are now being made to estimate astrocyte contamination from the noradrenaline-stimulated adenyl cyclase activity (Clark and Perkins, 1971; Gilman and Nirenberg, 1971a,b).

Calculating from physiological data (Harvey and McIlwain, 1969), a specific marker of the neuronal plasma membrane should be 10- to 15-fold enriched in a pure preparation (Morgan et al., 1971). Unfortunately, absolutely specific markers are not known, but gangliosides (Lowden and Wolfe, 1964; Spence and Wolfe, 1967; Derry and Wolfe, 1968) and [Na + K]-ATPase (Bonting, Caravaggio, and Hawkins, 1962; Cotman, Herschman, and Taylor, 1971a) may be sufficiently concentrated in the neuronal plasma membrane to serve as satisfactory markers. They are enriched 10- to

12-fold in the membrane preparations (Table 4), confirming the predominantly neuronal (or synaptosomal) origin of the plasma membranes. There is a corresponding enrichment of neuraminidase in the membranes (Tettamanti, Morgan, Gombos, Vincendon, and Mandel, 1972), which may be of some importance for glycolipid and glycoprotein metabolism.

TABLE 4. *Enrichments of putative plasma membrane markers in synaptic vesicles and synaptosomal plasma membranes*

Marker	Synaptic vesicles	Synaptosomal plasma membranes
[Na + K]-ATPase	0.50	11.6
Ganglioside sialic acid	0.53	11.1
Neuraminidase	0.32	10.0
K-Stimulated, ouabain-inhibited	0.39	9.8
p-Nitrophenyl phosphatase	0.48	10.8
Thiamine pyrophosphatase	0.43	6.8
5'-Nucleotidase	0.31	1.2
Alkaline phosphatase	1.62	2.3
Acetylcholinesterase	0.05	0.85

Thiamine diphosphatase is also concentrated in the membranes (Reith, Morgan, Gombos, Breckenridge, and Vincendon, 1972), although this enzyme is often regarded as a Golgi apparatus marker (Novikoff and Goldfischer, 1961). In the nervous system, thiamine diphosphatase activity is found histochemically both in the Golgi apparatus and on plasma membranes (Lane, 1968; Tanaka, Barrnett and Cooper, *unpublished results*). This activity may be only one manifestation of a general nucleoside diphosphatase activity (Barchi and Braun, 1972), and, in fact, UDPase activity is also concentrated in synaptosomal plasma membranes (Cotman, *personal communication*). This may indicate that the build-up of thiamine diphosphatase in constricted axons (Pellegrino de Iraldi and Rodriguez de Lores Arnaiz, 1970) reflects the flow of plasma membrane precursors rather than Golgi apparatus, in accord with the flow of other plasma membrane components, such as adenyl cyclase (Bray, Kon, and Breckenridge, 1971) and glycoproteins (Elam, Goldberg, Radin, and Agranoff, 1970; Bondy, 1971; Forman, McEwen, and Grafstein, 1971; Karlsson and Sjöstrand, 1971).

Two common plasma membrane markers (5'-nucleotidase and alkaline phosphatase) were not enriched in the preparations. Nor was acetylcholinesterase, in contrast to the observations of many others. Histochemically, acetylcholinesterase is neither exclusively nor even predominantly located in the synaptosomal plasma membrane (Kokko, Mautner, and Barrnett,

1969), and the low levels of acetylcholinesterase in our membranes could simply reflect lower microsomal contamination of our fractions. However, McBride and Cohen (1972) have shown that acetylcholine is overwhelmingly concentrated in the postsynaptic membrane. Since we see very little postsynaptic membrane (Fig. 2), possibly because postsynaptic material detaches in Ficoll-sucrose (Garey et al., 1972), it is possible that the low acetylcholinesterase activity is due to the predominantly presynaptic nature of the membranes.

Overall, the preparations are 85 to 90% plasma membrane, of which less than 10% seems to be of glial origin. The membranes are primarily synaptosomal, rather than cell body, and seem to be overwhelmingly presynaptic. They are probably derived from the range of neuronal types found in the central nervous system, and are thus intrinsically heterogeneous. Similar preparations can probably be obtained using the method of Cotman and Matthews (1971).

E. Preparation of Synaptic Vesicles

The standard methods (De Robertis, Rodriguez de Lores Arnaiz, Salganicoff, Pellegrino de Iraldi, and Zieher, 1963; Whittaker et al., 1964; Lapetina, Soto, and De Robertis, 1967) give preparations which are highly enriched, but variably contaminated. Up to 30% of the fraction can be derived from the synaptosomal plasma membrane, myelin, and the endoplasmic reticulum. Most of the contamination can be eliminated by passing the crude vesicles through Millipore filters of pore size 4,500, 3,000, and 2,200 Å (Fig. 3).

Such preparations are almost free of contamination (Table 5). Only 5 to 10% of the protein could be accounted for by contamination with fragments of the synaptosomal plasma membrane, more than 90% of the preparation consisting of vesicles. The preparations consisted primarily of small round particles of approximately 500 Å diameter (Fig. 4), with a limited amount of membranous contamination.

The transmitter content of these vesicles is not known, but analogous preparations contain acetylcholine (De Robertis et al., 1963; Whittaker et al., 1964) and perhaps catecholamines (Michaelson, Whittaker, Laverty, and Sharman, 1963; Maynert, Levi, and De Lorenzo, 1964; De Robertis, Pellegrino de Iraldi, Rodriguez de Lores Arnaiz, and Zieher, 1965), but do not appear to concentrate the putative amino acid transmitters (Rassin, 1972). The yield of vesicles is 25 to 30% of the theoretical amount, and thus it is possible that only certain types of vesicles are isolated. However, it seems more likely that the vesicles are internally heterogeneous, being derived from a range of transmitter-containing neurons.

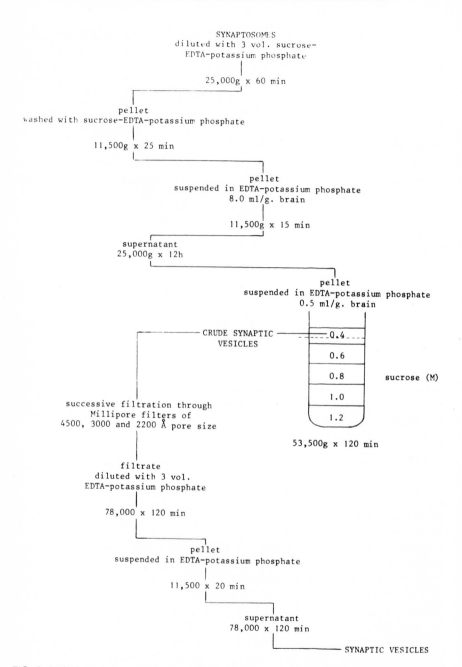

FIG. 3. Isolation of the synaptic vesicles from rat brain. Passage of the vesicle fraction from the sucrose gradient through Millipore filters reduced the level of contamination from 20 to 30% to 5% (Table 5).

TABLE 5. *Contamination of synaptic vesicles*

Contaminant	Marker	% Contamination
Soluble proteins	Lactate dehydrogenase	<1
Lysosomes	β-Galactosidase	
	β-Glucosidase	<1
Rough endoplasmic reticulum	RNA	<1
Smooth endoplasmic reticulum	NADPH: Cytochrome c reductase	
	PAPS: Cerebroside	
	sulfotransferase	
	UDP-glucose: Ceramide glucosyl	
	transferase	
	CDP-choline: Diglyceride	
	phosphocholine transferase	<1
Golgi apparatus	UDP-galactose:	
	N-acteylglucosamine	
	Galactosyl transferase	<1
Inner mitochondrial membrane	Succinate dehydrogenase	
	Cytochrome c oxidase	<1
Outer mitochondrial membrane	Monoamine oxidase	
	NADH: Cytochrome c reductase	<1
Myelin	Cerebrosides and sulfatides	
	Myelin-specific proteins	<1
Synaptosomal plasma membrane	[Na + K]-ATPase	
	Gangliosides	
	Neuraminidase	
	Acetylcholinesterase	<10

III. PROTEIN COMPOSITION OF THE FRACTIONS

Protein profiles of the two systems were examined by polyacrylamide gel electrophoresis in the presence of SDS. The synaptosomal plasma membrane (Fig. 5) showed 12 major bands, with three predominant constituents. The molecular weights of these bands were determined from a calibration curve of proteins of known molecular weight (Table 6). The three major constituents had molecular weights of 93,000, 52,000, and 39,000. These values are in substantial agreement with the estimations of Banker, Crain, and Cotman (1972). The 93,000 and 52,000 molecular weight bands accounted for 10 to 20% of the protein by densitometry, and it may be significant that isolated canine kidney [Na + K]-ATPase consists of two polypeptide chains of molecular weight 90,000 and 57,000 (Kyte, 1971*b*). In a number of systems, the phosphorylated subunit of [Na + K]-

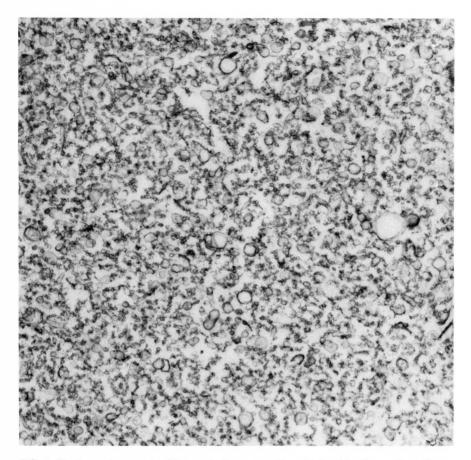

FIG. 4. Electron micrograph of the vesicular preparation obtained by the method shown in Fig. 3. The preparation primarily consists of very small vesicular structures, but small amounts of the contaminating membrane structures which contain the synaptosomal plasma membrane markers are also present.

ATPase has been shown to have a molecular weight of 90,000 to 100,000 (Kyte, 1971a; Uesugi, Dulac, Dixon, Hexum, Dahl, Perdue, and Hokin, 1971; Collins and Albers, 1972). Since the purified enzyme had an activity of 800 μmole P_i liberated/mg protein/hr (Kyte, 1971b) and the membranes had an activity of 100 to 120 μmole P_i liberated/mg protein/hr (Morgan et al., 1971), 10 to 15% of the membrane protein could be [Na + K]-ATPase.

When stained for carbohydrate by the method of Zacharius, Zell, Morrison, and Woodlock (1969) or Glossmann and Neville (1971), five prominent

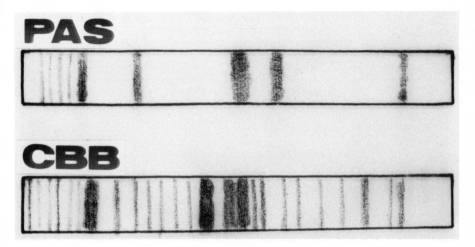

FIG. 5. Line drawings of the protein (CBB) and glycoprotein (PAS) profiles of the synaptosomal plasma membrane. Proteins were dissolved in 1% SDS, 1% β-mercaptoethanol, 2 M urea, and carboxymethylated before electrophoresis.

glycoprotein bands were seen (Fig. 5). Their molecular weights were determined from the molecular weight calibration curve, which is probably valid, since most glycoproteins seemed to fall on the curve (Glossmann and Neville, 1971). It may be only glycoproteins with a very high carbohydrate content which behave abnormally (Bretscher, 1971; Marchesi, Tillack, Jackson, Segrest, and Scott, 1972).

The synaptic vesicles contained seven major bands (Fig. 6). The predominant band appeared to consist of two very closely migrating bands after closer inspection. When parallel gels were stained for carbohydrate, one major band and several minor bands were detected, including two very closely migrating bands. The molecular weights of these bands were determined (Table 6).

From the molecular weights it seemed that protein and glycoprotein bands similar to those of the synaptic vesicles could also be observed in the synaptosomal plasma membranes, and that the synaptic vesicles did not appear to contain unique constituents. This was confirmed for the glycoproteins by mixing experiments which showed that the glycoprotein bands of the two membranes superimposed (Breckenridge and Morgan, 1972). This contrasts with the observations of McBride and Van Tassel (1972), who found that the synaptic vesicles contain unique protein bands not found in the synaptosomal plasma membrane, although they also observed a number of common proteins. Previous studies (Cotman and Mahler, 1967; Mehl, 1967; Bosmann, Case, and Shea, 1970) were not able to determine

TABLE 6. *Molecular weights of synaptosomal plasma and synaptic vesicle membrane proteins and glycoproteins*
(Determined in 12 × 2.5 acrylamide gels in 0.2% SDS)

Synaptosomal plasma membranes		Synaptic vesicles	
Proteins	Glycoproteins	Proteins	Glycoproteins
210,000			
180,000			
160,000			
125,000	120,000	128,000	120,000
98,000		96,000	
93,000			
64,000	66,000	64,000	68,000
58,000		58,000	
53,000		53,000	
52,000			
49,000		48,000	
42,000	43,000	41,500	45,000
39,000			
37,500		37,500	
35,700	34,000	35,800	
32,500		32,500	
30,300			
29,200		29,600	
24,800		24,500	
22,500	23,000	21,100	
20,800			
18,100		18,200	
16,100			
14,000		13,800	
12,000		12,000	

the existence of common constituents due to the impurity of the fractions.

There is now clear evidence from our studies and those of McBride and Van Tassel (1972) that the two membrane systems have electrophoretically common constituent proteins. It is possible that the common constituents have no functional or physiological role in the synaptosomal plasma membrane, but they may be due to the fusion of the synaptic vesicle into the plasma membrane during exocytosis of the transmitter content of the vesicles. Exocytosis is now well established as the secretory mechanism in a number of tissues (Smith, 1971), and there is increasing evidence that it is the mechanism of release for adrenergic nerves (Smith, De Potter, Moerman, and De Schaepdryver, 1970), the neuromuscular junction (Clark, Hurlbut, and Mauro, 1972), and other synapses (Pysh and Wiley, 1972). Common constituents would be in accord with such a process, although the observation of unique components in the synaptic vesicles needs to be

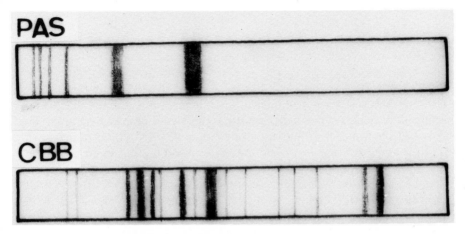

FIG. 6. Line drawings of the protein (CBB) and glycoprotein (PAS) profiles of the synaptic vesicles. Proteins were dissolved in 1% SDS, 1% β-mercaptoethanol, 2 M urea, and carboxymethylated before electrophoresis.

explained. In another secretory system, the pancreas, there is some evidence of common constituents between the plasma membrane and the secretory granule membrane (Meldolesi and Cova, 1972).

The subsequent fate of the vesicles incorporated into the membrane remains to be determined, but the observation that the common constituents account for a significant part of the plasma membrane proteins would suggest that the fusion may be long lasting. However, Bittner and Kennedy (1970) have calculated that the rate of release of transmitter in the opener-stretcher motor neuron of the crayfish is such that vesicle reutilization is almost certain. Morphological evidence of the reformation of vesicles by pinocytosis from the plasma membrane has been reported frequently (Andres, 1964; Kanaseki and Kadota, 1969; Gray and Willis, 1970; Holtzmann, Freeman, and Kashner, 1971; Jones and Bradford, 1971). The relationship of the common constituents to complex vesicles (Kanaseki and Kadota, 1969; Gray and Willis, 1970) and presynaptic densities (Bloom and Aghajanian, 1966, 1968; Akert, Moore, Pfenninger, and Sandri, 1969) must also be investigated.

The importance of these observations for membrane models is evident. The process of exocytosis-pinocytosis is not consistent with a uniform membrane model. The membrane must be composed of a mosaic in order to account for the facts that the protein profile of the vesicles is simpler than that of the membranes and that the vesicles do not contain gangliosides, whereas the membranes do (Breckenridge, Gombos, and Morgan, 1972*b,c, unpublished results*).

IV. LOCALIZATION OF SYNAPTOSOMAL PLASMA MEMBRANE PROTEINS

De Robertis, Azcurra, and Fiszer (1967) reported that the detergent Triton X-100 selectively solubilized the nonjunctional parts of the synaptic complex, leaving an insoluble pellet enriched in junctional material. This has been confirmed to some extent by Cotman, Levy, Banker, and Taylor (1971*b*) and McBride and Van Tassel (1972). Differences in the protein and glycoprotein composition of the Triton-soluble and insoluble material have been reported (Waehneldt, Morgan, and Gombos, 1971; Breckenridge and Morgan, 1972; Levitan et al., 1972; McBride and Van Tassel, 1972). The Triton-insoluble material appears to contain several components which are not found in the Triton-soluble material, but it is premature to attempt to relate them to components of the junctional complex in view of the differential solubilities of proteins in detergents and of the heterogeneity of the Triton-insoluble material. The Triton-insoluble material is enriched in glycoproteins which do not contain sialic acid (Breckenridge, Breckenridge, and Morgan, 1972*a*), which may be related to the staining properties of the junctional material (McBride, Mahler, Moore, and White, 1970).

CONCLUSIONS

A number of problems concerning the proteins and glycoproteins of synaptic structures remain unsolved. In particular, it is necessary to define more closely the localization of the proteins within the plasma membrane and the junctional complex. This will require the isolation and structural characterization of the polypeptide chains.

Another area which remains to be investigated is that of the synthesis of these proteins. After a series of negative experiments (Morgan, 1970; Cotman and Taylor, 1971; Gambetti, Autilio-Gambetti, Gonatas, and Shafer, 1972), the possibility of local synthesis of polypeptide chains has been reopened (Ramirez et al., 1972). A similar confusion concerns the synthesis of the carbohydrate chains of synaptic glycoproteins (Barondes, 1968; Marinari, Morgan, Mack, and Gombos, 1972). However, a synthetic view of the data already available suggests that the majority of the components of the synaptic vesicles and the synaptosomal plasma membrane are synthesized in the cell body, and flow to the synapse in a particulate form as part of the fast axonal flow process.

The possible roles of the proteins and glycoproteins in the more complex functions of the nervous system remain to be established. In the case of the glycoproteins, there is now suggestive evidence that they may have a role in controlling neuronal differentiation (Treska-Ciesielski, Gombos, and Morgan, 1971; Gombos, Hermetet, Reeber, Zanetta, and Treska-Ciesielski, 1972), although relating these observations to cell-contact specification is still speculative.

However, the results already obtained show that preparations of sufficient purity are now available, and that the composition, metabolism, and functioning of the synaptic region can be realistically studied at a chemical level.

ACKNOWLEDGMENT

The work reported here was in part supported by grants from the Fondation pour la Recherche Médicale Française and the Institut National de la Santé et de la Recherche Médicale (No. 7111698). WCB was recipient of a fellowship from the Medical Research Council of Canada. IGM is Attaché and GG Chargé de Recherche of the Centre National de la Recherche Scientifique.

REFERENCES

Abdel-Latif, A. A. (1966): A simple method for the isolation of nerve-ending particles from rat brain. *Biochimica et Biophysica Acta,* 121:403–406.

Akert, K., Moore, H., Pfenninger, K., and Sandri, C. (1969): Contributions of new impregnation methods and freeze-etching to the problems of synaptic fine structure. In: *Mechanism of Synaptic Transmission—Progress in Brain Research,* Vol. 31, edited by K. Akert and P. G. Wazer, pp. 223–240. American Elsevier, New York.

Andres, K. H. (1964): Micropinozytose im Zentralnervensystem. *Zeitschrift für Zellforschung und Mikroskopische Anatomie,* 64:63–73.

Autilio, L. A., Appel, S. H., Pettis, P., and Gambetti, P. L. (1968): Biochemical studies of synapses *in vitro.* I. Protein synthesis. *Biochemistry,* 7:2615–2622.

Banker, G., Crain, B., and Cotman, C. W. (1972): Molecular weights of the polypeptide chains of synaptic plasma membranes. *Brain Research,* 42:508–513.

Barchi, R. L., and Braun, P. E. (1972): Thiamine in neural membranes. Enzymic hydrolysis of thiamine diphosphate. *Journal of Neurochemistry,* 19:1039–1048.

Barondes, S. H. (1968): Incorporation of radioactive glucosamine into macromolecules at nerve endings. *Journal of Neurochemistry,* 15:699–706.

Bittner, G. D., and Kennedy, D. (1970): Quantitative aspects of transmitter release. *Journal of Cell Biology,* 47:585–592.

Bloom, F. E., and Aghajanian, G. K. (1966): Cytochemistry of synapses: Selective staining for electron microscopy. *Science,* 154:1575–1577.

Bloom, F. E., and Aghajanian, G. K. (1968): Fine structural and cytochemical analysis of the staining of synaptic junctions with phosphotungstic acid. *Journal of Ultrastructure Research,* 22:361–375.

Bondy, S. C. (1971): Axonal transport of macromolecules. I. Protein migration in the central nervous system. *Experimental Brain Research,* 13:127–134.

Bonting, S. L., Caravaggio, L. L., and Hawkins, N. M. (1962): Studies on sodium-potassium-activated adenosine-triphosphatase. IV. Correlation with cation transport sensitive to cardiac glycosides. *Archives of Biochemistry and Biophysics,* 98:413–419.

Bosmann, H. B. (1972): Synthesis of glycoproteins in brain: identification, purification and properties of glycosyl-transferases from purified synaptosomes of guinea pig cerebral cortex. *Journal of Neurochemistry,* 19:763–778.

Bosmann, H. B., Case, K. R., and Shea, M. B. (1970): Proteins and glycoproteins of rat cerebral cortex subsynaptosomal fractions: Extraction with sodium dodecylsulphate and analytic electrophoresis. *Federation of European Biochemical Societies. Letters,* 11:261–264.

Bray, J. J., Kon, C. M., and Breckenridge, B. McL. (1971): Adenylcyclase, cyclic nucleotide phosphodiestearase and axoplasmic flow. *Brain Research,* 26:385–394.

Breckenridge, W. C., Breckenridge, J. E., and Morgan, I. G. (1972a): Glycoproteins of the synaptic region. In: *Functional and Structural Proteins of the Nervous System,* edited by A. N. Davison, P. Mandel, and I. G. Morgan, pp. 135–153. Plenum Press, New York.

Breckenridge, W. C., Gombos, G., and Morgan, I. G. (1972b): The decosahexaenoic acid of the phospholipids of synaptic membranes, vesicles and mitochondria. *Brain Research,* 33:581–583.

Breckenridge, W. C., Gombos, G., and Morgan, I. G. (1972c): The lipid composition of adult rat brain synaptosomal plasma membranes. *Biochimica et Biophysica Acta,* 266:695–707.

Breckenridge, W. C., and Morgan, I. G. (1972): Common glycoproteins of synaptic vesicles and the synaptosomal plasma membranes. *Federation of European Biochemical Societies. Letters,* 22:253–256.

Bretscher, M. S. (1971): Major human erythrocyte glycoprotein spans the cell membrane. *Nature,* 231:229–232.

Broquet, P., and Louisot, P. (1971): Biosynthèse des glycoprotéines cérébrales. II. Localisation subcellulaire des transglycosylases cérébrales. *Biochimie* (Paris), 53:921–927.

Clark, A. W., Hurlbut, W. P., and Mauro, A. (1972): Changes in the fine structure of the neuromuscular junction of the frog caused by black widow spider venom. *Journal of Cell Biology,* 52:1–14.

Clark, R. B., and Perkins, J. P. (1971): Regulation of adenosine 3'-5'-cyclic monophosphate concentrations in cultured human astrocytoma cells by catecholamines and histamine. *Proceedings of the National Academy of Sciences,* 68:2757–2760.

Collins, R. C., and Albers, R. W. (1972): The phosporyl acceptor protein of Na-K-ATPase from various tissues. *Journal of Neurochemistry,* 19:1209–1213.

Cotman, C. W., Blank, M. L., Moehl, A., and Snyder, F. (1969): Lipid composition of synaptic plasma membranes isolated from rat brain by zonal centrifugation. *Biochemistry,* 8:4606–4612.

Cotman, C. W., Brown, D. H., Harrell, B. W., and Anderson, N. G. (1970): Analytical differential centrifugation: An analysis of the sedimentation properties of synaptosomes, mitochondria, and lysosomes from rat brain homogenates. *Archives of Biochemistry and Biophysics,* 136:436–447.

Cotman, C. W., Herschman, H., and Taylor, D. (1971a): Subcellular fractionation of cultured glial cells. *Journal of Neurobiology,* 2:169–180.

Cotman, C. W., Levy, W., Banker, G., and Taylor, D. (1971b): An ultrastructural and chemical analysis of the effect of Triton X-100 on synaptic plasma membranes. *Biochimica et Biophysica Acta,* 249:406–418.

Cotman, C. W., and Mahler, H. R. (1967): Resolution of insoluble proteins in rat brain subcellular fractions. *Archives of Biochemistry and Biophysics,* 120:384–396.

Cotman, C. W., and Matthews, D. A. (1971): Synaptic plasma membranes from rat brain synaptosomes. Isolation and partial characterization. *Biochimica et Biophysica Acta,* 249:380–394.

Cotman, C. W., and Taylor, D. A. (1971): Autoradiographic analysis of protein synthesis in synaptosomal fractions. *Brain Research,* 29:366–372.

Den, H., Kaufman, B., and Roseman, S. (1970): Properties of some glycosyltransferases in embryonic chicken brain. *Journal of Biological Chemistry,* 245:6607–6615.

De Robertis, E., Azcurra, J. M., and Fiszer, S. (1967): Ultrastructure and cholinergic binding capacity of junctional complexes isolated from rat brain. *Brain Research,* 5:45–56.

De Robertis, E., Pellegrino de Iraldi, A., Rodriguez de Lores Arnaiz, G., and Salganicoff, L.

(1962): Cholinergic and non-cholinergic nerve endings in rat brain. I. Isolation and sub-cellular distribution of acetylcholine and acetylcholine esterase. *Journal of Neurochemistry*, 9:23–35.

De Robertis, E., Pellegrino de Iraldi, A., Rodriguez de Lores Arnaiz, G., and Zieher, L. M. (1965): Synaptic vesicles from rat hypothalamus. Isolation and norepinephrine content. *Life Sciences*, 4:193–201.

De Robertis, E., Rodriguez de Lores Arnaiz, G., Salganicoff, L., Pellegrino de Iraldi, A., and Zieher, L. M. (1963): Isolation of synaptic vesicles and structural organization of the acetyl-choline system within brain nerve-endings. *Journal of Neurochemistry*, 10:225–235.

Derry, D. M., and Wolfe, L. S. (1968): Gangliosides in isolated neurons and glial cells. *Science*, 158:1450–1452.

Doyle, L. C., and Cotman, C. W. (1972): Analysis of myelin-synaptosomal interactions in sucrose and Ficoll-sucrose gradients. *Analytical Biochemistry*, 49:29–36.

Elam, J. S., Goldberg, J. M., Radin, N. S., and Agranoff, B. W. (1970): Rapid axonal transport of sulphated mucopolysaccharide proteins. *Science*, 170:458–460.

Festoff, B. W., Appel, S. H., and Day, E. (1971): Incorporation of [^{14}C] glucosamine into synaptosomes *in vitro*. *Journal of Neurochemistry*, 18:1871–1886.

Fewster, M. E., and Mead, J. F. (1968): Fatty acid and fatty aldehyde composition of glial cell lipids isolated from bovine white matter. *Journal of Neurochemistry*, 15:1303–1312.

Forman, D. S., McEwen, B. S., and Grafstein, B. (1971): Rapid transport of radioactivity in goldfish optic nerve following injections of labelled glucosamine. *Brain Research*, 28:119–130.

Gambetti, P., Autilio-Gambetti, L. A., Gonatas, N. K., and Shafer, B. (1972): Protein synthesis in synaptosomal fractions. Ultrastructural radioautographic study. *Journal of Cell Biology*, 52:526–535.

Garey, R., Harper, J., Best, J. B., and Goodman, A. B. (1972): Preparative resolution and identification of synaptic components of rat neocortex. *Journal of Neurobiology*, 3:163–195.

Gilman, A. G., and Nirenberg, M. (1971a): Effect of catecholamines on adenosine 3'-5'-cyclic monophosphate concentrations of clonal satellite cells of neurons. *Proceedings of the National Academy of Sciences*, 68:2165–2168.

Gilman, A. G., and Nirenberg, M. (1971b): Regulation of adenosine 3'-5'-cyclic monophos-phate metabolism in cultured neuroblastoma cells. *Nature*, 234:356–358.

Glossmann, H., and Neville, D. M. (1971): Glycoproteins of cell surfaces. A comparative study of three different cell surfaces of the rat. *Journal of Biological Chemistry*, 246:6339–6346.

Gombos, G., Hermetet, J. C., Reeber, A., Zanetta, J. P., and Treska-Ciesielski, J. (1972): The composition of glycopeptides, derived from neural membranes, which affect neurite growth *in vitro*. *Federation of European Biochemical Societies. Letters*, 24:247–250.

Gray, E. G., and Whittaker, V. P. (1962): The isolation of nerve endings from brain: An electron-microscopic study of cell fragments derived by homogenization and centrifugation. *Journal of Anatomy*, 96:79–88.

Gray, E. G., and Willis, R. A. (1970): On synaptic vesicles, complex vesicles and dense projections. *Brain Research*, 24:149–168.

Harvey, J. A., and McIlwain, H. (1969): Electrical phenomena and isolated tissues from the brain. In: *Handbook of Neurochemistry*, Vol. II, edited by A. Lajtha, pp. 115–136. Plenum Press, New York.

Holtzmann, E., Freeman, A. R., and Kashner, L. A. (1971): Stimulation-dependent alterations in peroxidase uptake at lobster neuromuscular junctions. *Science*, 173:733–736.

Jones, D. G., and Bradford, H. F. (1971): The relationship between complex vesicles, dense-cored vesicles and dense projections in cortical synaptosomes. *Tissue & Cell*, 3:177–190.

Kanaseki, T., and Kadota, K. (1969): The "vesicle in a basket." A morphological study of the coated vesicle isolated from the nerve endings of the guinea pig brain, with special reference to the mechanism of membrane movements. *Journal of Cell Biology*, 42:202–220.

Karlsson, J. O., and Sjöstrand, J. (1971): Rapid intracellular transport of fucose-containing glycoproteins in retinal ganglion cells. *Journal of Neurochemistry*, 18:2209–2216.

Kishimoto, Y., Agranoff, B. W., Radin, N. S., and Burton, R. M. (1969): Comparison of the fatty acids of lipids of subcellular brain fractions. *Journal of Neurochemistry,* 16:397–404.

Kokko, A., Mautner, H. G., and Barrnett, R. J. (1969): Fine structural localization of acetyl-cholinesterase using acetyl-β-methylcholine and acetylselenotholine as substrates. *Journal of Histochemistry and Cytochemistry,* 17:625–640.

Kornguth, S. E., Anderson, J. W., and Scott, G. (1969): Isolation of synaptic complexes in a cesium chloride density gradient. Electron microscopic and immunohistochemical studies. *Journal of Neurochemistry,* 16:1017–1024.

Kornguth, S. E., Flangas, A., Perrin, J., Geison, R., and Scott, G. (1972): Isolation of synaptic complexes in a CsCl gradient: Conditions for maximal resolution in the zonal rotor B-XIV and circular dichroism patterns. *Preparative Biochemistry,* 2:167–192.

Kornguth, S. E., Flangas, A., Siegel, F., Geison, R., O'Brien, J., Lamar, C., and Scott, G. (1971): Chemical and metabolic characteristics of synaptic complexes from brain isolated by zonal centrifugation in a cesium chloride gradient. *Journal of Biological Chemistry,* 246: 1177–1184.

Kurihara, T., and Tsukada, Y. (1967): The regional and subcellular distribution of 2′,3′-cyclic nucleotide 3′-phosphohydrolase in the central nervous system. Journal of Neurochemistry, 14:1167–1174.

Kurihara T., and Tsukada, Y. (1968): 2′,3′-Cyclic nucleotide 3′-phosphohydrolase in the developing chick brain and spinal cord. *Journal of Neurochemistry,* 15:827–832.

Kurokawa, M., Sakamoto, T., and Kato, M. (1965): Distribution of sodium-plus-potassium-stimulated adenosine triphosphatase activity in isolatiod nerve-ending particles. *Biochemical Journal,* 97:833–844.

Kyte, J. (1971a): Phosphorylation of a purified ($Na^+ + K^+$) adenosine triphosphatase. *Biochemical and Biophysical Research Communications,* 43:1259–1265.

Kyte, J. (1971b): Purification of the sodium- and potassium-dependent adenosine triphosphatase from canine renal medulla. *Journal of Biological Chemistry,* 246:4157–4165.

Lane, N. J. (1968): Distribution of phosphatases in the Golgi region and associated structures of the thoracic ganglionic neurons in the grasshopper, *Melanoplus differentialis. Journal of Cell Biology,* 37:89–104.

Lapetina, E. G., Soto, E. F., and De Robertis, E. (1967): Gangliosides and acetylcholin-esterase in isolated membranes of the rat-brain cortex. *Biochimica et Biophysica Acta,* 35:33–43.

Lemkey-Johnston, N., and Dekirmenjian, H. (1970): The identification of fractions enriched in nonmyelinated axons from rat whole brain. *Experimental Brain Research,* 11:392–410.

Lemkey-Johnston, N., and Larramendi, L. M. H. (1968): The separation and identification of fractions of non-myelinated axons from the cerebellum of the Cat. *Experimental Brain Research,* 5:326–340.

Levitan, I. B., Mushynski, W. E., and Ramirez, G. (1972): Highly purified synaptosomal membranes from rat brain. Isolation and characterization. *Journal of Biological Chemistry,* 247:5376–5381.

Lowden, J. A., and Wolfe, L. S. (1964): Brain gangliosides. III. Evidence for the location of gangliosides specifically in neurons. *Canadian Journal of Biochemistry,* 42:1587–1594.

Marchesi, V. T., Tillack, T. W., Jackson, R. L., Segrest, J. P., and Scott, R. E. (1972): Chemical characterization and surface orientation of the major glycoprotein of the human erythrocyte membrane. *Proceedings of the National Academy of Sciences,* 69:1445–1449.

Marinari, U. M., Morgan, I. G., Mack, G., and Gombos, G. (1972). Synthesis of the synaptic glycoproteins. II. Delayed labelling of the glycoproteins of synaptic vesicles and synaptosomal plasma membranes. *Neurobiology,* 2:176–182.

Maynert, E. W., Levi, R., and De Lorenzo, A. J. (1964): The presence of norepinephrine and 5-hydroxytryptamine in vesicles from disrupted nerve-ending particles. *Journal of Pharmacology and Experimental Therapeutics,* 144:385–392.

McBride, W. J., and Cohen, H. (1972): Cytochemical localization of acetylcholinesterase on isolated synaptosomes. *Brain Research,* 41:489–493.

McBride, W. J., Mahler, H. R., Moore, W. J., and White, F. P. (1970): Isolation and characterization of membranes from rat cerebral cortex. *Journal of Neurobiology,* 2:73–92.

McBride, W. J., and Van Tassel, J. (1972): Resolution of proteins from subfractions of nerve-endings. *Brain Research*, 44:177–187.

Mehl, E. (1967): Electrophoresis of membrane proteins from brain. In: *Macromolecules and the Function of the Neuron*, edited by Z. Lodin and S. P. R. Rose, pp. 22–32. Excerpta Medica Foundation, Amsterdam.

Meldolesi, J., and Cova, D. (1972): Composition of the cellular membranes in the pancreas of the guinea pig. *Journal of Cell Biology*, 55:1–18.

Michaelson, I. A., Whittaker, V. P., Laverty, R., and Sharman, D. F. (1963): Localization of acetylcholine, 5-hydroxytryptamine and noradrenaline within subcellular particles derived from guinea pig subcortical brain tissue. *Biochemical Pharmacology*, 12:1450–1453.

Morgan, I. G. (1970): Protein synthesis in brain mitochondrial and synaptosomal preparations. *Federation of European Biophysical Societies. Letters*, 10:273–275.

Morgan, I. G., Reith, M., Marinari, U., Breckenridge, W. C., and Gombos, G. (1972): The isolation and characterization of synaptosomal plasma membranes. In: *Glycolipids, Glycoproteins and Mucopolysaccharides of the Nervous System*, edited by V. Zambotti, G. Tettamanti, and M. Arrigoni, pp. 209–228. Plenum Press, New York.

Morgan, I. G., Wolfe, L. S., Mandel, P., and Gombos, G. (1971): Isolation of plasma membranes from rat brain. *Biochimica et Biophysica Acta*, 241:737–751.

Novikoff, A. B., and Goldfischer, S. (1961): Nucleoside diphosphatase activity in the Golgi apparatus and its usefulness for cytological studies. *Proceedings of the National Academy of Sciences*, 47:802–810.

O'Brien, J. S., and Sampson, E. L. (1965): Fatty acid and fatty aldehyde composition of the major brain lipids in normal human gray matter, white matter, and myelin. *Journal of Lipid Research*, 6:545–551.

Pellegrino de Iraldi, A., and Rodriguez de Lores Arnaiz, G. (1970): Thiamine pyrophosphatase activity in a fraction rich in Golgi-like structures from crushed sciatic nerve of the cat. *Journal of Neurochemistry*, 17:1601–1606.

Pfeiffer, S. E., and Wechsler, W. (1972): Biochemically differentiated neoplastic clone of Schwann cells. *Proceedings of the National Academy of Sciences*, 69:2885–2889.

Poduslo, S. E., and Norton, W. T. (1972): Isolation and some chemical properties of oligodendroglia from calf brain. *Journal of Neurochemistry*, 19:727–736.

Pomazanskaya, L. F., Freysz, L., and Mandel, P. (1969): Fatty acids of some phospholipids in neurons and glial cells isolated from rat cerebral cortex. *Zh. Evol. Biokhim. Fiziol.*, 5:523–528.

Pysh, J. J., and Wiley, R. G. (1972): Morphological alterations of synapses in electrically stimulated superior ganglia of the cat. *Science*, 176:191–193.

Ramirez, G., Levitan, I. B., and Mushynski, W. E. (1972): Highly purified synaptosomal membranes from rat brain. Incorporation of amino acids into membrane proteins *in vitro. Journal of Biological Chemistry*, 247:5382–5390.

Rassin, D. K. (1972): Amino acids as putative transmitters: Failure to bind synaptic vesicles of guinea pig cerebral cortex. *Journal of Neurochemistry*, 19:139–148.

Reith, M., Morgan, I. G., Gombos, G., Breckenridge, W. C., and Vincendon, G. (1972): Biosynthesis of synaptic glycoproteins. I. The distribution of UDP-galactose N-acetylglucosamine galactosyl transferase and thiamine diphosphatase in adult rat brain subcellular fractions. *Neurobiology*, 2:169–175.

Smith, A. D. (1971): Summing up: Some implications of the neuron as a secreting cell. *Philosophical Transactions of the Royal Society of London. Biological Sciences*, 261:423–437.

Smith, A. D., De Potter, W. P., Moerman, E. J., and De Schaepdryver, A. F. (1970): Release of dopamine-β-hydroxylase and chromogranin A upon stimulation of the splenic nerve. *Tissue & Cell*, 2:547–568.

Spence, M. W., and Wolfe, L. S. (1967): Gangliosides in developing rat brain. Isolation and composition of subcellular membranes enriched in gangliosides. *Canadian Journal of Biochemistry*, 45:671–688.

Svennerholm, E., Ställberg-Stenhagen, S., and Svennerholm, L. (1966): Fatty acid composition of sphingomyelins in blood, spleen, placenta, liver, lung, and kidney. *Biochimica et Biophysica Acta*, 125:60–69.

Tanaka, R., and Abood, L. G. (1963): Isolation from rat brain of mitochondria devoid of glycolytic activity. *Journal of Neurochemistry,* 10:571–576.

Tettamanti, G., Morgan, I. G., Gombos, G., Vincendon, G., and Mandel, P. (1972): Sub-synaptosomal localization of brain particulate neuraminidase. *Brain Research,* 47:515–518.

Treska-Ciesielski, J., Gombos, G., and Morgan, I. G. (1971): Effet de la concanavaline A sur les neurones de ganglions spinaux d'embryons de Poulet en culture. *Comptes Rendus Hebdomadaires de l'Academie des Sciences* (Paris), 273:1041–1043.

Uesugi, S., Dulac, N. C., Dixon, J. F., Hexum, T. D., Dahl, J. L., Perdue, J. F., and Hokin, L. E. (1971): Studies on the characterization of the sodium-potassium transport adenosine triphosphatase. VI. Large scale partial purification and properties of a Lubrol-solubilized bovine brain enzyme. *Journal of Biological Chemistry,* 246:531–543.

Waehneldt, T. V., Morgan, I. G., and Gombos, G. (1971): The synaptosomal plasma membrane: Protein and glycoprotein composition. *Brain Research,* 34:403–406.

Whittaker, V. P. (1968): The morphology of fractions of rat forebrain synaptosomes separated on continuous sucrose density gradients. *Biochemical Journal,* 106:412–417.

Whittaker, V. P., Michaelson, I. A., and Kirkland, R. J. A. (1964): The separation of synaptic vesicles from nerve-ending particles ("synaptosomes"). *Biochemical Journal,* 90:293–303.

Zacharius, R. M., Zell, T. E., Morrison, J. H., and Woodlock, J. J. (1969): Glycoprotein staining following electrophoresis on acrylamide gels. *Analytical Biochemistry,* 30:148–152.

Zanetta, J. P., Benda, P., Gombos, G., and Morgan, I. G. (1972): The presence of 2′,3′-cyclic AMP 3′-phosphohydrolase in a glial cell tumor. *Journal of Neurochemistry,* 19:881–883.

Proteins of the Nervous System
Raven Press, New York © 1973

Synthesis and Degradation of Synaptic Membrane Proteins

Walter J. Moore

I. INTRODUCTION

Our interest in brain proteins is the result of the concept that the synapse and its components may be a site of changes which underlie memory and brain plasticity. This concept can be traced from Descartes in 1650 to the present, and presumes that sensory input produces a modification of synaptic connections that in turn produces a record or memory of the event. The answers to many of the most interesting questions about the plasticity of neurons and the ways in which chemical reactions in brain cells are influenced or controlled by electrical phenomena may best be found by careful investigation of the *in vivo* synthesis and breakdown of brain proteins.

This field is experimentally difficult because many kinds of heterogeneity can influence the rate constants involved, including differences between brain regions, cellular types, cellular regions and organelles, and circadian rhythms. Little quantitative data are available for the rate constants of both synthesis and decay in brain tissue. Much more data are available for liver, where a wide spectrum of turnover rates has been established (Rechcigl, 1971), and changes in the steady-state concentrations of enzymes have been found to be controlled by their specific rates of synthesis and breakdown.

Measurement of the dynamics of brain proteins is usually based on either the specific activities of amino acids in the protein and in precursor pools or the enzyme activities. The calculation of the specific rates of synthesis and degradation is based on the choice of a model for the relationship between the amino acid pool and the protein. These models are usually simplified by neglecting intracellular transport, and consist of a single plasma pool and a single extracellular pool. This approach has been criticized in recent years, even for organs less complex than the brain (Hider, Fern, and London, 1971; Mortimore, Woodside, and Henry, 1972).

193

II. THE USE OF SUBCELLULAR FRACTIONATION METHODS TO EXAMINE STRAIN DIFFERENCES

We have been particularly interested in the synthesis of membrane proteins and the assembly of these proteins into the membranes of nerve endings. Our first extension of the early methods for the subcellular fractionation of brain homogenates (Whittaker, Michaelson, and Kirkland, 1964) was to introduce the use of continuous sucrose density gradients in zonal rotors (Cotman, Mahler, and Anderson, 1968), which permitted a quantitative reproducibility in the specification of the isopycnic densities of the various fractions. Gurd, Mahler, and Moore (1972) have used this method to examine genetic differences in the polyacrylamide gel patterns of proteins from the synaptic regions of brain tissue from C57 and DBA mice. These strains were chosen because they show interesting behavioral differences and respond differently to drugs such as chlorpromazine, which may act on neuronal membranes. A preliminary survey showed that the largest strain differences occurred in the brainstem, and this region was therefore used in subsequent studies. No difference was observed in the gel patterns for the two species except for those fractions that were highly enriched in synaptic membranes (Fig. 1*b*).

The separation of proteins on these acidic gels is a function of both molecular weight and the effective charge on the migrating proteins. No difference between the strains was detected when they were subsequently compared on SDS gels, which under appropriate conditions separate molecules solely on the basis of molecular weight (Gurd, *unpublished observation*). This result indicates that the strain differences observed on polyacrylamide gel separation may represent the type of difference in charge that would be expected from genetically determined amino acid substitutions in the polypeptide chains of specific proteins. This conclusion must be verified by the isolation and identification of the specific proteins involved.

Our more recent work has utilized the Ficoll gradient technique described elsewhere in this volume by Dr. Morgan. This technique is currently in wide use for the preparation of purified synaptic membranes. Maguire and McGovern *(unpublished observations)* have utilized this technique to study the incorporation of transmitter precursors into rat cortex slices. Two separate synaptosomal fractions, B_2 and B_3, can be obtained by a second Ficoll gradient fractionation of the crude synaptosomal fraction obtained by discontinuous fractionation of tissue homogenate. The less dense B_2 fraction is enriched in adrenergic endings compared to the more dense B_3 fraction. Dopamine accumulates preferentially in the B_2 fraction, which has been shown to contain a sevenfold greater concentration of catechol-O-methyltransferase than the B_3 fraction, and the choline is more evenly distributed (Fig. 2). The norepinephrine concentration in B_2 is seven times that in B_3, whereas the acetylcholine concentration is four times higher in B_3 than in B_2.

Both synaptosomal fractions are easily lysed by osmotic shock, and yield preparations of vesicles and synaptic membranes. Although this fractionation procedure does not yield fractions that are completely specific for single transmitters, it appears that this is a reasonable goal, and in future studies we shall examine the distribution of proteins in the membrane and vesicle populations of each fraction.

III. DETERMINATION OF PROTEIN TURNOVER RATES

Our first *in vivo* studies (Von Hungen, Mahler, and Moore, 1968) were attempts to determine the relative turnover rates of vesicle and membrane protein, in order to distinguish between three possible mechanisms of transmitter release: 1) transmitter release that results in destruction of the vesicle, which then has to be replaced by axoplasmic flow; 2) fusion of the vesicles with the membrane in order to release transmitter, so that the vesicle membrane protein is in constant exchange with the presynaptic membrane protein; or 3) that the vesicles release transmitter and are then refilled, which appeared the most likely situation in 1968. The first possibility would result in a rapid turnover of vesicle protein relative to membrane protein, whereas the latter two would not. This possibility was eliminated by the demonstration that the half-lives for both synaptic membranes and synaptic vesicles were approximately 20 days (Fig. 3). These values are in good agreement with those of Morris, Ralston, and Shooter (1971), who calculated turnover times for the synaptic vesicle and membrane proteins of 15.6 and 17 days, respectively.

Fusion of the vesicle with the presynaptic membrane at the time of transmitter release does not seem likely, since the half-life of this exchange would have to be approximately 60 sec. In conjunction with the data presented by Whittaker in this volume, these half-lives suggest that some vesicles are refilled after the release of transmitter.

Studies such as this utilize an extremely simplified model with a single plasma pool and a single extracellular pool. The mathematical treatment of this model ignores the reutilization of radioactive amino acid derived from the breakdown of protein, which is necessary in order to obtain one simple rate constant. Garlick and Marshall (1972) have examined the problem of reutilization by retaining a relatively simple model. They found that 40%

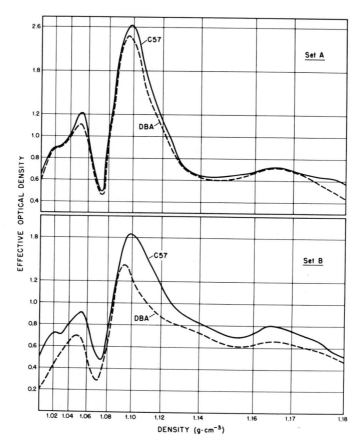

FIG. 1. The detection of strain differences in the synaptosomal proteins of DBA and C57 mice (Gurd, Mahler, and Moore, 1972). *(Left):* Zonal centrifugation of lysed crude mito-chondrial fractions from the two strains. *(Right):* Fractions shown to be highly enriched

of the tyrosine pool in mouse brain is derived from the breakdown of brain protein.

The effect of reutilization is most important when dealing with proteins whose half-lives are short. The neglect of this factor has resulted in most of the recently reported turnover rates being too slow. For example, Poole (1971) has shown that simplistic treatment of the data for liver catalase gives a half-life for this protein of 3.5 days, whereas a more correct model which incorporates the effects of reutilization gives a half-life of 1.5 days. The available figures on half-lives of synaptic vesicle and membrane proteins may likewise be too high by a factor of two.

Interpretation of incorporation data becomes extremely difficult when one

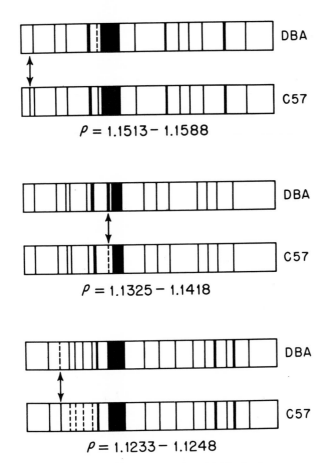

$P = 1.1513 - 1.1588$

$P = 1.1325 - 1.1418$

$P = 1.1233 - 1.1248$

in synaptic membranes were compared by acidic polyacrylamide gel electrophoresis and shown to possess several marked differences.

deals with the average rate of turnover of a group of proteins rather than with the turnover of a specific protein. Garlick, Waterlow, and Millward (1973 and *personal communication*) have demonstrated that mean turnover rates calculated from a population of sets of proteins with different turnover rates will probably be far from accurate. An averaging of the initial *uptake rate* does actually represent the true mass average. However, the situation for *decay rates* is far more complex, because the extent of initial labeling of a given protein is dependent on its rate of synthesis. They have found that valid mean turnover rates can only be calculated at times of approximately three half-lives.

These results indicate that accurate mean turnover rates cannot be ob-

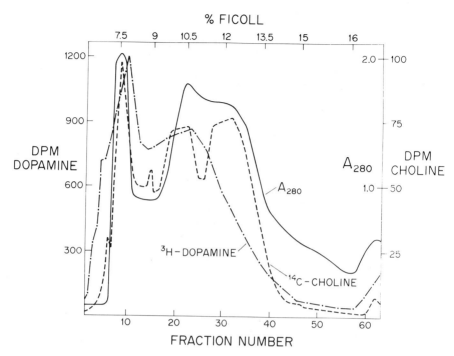

FIG. 2. Separation of a crude synaptosomal fraction from rat cerebral cortex on continuous linear isotonic Ficoll gradients. Rat cortex slices (McIlwain and Rodnight, 1962) were incubated with ^{14}C-choline and ^{3}H-dopamine. The incubated material was fractionated on continuous Ficoll gradients, and the distribution of label and effective absorbance (A_{280}) determined for each gradient fraction.

tained by determining the slope of decline in radioactivity after only one or two half-lives. Many studies in which the effects on protein synthesis of specific behaviors, such as learning or imprinting, have been examined have not only neglected the quantitative analysis necessary to obtain such rates, but in some cases have entirely neglected the measurement of amino acid pools and reported only the amount of label incorporated into the protein or nucleic acid. Such experiments are therefore of limited value.

IV. THE SPECTRUM OF TURNOVER RATES IN MEMBRANE PROTEINS

In order to avoid the problems inherent in determining an average turnover rate for a protein population, we next attempted to determine turnover rates for individual proteins. One approach to this problem would be the isolation of individual proteins that can be characterized as well-defined entities. However, this has not yet been achieved for most membrane proteins, and we have been forced to rely on the as yet uncharacterized fractions that can be obtained by polyacrylamide gel fractionation.

Merel *(unpublished observations)* has recently applied the double-labeling technique of Arias, Schimke, and Doyle (1969) to a determination of the individual turnover rates of such fractionated proteins (Fig. 4). ^{14}C-labeled amino acid is administered intraventricularly at time 0, followed by ^{3}H-amino acid at time τ. At time τ' the animals are killed and the protein extracted and fractionated on polyacrylamide gels. The ^{3}H/^{14}C ratio is then determined for each gel band. If the decline in specific activity of the protein follows first-order kinetics, with a rate constant k_d, the logarithm of the ratio of ^{3}H/^{14}C in protein 1 to that of protein 2 is proportional to the difference in the rate constants for the decomposition of the two proteins. These measurements can be combined with determinations of absolute rate constants to yield separate turnover times for the two proteins.

As expected, when $\tau = 0$ there is no significant difference between gel fractions. The soluble protein fraction shows marked heterogeneity when $\tau = 25$ days. In contrast to this heterogeneous turnover for the soluble proteins, the proteins obtained from the synaptic membrane fraction show only a limited heterogeneity of turnover, with the higher molecular weight proteins turning over slightly more rapidly than those of low molecular weight, with a range in turnovers of 16 to 20 days. (Results from this method are, however, not corrected for reutilization.)

Arias et al. (1969) suggested that there are two basic possibilities for membrane synthesis: 1) synchronous, with the membrane synthesized as a unit, and 2) asynchronous, with the individual components synthesized at different rates before incorporation into the membrane structure. Dehlinger and Schimke (1971) observed a marked heterogeneity in the synthesis of liver membrane proteins that appeared inconsistent with the possibility of synchronous behavior. The lack of such marked heterogeneity in the brain synaptic membrane proteins suggests that synchronous synthesis may occur in this fraction.

One difficulty with this approach is that it is entirely possible that the individual acrylamide gel bands used in these studies may contain multiple proteins with heterogeneous turnover rates. This problem will only be solved by more detailed analysis of the individual bands.

V. *IN VITRO* PROTEIN SYNTHESIS IN SLICED RAT BRAIN TISSUE

The use of tissue slices essentially represents an intermediate level of complexity between the *in vivo* situation and that of cell-free systems. Yamomoto and McIlwain (1966) have shown that electrical stimulation

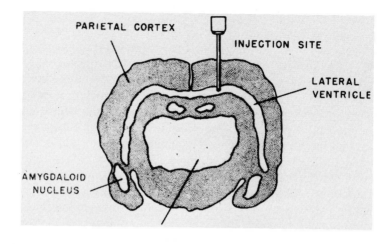

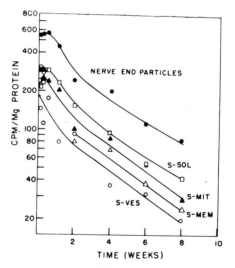

FIG. 3. Determination of the average turnover rates of proteins and RNA in subcellular fractions of rat cerebral cortex (Von Hungen et al., 1968). *(Upper left):* Thalamic injection site of ³H-leucine and ¹⁴C-orotic acid. *(Upper right):* Time course of leucine radioactivities following a single injection of label. *(Lower left):* Time course of the radioactivity in the

produces volleys of nerve impulses through tissue slices, and Orrego and Lipmann (1967) demonstrated an inhibition of protein synthesis in response to such stimulation, indicating that at least some of the physiological responses of the *in vivo* system are preserved.

The major advantage to the use of tissue slices is that it is possible to

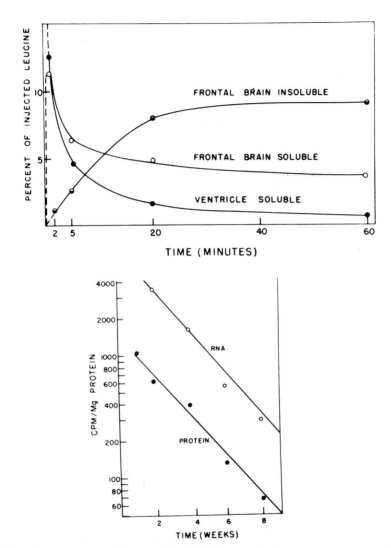

proteins of various subcellular fractions derived from nerve endings. The half-lives for proteins in both the synaptic membrane and synaptic vesicles were calculated to be approximately 20 days. *(Lower right):* Semilogarithmic plot of radioactivities in ribosomal proteins and RNA. The parallel decrease indicates that the ribosomes turn over as entities.

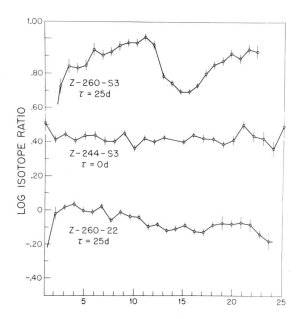

FIG. 4. Heterogeneity of turnover rates among various classes of rat brain proteins (Merel, *personal communication*), determined by the method of Arias, Doyle, and Schimke (1969). Each rat was injected intraventricularly with 5 μC ^{14}C-arginine at time 0, and with 20 μC ^{3}H-arginine at time τ, comparable to the average half-life of membrane proteins. The animals were killed at $\tau + 3$d, the brain tissue was fractionated, and the fractions were solubilized in SDS and analyzed on polyacrylamide gels. The gels were sectioned and the ratio of ^{3}H/^{14}C determined for each section. A high ratio corresponds to a high turnover rate. Z260-S3 and Z244-S3 were determinations on the soluble protein fractions S3 at $\tau = 25$d and $\tau = 0$d, whereas Z-260-22 is a determination on a synaptic membrane fraction with $\tau = 25$d. Membrane fractions with $\tau = 0$d are essentially similar to the $\tau = 0$d determination for the S3 fraction. Molecular weights decrease from left to right.

control the incubation medium and thus to examine the effects of drugs and environmental variables. In studies of protein synthesis, the level of precursor can be controlled, and the problems of pools and uneven distribution are to some extent relieved. The major disadvantage is that the system is far from a stationary state of macromolecular synthesis and degradation. For example, Jones and McIlwain (1971) demonstrated a large net proteolysis during incubation. Even if it were possible to determine absolute rates of protein synthesis and degradation in brain tissue slices, such values would probably be of quite limited relevance to any physiological situation.

White, McBride, Mahler, and Moore (1972) utilized a modified slice technique to examine the synthesis of membrane proteins (Fig. 5). After incubation for 15 min in the standard protein synthetic medium, 100 μg/ml cycloheximide was added to stop cytoplasmic protein synthesis, and radioactivity incorporation was determined at various time intervals. The

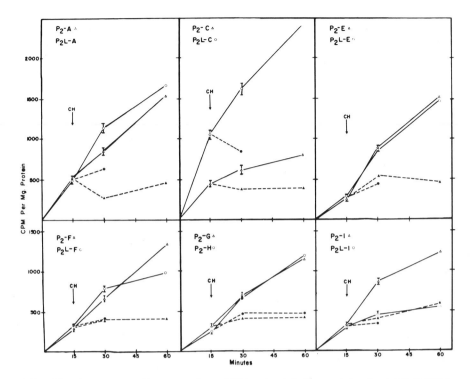

FIG. 5. The time course of incorporation of ³H-leucine into the protein of subcellular fractions of chopped rat cerebral cortex. The incubations were carried out either in the absence (——) or presence (----) of 100 μg/ml cycloheximide, added at τ = 15 min. Fractions P2-E to P2-H are enriched in synaptic membranes, P2-A is soluble protein, P2-C is primarily myelin, and P2-I is primarily mitochondria.

membrane fractions continued to show increasing specific activity for 15 to 30 min after the cycloheximide block, while no further increase occurred in the soluble fraction and myelin. Only the cell-body mitochondrial fraction showed a continued protein synthesis up to 60 min. Although these experiments are based on rather complex systems, a reasonable interpretation of the data is that the continued increase of protein radioactivity in the membrane fractions after complete inhibition in the cytoplasmic fraction is the result of rapid transport to the membranes of proteins that were synthesized elsewhere in the initial 15-min period.

VI. ACETYLCHOLINESTERASE AND THE ACETYLCHOLINE RECEPTOR

We have recently focused our attention on the two membrane proteins, acetylcholinesterase and the receptor for acetylcholine, both of which are found in the postsynaptic membrane (Fig. 6). Chan, Shirachi, and Trevor (1972) have observed three oligomers for the purified acetylcholinesterase of the bovine caudate nucleus, with molecular weights of 130,000, 270,000, and 390,000. It is not yet known whether these represent polymers of an

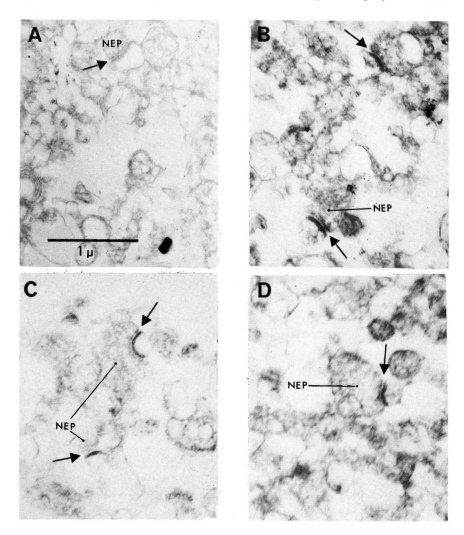

FIG. 6. Cytochemical localization of acetylcholinesterase (ACHase) on isolated synaptosomes (McBride and Cohen, 1972). The pellets were fixed in formaldehyde and stained for ACHase (Kasa and Csillik, 1966). (A): An example of a postsynaptic membrane that did not stain for ACHase. (B–D): Examples of postsynaptic membrane stained for ACHase.

identical subunit, but, by analogy with the observations of Leuzinger (1971) for the eel enzyme, they may represent $(\alpha\beta)_1$, $(\alpha\beta)_2$, and $(\alpha\beta)_3$.

Wenthold *(personal communication)* has examined the properties of ACHase from subcellular regions of rat brain. Extracts of purified ACHase from the synaptic membrane fractions of rat brain contain five distinct isoenzymes as determined by isoelectric focusing in polyacrylamide gels, but the enzymes extracted from the microsomal or soluble fractions of rat cortex contain only three isoenzymes. Although it is possible that such isoenzymes are formed during the extraction procedure, controls indicate that it is more likely that the enzyme is synthesized in one isoenzymic form and undergoes reaction after transport to the membrane to yield different forms, which are only partially dissociated upon extraction. Such a mechanism might be of general importance in membrane assembly. ACHase represents a type of protein intermediate to the more soluble hydrophilic proteins of the cytoplasm and the nonsoluble lipophilic proteins that constitute much of the membrane.

Study of the acetylcholine receptor protein (ACH—R) has been facilitated by the discovery that α-bungarotoxin and similar toxins bind to the R protein, even in its membrane-bound form, with a very low dissociation constant ($\sim 10^{-8}$ M). *Torpedo* tissue is the richest known source of this protein, as described elsewhere in this volume by Dr. Whittaker, and a great deal of work has been devoted to its isolation (Meunier and Olsen, 1971; Miledi and Potter, 1971; Raftery, Schmidt, Clark, and Wolcott, 1971).

Research on the acetylcholine receptor has been made difficult by the problem of distinguishing a small amount of specific binding with a low dissociation constant from a much larger amount of nonspecific binding with a much higher dissociation constant. A Scatchard plot of measurements of the adsorption of ^{14}C-acetylcholine on a proteolipid fraction extracted from eel electroplax (De Robertis, 1971) indicated that there was a small number of adsorbent sites with a dissociation constant of $\sim 10^{-7}$ M, but a much larger number with a considerably higher dissociation constant of $\sim 10^{-5}$ M. This same pattern appears repeatedly in studies of the binding of the various acetylcholine agonists and antagonists on synaptic membrane fractions. It is likely that the so-called "receptor proteins" of Bosmann (1972) and De Robertis (1971) belong to the group of membrane proteins having moderate affinities for bungarotoxin and acetylcholine, respectively, and do not represent the high-affinity physiological receptor itself. An additional point in support of this view is that calculations based on the work of Chan et al. (1972) yield a value of 15×10^{-12} moles/g wet weight tissue of ACHase in the ox caudate nucleus, although the amount of

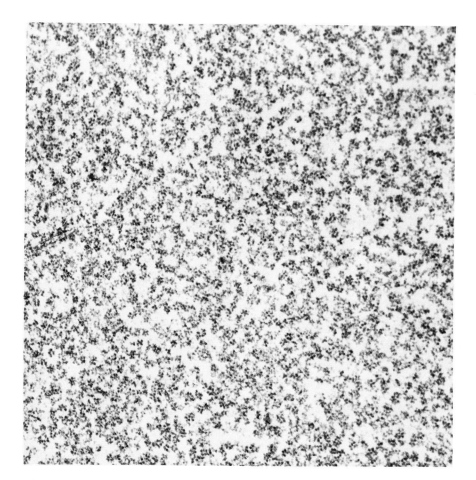

FIG. 7. Polysomes utilized for *in vitro* protein synthesis. It is possible to distinguish ribosomal chains, presumably linked by strands of messenger RNA.

receptor would be calculated to be 1,000 times greater based on the above data, a situation that appears highly unlikely.

We have found that at high concentrations ^{125}I-BTX is tenaciously held to intact membranes and is not removed by repeated washings with solutions of low ionic strength. Extraction with dilute detergent (e.g., 0.1% Triton X-100) removes most of the ^{125}I-BTX as free toxin, indicating that the toxin is only held tenaciously to an appreciable fraction of the membrane protein when the membrane is intact. In order to use ^{125}I-BTX to identify and titrate the ACH receptor, it is therefore necessary either to work at very low concentrations of BTX or to extract the receptor before studying its binding to the toxin.

TABLE 1. *Polysomal protein synthesizing systems*

	Munroe	Zomzely-Neurath, York, and Moore (1972)
NH_4Cl	105 m M	—
$MgCl_2$	6.25	5.0
KCl	6.25	100.0
(pH 7.6) Tris HCl	50.0	50.0
Dithiothreitol	0.75	1.0
ATP, Na salt	2.0	1.0
GTP, Na salt	1.0	1.0
Phosphocreatine	—	20.0
pH 5 enzymes	0.2 mg/ml	2.5
S-105 protein	1.0	1.3
Polysomes	0.1 mgP/ml	12 A_{260} units/ml
^{14}C amino acids	2.0 μC	1.0 μC

Like the esterase, the R protein readily polymerizes both in detergent and in the membrane matrix. This apparently insoluble lipophilic protein might be transported from its cytoplasmic site of synthesis to the synaptic membrane by carrier proteins that can temporarily solubilize such membrane proteins in monomeric form. Our results and those of Changeux, Meunier, and Huchet (1972) indicate that the monomer may have a molecular weight as low as 45,000, whereas the units extracted from the membrane have molecular weights of 180,000 or greater.

The systematic study of membrane proteins prepared in various detergents under various conditions of pH, ionic strength, and temperature is just beginning (Helenius and Simons, 1972). Detergent fractionations of this type should be valuable steps prior to analysis of the membrane proteins on polyacrylamide gels.

VII. SYNTHESIS OF BRAIN PROTEINS IN CELL-FREE SYSTEMS

The *in vitro* synthesis of membrane proteins in cell-free systems may lead to an understanding of the way in which these proteins are synthesized and are then altered or polymerized for incorporation into the membrane. The most striking achievement in this field to date is the recent synthesis of S-100 protein by Zomzely-Neurath, York, and Moore (1972), using a homologous preparation of brain ribosomes and messenger RNA. The approach taken by our laboratory has been to study the synthesis of tubulin, which is present in large amounts in brain protein extracts and which is analogous to the membrane proteins in displaying an assembly of subunits (Munroe, *personal communication*). The *in vitro* synthesis of tubulin has also been reported by Baxter and Raeburn (1971).

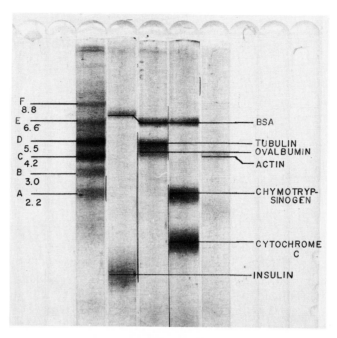

FIG. 8. Electrophoretic separation on SDS polyacrylamide gels of the vinblastine-precipitable material obtained from the supernatant of a rat brain cell-free protein synthesizing system. *(Left):* Polyacrylamide gel electrophoresis pattern of soluble proteins obtained

Munroe initially used the polysomal system of Campagnoni and Mahler (1967), but later included a supplement described by Zomzely-Neurath et al. (1972) which gave a higher activity. Figure 7 is an electron micrograph of the polysomes used in his protein synthesizing system, and the composition of the media used in our laboratory and by Zomzely-Neurath et al. is shown in Table 1. The polyribosomal preparation had an RNA/protein ratio of 0.61. This ratio and our electron micrographs indicate that any contamination with microsomal membranes is small.

The polysomal mixture is incubated for 1 to 2 hr at 37°C, then centrifuged to remove the polysomes. The supernatant is mixed with unlabeled supernatant that is dialyzed to remove sucrose and ions, and the tubulin is precipitated by 1 mM vinblastine. The vinblastine precipitable material represents approximately 30% of the TCA precipitable counts in the dialysate, and appears to represent the *in vitro* cell-free synthesis of tubulin (Fig. 8). Appreciable levels of other proteins are also present, one of which has some of the properties of nerve actin, whose synthesis has also been demonstrated in growing cultures of sympathetic neurons from chick embryo (Fine and Bray, 1971). Control experiments with liver polysomes do

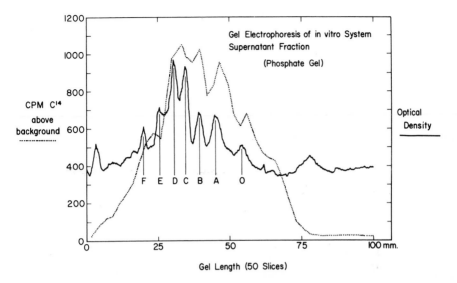

from a rat brain cell-free protein synthesizing system, with marker proteins to provide an approximate molecular weight scale. *(Right):* Radioactivity incorporation into the protein bands of the gel shown at left.

not show appreciable synthesis of either the tubulin-like or actin-like fractions.

APPENDIX A

THE EFFECT OF REUTILIZATION OF AMINO ACIDS FROM DEGRADATION OF BRAIN PROTEINS

Consider a simple pool model consisting of a single pool A of plasma amino acids and a single intracellular pool B in the brain.

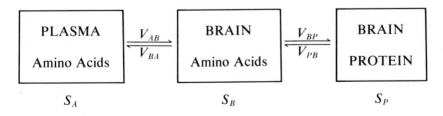

Let S denote specific activity and V rate of reaction as shown. The rate of change of radioactivity in the protein is

$$d(PS_p)/dt = V_{BP}S_B - V_{PB}S_P$$

In the stationary state $dP/dt = 0$ with protein concentration P,

$$V_{BP} = V_{PB} = k_{-1}P \qquad (1)$$

where k_{-1} is the specific rate of protein degradation. Hence,

$$dS_P/dt = k_{-1}P(S_B - S_P) \qquad (2)$$

The rate of change of labeled amino acid in pool B is

$$dB/dt = V_{AB}S_A - V_{BA}S_B - V_{BP}S_B + V_{PB}S_P \qquad (3)$$

In the stationary state,

$$V_{AB} - V_{BA} + V_{PB} - V_{BP} = 0 \qquad (4)$$

so that, from (1),

$$V_{AB} = V_{BA} \qquad (5)$$

Experimentally, the labels in A and B will often reach plateau values S_A^m and S_B^m while S_P is still negligible. Under these conditions, (1), (3) and (5) yield,

$$\frac{S_B^m}{S_A^m} = \frac{V_{AB}}{V_{AB} + V_{PB}} \qquad (6)$$

This is the expression used by Garlick and Marshall (1972) to estimate the fraction of the intracellular brain amino acid pool that comes from the plasma amino acids.

APPENDIX B

AVERAGING UPTAKE AND DECAY OF LABELED AMINO ACID OVER GROUPS OF PROTEINS

This analysis was given by Garlick and Millward as follows: the mass average specific turnover rate is

$$\bar{k} = \sum k_i m_i / M \qquad (1)$$

where m_i is the mass of protein i and $M = \sum m_i$ is the total mass of proteins in group. The increase in specific activity S_{Pi} in protein i is

$$dS_{Pi}/dt = k_i(S_B - S_{Pi}) \qquad (2)$$

where S_B is the specific activity of the amino acid in the intracellular pool. From (1) and (2),

$$\bar{k} = \sum \frac{dS_{Pi}}{dt} \frac{1}{S_B - S_{Pi}} \frac{m_i}{M} \qquad (3)$$

Initially $S_{Pi} = 0$ and (3) becomes

$$\bar{k} = \frac{1}{S_B} \sum \left(\frac{dS_{Pi}}{dt}\right)_{initial} \frac{m_i}{M} \tag{4}$$

Hence we see that the initial rate of uptake of label gives a true mass average specific turnover rate.

The initial label in a given protein is proportional to its specific turnover rate k_i, so that, with first order decay, the total label at time t becomes

$$C^*(t) = A \sum \frac{m_i}{M} k_i e^{-k_i t} \tag{5}$$

where A is a proportionality constant. This expression will not yield a linear plot of log C^* versus t unless all the k_i are the same.

APPENDIX C

THE DOUBLE-LABEL METHOD FOR DETERMINATION OF RELATIVE TURNOVER RATES OF PROTEINS (ARIAS ET AL., 1969)

Let t = time after administration of a given isotope. Let C_j and H_j refer to specific activities of ^{14}C and ^3H in a particular protein j.

Then the assumption of the Schimke method is that:

$$H_1(t) = \alpha \, C_1(t)$$
$$H_2(t) = \alpha \, C_2(t) \tag{1}$$

for any pair of proteins to be compared. In other words, since the proteins are all in steady states, the injection of the second isotope at time $t_2 > t_1$ (where t_1 is time of injection of first isotope) gives an activity proportional to an earlier point on the decay curve of the first isotope.

We measure

$$r_1 = H_1(t_1)/C_1(t_2)$$
$$r_2 = H_2(t_1)/C_2(t_2) \tag{2}$$

Therefore, from (1),

$$r_1 = \alpha \, C_1(t_1)/C_1(t_2)$$
$$r_2 = \alpha \, C_2(t_1)/C_2(t_2) \tag{3}$$

We take the ratio of ratios,

$$r_1/r_2 = \frac{C_1(t_1)/C_1(t_2)}{C_2(t_1)/C_2(t_2)} \tag{4}$$

But, assuming a pulse label has led to an initial activity C_0 at time $t_1 = 0$, the activity at any later time is:

$$C = C_0 e^{-k_0 t} \tag{5}$$

where k_0 is the degradation constant of the protein. Note also that in (4), since we take ratios, it makes no difference whether we take specific activity of tracer or total activity, since for a protein in a stationary state they remain always proportional.

Combining (4) and (5):

$$\frac{r_1}{r_2} = \frac{e^{-k_1 \Delta t}}{e^{-k_2 \Delta t}} = e^{-\Delta k_0 \Delta t} \tag{6}$$

or

$$\ln (r_1/r_2) = -\Delta k_0 \Delta t \tag{7}$$

Thus the log of a "Schimke ratio" for two proteins is proportional to the *difference* in the *rate constants* for degradation of the two proteins.

ACKNOWLEDGMENTS

This work has been supported by the National Institute of Neurological Diseases and Stroke (Grant NS08309) and the National Science Foundation (Grant GB17157). The research work from our laboratory is jointly directed with H. R. Mahler. I am indebted to Professor Mahler and Dr. R. Gurd for many useful discussions. I wish especially to thank our graduate students M. Maguire, S. Munroe, S. McGovern, A. Merel, and R. Wenthold, some of whose current research is included in this chapter.

REFERENCES

Arias, I. M., Doyle, D., and Schimke, R. T. (1969): Studies on the synthesis and degradation of proteins of the endoplasmic reticulum of rat liver. *Journal of Biological Chemistry,* 244:3303.

Baxter, C., and Raeburn, S. (1971): The synthesis *in vitro* of colchicine-binding protein. Paper presented at the 1971 meeting of the American Neurochemical Society.

Bosmann, H. B. (1972): Acetylcholine receptor. I. Identification and biochemical characteristics of a cholinergic receptor of guinea pig cerebral cortex. *Journal of Biological Chemistry,* 247:130.

Campagnoni, A. T., and Mahler, H. R. (1967): Isolation and properties of polyribosomes from cerebral cortex. *Biochemistry,* 6:956.

Chan, S. L., Shirachi, D. Y., and Trevor, A. J. (1972): Purification and properties of brain acetylcholinesterase. *Journal of Neurochemistry*, 19:437.

Changeux, J. P., Meunier, J.-C., and Huchet, M. (1972): Studies on the cholinergic receptor protein of *Electrophorus electricus*. *Molecular Pharmacology*, 7:538.

Cotman, C. W., Mahler, H. R., and Anderson, N. G. (1968): Isolation of a membrane fraction enriched in nerve-end membranes from rat brain by zonal centrifugation. *Biochimica et Biophysica Acta*, 163:272.

Dehlinger, P. J., and Schimke, R. T. (1971): Size distribution of membrane proteins of rat liver and their relative rates of degradation. *Journal of Biological Chemistry*, 246:2574.

De Robertis, E. (1971): Biology of synaptic receptors. *Science*, 171:963.

Fine, R. E., and Bray, D. (1971): Actin in growing nerve cells. *Nature New Biology*, 234:115.

Garlick, P. J., and Marshall, I. (1972): A technique for measuring brain protein synthesis. *Journal of Neurochemistry*, 19:577.

Garlick, P. J., Waterlow, J. C., and Millward, D. J. (1973): *Physiological Reviews, in press*.

Gurd, R. S., Mahler, H. R., and Moore, W. J. (1972): Differences in protein patterns on polyacrylamide-gel electrophoresis of neuronal membranes from mice of different strains. *Journal of Neurochemistry*, 19:553.

Helenius, A., and Simons, K. (1972): The binding of detergents to lipophilic and hydrophilic proteins. *Journal of Biological Chemistry*, 247:3656.

Hider, R. C., Fern, E. B., and London, D. R. (1971): The effect of insulin on free amino acid pools and protein synthesis in rat skeletal muscle *in vitro*. *Biochemical Journal*, 125:751.

Jones, D. A., and McIlwain, M. (1971): Amino acid production and translocation in incubated and superfused tissues from the brain. *Journal of Neurobiology*, 2:311.

Kasa, P., and Csillik, B. (1966): Electron microscopic localization of cholinesterase by a copper-lead-thiocholine technique. *Journal of Neurochemistry*, 13:1345.

Leuzinger, W. (1971): In: *Cholinergic Ligand Interactions*, edited by D. J. Triggle, J. F. Moran, and E. A. Barnard. Academic Press, New York.

McBride, W. J., and Cohen, H. (1972): Cytochemical localization of acetylcholinesterase on isolated synaptosomes. *Brain Research*, 41:489.

McIlwain, H., and Rodnight, R. (1962): *Practical Neurochemistry*. J. & A. Churchill, London.

Meunier, J. C., and Olsen, R. W. (1971): Some physical properties of the protein of the acetylcholine receptor studied by means of a radioactive neurotoxin. *Comptes Rendus de l'Academie des Sciences*, (Paris), D273:595.

Meunier, J. C., Olsen, R. W., Menez, A., Fromageot, P., and Boquet, P. (1972): Some physical properties of the cholinergic receptor protein from *Electrophorus electricus* revealed by a tritiated α-toxin from *Naja nigricollis* venom. *Biochemistry*, 11:1200.

Miledi, R., and Potter, L. T. (1971): Acetylcholine receptors in muscle fibres. *Nature*, 233:599.

Morris, S. J., Ralston, M. J., and Shooter, E. M. (1971): Effects of X-irradiation on the content of amino acids in the developing rat cerebellum. *Journal of Neurochemistry*, 18:2279.

Mortimore, G. E., Woodside, K. H., and Henry, J. E. (1972): Compartmentation of free valine and its relation to protein turnover in perfused rat liver. *Journal of Biological Chemistry*, 247:2776.

Orrego, F., and Lipmann, F. (1967): Protein synthesis in brain slices. *Journal of Biological Chemistry*, 242:665.

Poole, B. (1971): The kinetics of disappearance of labeled leucine from the free leucine pool of rat liver and its effect on the apparent turnover of catalase and other hepatic proteins. *Journal of Biological Chemistry*, 246:6587.

Raftery, M. A., Schmidt, J., Clark, D. G., and Wolcott, R. G. (1971): Demonstration of a specific α-bungarotoxin binding component in *Electrophorus electricus* electroplax membranes. *Biochemical and Biophysical Research Communications*, 45:1622.

Rechcigl, M. (1971): *Enzyme Synthesis and Degradation in Mammalian Systems*. S. Karger, Basel.

Von Hungen, K., Mahler, H. R., and Moore, W. J. (1968): Turnover of protein and ribonucleic acid in synaptic subcellular fractions from rat brain. *Journal of Biological Chemistry*, 243:1415.

White, F. P., McBride, W. J., Mahler, H. R., and Moore, W. J. (1972): Subcellular distribution of proteins synthesized in slices of rat cerebral cortex. *Journal of Biological Chemistry,* 247:1247.

Whittaker, V. P., Michaelson, I. A., and Kirkland, R. J. A. (1964): The separation of synaptic vesicles from nerve-ending particles ("synaptosomes"). *Biochemical Journal,* 90:293.

Yamamoto, C., and McIlwain, H. (1966): Electrical activities in thin sections from the mammalian brain maintained in chemically-defined media *in vitro. Journal of Neurochemistry,* 13:1333.

Zomzely-Neurath, C., York, C., and Moore, B. (1972): Synthesis of a brain-specific protein (S100 protein) in a homologous cell-free system programmed with cerebral polysomal messenger RNA. *Proceedings of the National Academy of Sciences,* 69:2326.

Proteins of the Nervous System
Raven Press, New York © 1973

Neuronal Proteins: Synthesis, Transport, and Neuronal Regulation

Samuel H. Barondes

The most common method of regulating cellular functions is to alter the activity of specific proteins within those cells. Although most known proteins are enzymes, others function as receptors, contractile proteins, regulators of gene expression, etc. Our knowledge of the mechanisms for changing the functional levels of cellular proteins is derived from general biological studies. Since it is clear that similar mechanisms are employed in the nervous system, these will first be reviewed as background for the more specialized studies which will be considered.

I. GENERAL MECHANISMS FOR CHANGING THE FUNCTIONAL LEVEL OF A PROTEIN

Five general ways of changing the activity of cellular proteins have been identified. The one which has received the greatest attention is to increase the actual amount of a given protein by increasing its rate of synthesis. A classic example of this type of regulation is the induction of an enzyme such as β-galactosidase in *Escherichia coli* (Watson, 1970), in which an inducer, lactose, initiates the synthesis of the messenger RNA which directs the synthesis of this particular enzyme. There is a great deal of evidence that mammalian cells also utilize this method of regulation, and that specific inducers may initiate or increase the synthesis of specific proteins, thus altering cellular function. In some cases the inducer may direct increased translation of an existent messenger RNA, which also leads to greater synthesis of the specific protein (Tomkins, Gelehrten, Granner, Martin, Samuels, and Thompson, 1969).

It is also possible to alter the functional activity of cellular proteins which have already been synthesized by inducing reversible or irreversible structural changes. Thus the second regulatory mechanism which will be considered involves reversible "allosteric" changes, in which the structure of a protein is transiently altered by its combination with a small molecule. The latter may be a product of a late step in a sequence of enzyme reactions and may influence an enzyme which catalyzes an early step. The reactivity of an enzyme toward its substrate is altered by the regulatory molecule. An example of such regulation in nervous system tissue is the feedback inhibition by norepinephrine of the enzyme tyrosine hydroxylase, which catalyzes the rate-limiting step in the biosynthesis of norepinephrine (Weiner, 1970). Norepinephrine thus regulates its own rate of synthesis. This method of regulation does not require protein synthesis and is characterized by a high degree of reversibility.

A third method for controlling protein activity is the irreversible cleavage of an inactive protein to produce an active molecule, as in the conversion of a proenzyme such as trypsinogen to trypsin. The residual protein undergoes an irreversible conformational change resulting in its activation.

Covalent addition of residues to a preexisting protein molecule is a fourth method of controlling function. This frequently alters the enzymatic action of the protein, and this mechanism undoubtedly operates in the nervous system. An example is protein phosphorylation in response to cyclic AMP, which results in enzyme activation (Walsh, Krebs, Reimann, Brostrom, Crobin, Hickenbottom, Soderling, and Perkins, 1970). The activation in this case is rapidly reversible. The addition of sugars to glycoproteins is another example of this type of regulation. It is not yet known if reversal of glycosylation plays a regulatory role.

The fifth known means of regulating the functional level of proteins is by changes in their rate of degradation (Schimke and Doyle, 1970) as described elsewhere in this volume by Dr. Walter Moore. Until recently, the process of degradation was ignored and it was assumed that regulation of the amount of a given protein occurred exclusively by alterations in synthesis.

II. METHODS FOR DETERMINING CHANGES IN THE FUNCTIONAL AND PHYSICAL AMOUNT OF A PROTEIN

The simplest and most specific method of studying such regulatory processes is by enzymatic assay. The activity of an enzyme can readily be measured in a crude mixture of proteins, and one can attempt to determine the functional activity of this enzyme under various conditions by purely enzymological methods. Various types of binding assays are also of great importance for such determinations. For example, the protein tubulin may have an enzymatic function, but it is best known by its ability to bind colchicine (Borisy and Taylor, 1967).

For proteins with no known enzymatic function, amount (but not state of activity) can be determined by taking advantage of a specific physical property. This approach has a long history in protein chemistry. For example, the gamma globulins were first discovered as an entity on the basis of their characteristic electrophoretic migration pattern. The S-100 protein described by Drs. Moore and Calissano in this volume was identified in much the same way. The use of a specific physical property such as electrophoretic mobility is frequently an excellent way to identify a particularly abundant protein, such as microtubular protein (Feit, Dutton, Barondes, and Shelanski, 1971), or one with an unusual physical property such as S-100.

Immunological methods are currently being widely used for the determination of protein levels. The preparation of an antibody to a highly purified protein can be used to assay the levels of protein available under specific circumstances. The availability of a precipitating antibody makes it possible to assay the relative amount of a protein which a tissue synthesizes in a given time period by exposing the tissue to radioactive amino acid, then precipitating the specific protein, and determining the amount of radioactivity which was incorporated. By comparing the relative amount of radioactive amino acid incorporated into the specific protein with that into all the other proteins of the tissue, its relative rate of synthesis can be determined (for a recent example see Levitan and Webb, 1970). The relative rate of synthesis can be compared in various experimental conditions.

III. THE DETERMINATION OF WHETHER PROTEIN SYNTHESIS PARTICIPATES IN A REGULATORY PROCESS

One reason that regulation of the nervous system by protein synthesis rather than by structural modification of proteins has received so much attention is that the technology for studying the general participation of protein synthesis in a specific regulatory response has been well developed. This is largely due to the availability of several highly potent inhibitors of protein synthesis which are as active in the brain as in other organs. Very extensive inhibition of brain protein synthesis is produced by the administration of cycloheximide or puromycin (Barondes, 1970). Cycloheximide is particularly favorable, since it is quite effective when administered subcutaneously, and in large doses it inhibits more than 95% of cerebral protein synthesis. It has therefore been possible to determine whether cerebral protein synthesis is required in such processes as memory storage, with no knowledge at all of which proteins might be involved. Potent inhibitors of RNA synthesis are also available. These include actinomycin-D, which inhibits all types of RNA synthesis (Barondes, 1970), and alpha amanitin, which inhibits the RNA polymerase II which participates in the synthesis of messenger RNA (Montanaro, Novello, and Stirpa, 1971). Both these antibiotics must be administered intracerebrally for maximal effect. As indicated above, regulation by means of protein synthesis may not be dependent on RNA synthesis, since the regulation may be at the level of translation of messenger RNA already present on ribosomes (Tomkins et al., 1969).

The use of inhibitors for studying the participation of protein synthesis in regulation of the brain is limited by the fact that the synthesis of all proteins is affected by these agents. What one would like to know is whether or not the synthesis of specific proteins is involved in a specific regulatory response. This can only be determined by examining the increased synthesis of the specific protein in question. Studies of this type have been useful primarily with enzymes, since a change in enzyme activity in a particular circumstance can be readily detected. Blockage of the change in the presence of a protein synthesis inhibitor is good evidence that the rate of synthesis of the enzyme has changed. Studies of rates of synthesis of specific proteins without known enzymatic function have been attempted by determining the incorporation of radioactive amino acid into them. Such studies are very difficult because radioactive amino acids are incorporated into a vast number of brain proteins, and the proteins in question may represent only a very small percentage of the total. Furthermore, the brain consists of a heterogeneous population of neuronal and glial cells, many of which may not be involved in the process of interest. For these reasons, most studies of brain protein synthesis as a regulatory response have looked at changes in overall levels of brain protein synthesis rather than at the synthesis of specific proteins. Although popular, such studies are difficult to interpret. If no change is found, it may be due to the fact that only a single protein or a group of proteins in a small number of cells are involved. Alternatively, if a change is found, one must take great care to be sure that it is not an artifact due to a change in the specific activity of the radioactive amino acid pool, as considered below.

IV. ESTIMATING THE RATE OF SYNTHESIS OF A BRAIN PROTEIN

The rate of brain protein synthesis can be examined following either intracerebral or subcutaneous administration of radioactive precursor. Intracerebral administration has the advantage of producing high levels of incorporation, and is of particular usefulness for pulse labeling studies, since the radioisotope level falls rapidly due to egress from the brain and cerebrospinal fluid, and rapid incorporation into protein (Barondes, 1968). However, this approach further increases nonuniform incorporation already present in brain tissue, because some regions are exposed to high concentrations of labeled amino acid while others are not exposed to the precursor to any significant extent. In addition, there is really no way to estimate the specific activity of the precursor pool, because the amount of the injected material that leaves the cerebrospinal fluid or the interstitial space and actually enters the brain cells is unknown.

Administration of radioactive amino acid via the subcutaneous, intravenous, or intraperitoneal route results in a gradually increasing brain level over a relatively long time period rather than an initial pulse. The major disadvantage of this method is that there is relatively little incorporation of label into brain protein, due to the blood-brain barrier and the enormous dilution in the whole body. The specific activity of the precursor pool can only be obtained from multiple determinations at many time points after administration of precursor. Ideally, the specific activity of radioactive amino acid incorporated in transfer-RNA (which is the immediate precursor of protein) should be determined at many time points. To facilitate studies of the specific activity of the precursor pool, it is preferable to use ^{14}C-labeled amino acid rather than ^{3}H-labeled precursors, due to extensive tritium exchange (Banker and Cottman, 1971). It is also preferable to use carboxyl-labeled ^{14}C precursors rather than uniformly labeled ^{14}C amino acids, because the initial step in amino acid metabolism is usually decarboxylation, and the label will be lost as CO_2 rather than complicating the data by its presence in many metabolites.

Because of the many limitations of these types of studies, convincing results can only be obtained by showing *relative* changes in the rates of synthesis of different classes of brain proteins. Such classes can be crudely separated by subcellular fractionation and then further fractionated on the basis of their size or charge by gel filtration, column chromatography, electrophoresis, and other means of protein fractionation. The finding of increased incorporation of radioactive amino acid into a restricted class of products and no change in others argues strongly against the change being due to an alteration in the specific radioactivity of the amino acid pool. Furthermore, such studies may lead to the identification of the proteins whose synthesis is affected. Work of this type will certainly be more productive than measurement of the incorporation of radioactive amino acid into brain proteins as a whole.

V. THE REGULATION OF INTERNEURONAL RELATIONSHIPS BY PROTEIN METABOLISM

A. The Problem of Regulation of Specific Regions of a Single Neuron

Although the greater part of neuronal protein metabolism is undoubtedly involved with maintaining the life of the cell, the aspects of brain protein metabolism that are most pertinent to specialized brain functions are involved in regulating interneuronal relationships and synaptic efficacy. Since some neurons have thousands of nerve terminals and thousands of dendrite sites for synapses, the special problem is posed of regulation of *specific regions* of a neuron, i.e., of specific terminals or dendritic patches. Let us consider two neurons, A and B, and the case in which a nerve terminal from A forms a synapse on a dendrite of B. Induction of synthesis of a specific protein in cell A might alter the concentration of this protein in its cell body, dendrites, and nerve terminals after the new protein had been distributed throughout the cell. To increase the specific consequences of increased synthesis of this protein, it is possible that it would be preferentially transported in the axon and localized primarily in the nerve terminals. However, it is difficult to imagine this as being specific for the one of many terminals of cell A. The same two alternatives hold for cell B, i.e., either a general or localized alteration in the cellular protein composition. In this case one would most likely be concerned with the biosynthesis of a specific dendritic protein, possibly part of the receptor mechanism. Again, it is difficult to imagine how such a change in the cell body of B could be made specific for the A → B contact without also affecting other synaptic connections.

This has led to a consideration of ways in which greater selectivity could be incorporated into a response to a changing environment, either by biosynthesis of material at the appropriate nerve terminal in cell A or in the dendrite of cell B. Of these, the dendrite appears to be a much more likely site of local protein synthesis, since ribosomes are present in this region. The protein synthetic machinery associated with these ribosomes could be activated without new RNA synthesis and participation of the nucleus. There are numerous examples in mammals of increased protein synthesis that utilizes stable messenger RNA (Tomkins et al., 1969) without the concurrent induction of new messenger RNA that is characteristic of bacterial systems. Because the axon and nerve terminal appear to be completely devoid of ribosomes, presynaptic regulation of synaptic function by protein synthesis at nerve terminals would seem unlikely. It remains possible that there are ribosomes in the synaptic membrane that are concealed in some as yet unknown manner, but there is no convincing evidence to support such a possibility. The status of studies of protein synthesis at nerve endings will be considered below.

It should also be pointed out that the type of specificity which is being considered may not be required for regulation of specific interneuronal pathways. These are characterized by considerable overlap. If the problem is reformulated as one in which there is an alteration in the relationship between a *class* of cells A to that of a *class* of cells B, then each of the cells in one or the other class may show changes in the protein composition of all its nerve terminals or dendrites although still selectively facilitating its relationship. This can occur because the *net* relationship between A and B will be greatly facilitated, due to the overlap of many members of A on B. However, the relationship of all the A cells or B cells to others may not be significantly changed since they may represent only occasional members of many other classes.

B. Axoplasmic Transport

Although local protein synthesis at nerve terminals could have important regulatory consequences, it is clear that the nerve cell body is presently the only established source of nerve ending proteins. These are transported in the axoplasm. Several methods have been used for studying this process (Barondes, 1969).

The first method used for this purpose was the axonal ligation technique, in which studies were made of the rate and composition of material which accumulates at the proximal side of the ligated axon. This approach has been useful for the study of enzymes and organelles. Since ligation is disruptive and could produce artifacts, it has been avoided (and is unnecessary) in studies in which radioactive labeling techniques are used (Barondes, 1969). These techniques all involve injection of a radioactive substance, usually an amino acid, into the region of nerve cell bodies and subsequent observation of the migration of radioactive products, such as proteins, into the axon and to the nerve terminals. A favorite site of injection is the eye, since this permits labeling of retinal ganglion cells and studies of transport of protein through the optic nerve to the optic tectum. The rate of appearance of products along the nerve and at the nerve terminals can be followed, and the radioactive proteins can be fractionated by electrophoresis, gel filtration, chromatography, or other methods.

Most studies of axoplasmic transport have been made with cranial nerves or peripheral nerves, since long nerve segments are readily accessible. Studies of axoplasmic transport in the central nervous system are more difficult but the conceptual basis is quite similar. Droz (1969) examined the migration of proteins along the axons of specified neurons using autoradiography. Other studies have been based on isolation of nerve ending particles from brain at various times after the injection of radioactive precursor to determine the arrival of proteins of various kinds (Barondes, 1969). Since the nerve terminals and cell bodies are both exposed to precursor, this technique permits evaluation both of transport of protein to nerve terminals and also of local synthesis of protein at nerve terminals. Unfortunately, the latter is particularly difficult to evaluate, because nerve ending fractions are contaminated by other brain components.

An adaptation of the techniques used in the peripheral nervous system was recently described (Fibiger, Pudritz, McGeer, and McGeer, 1972) in which a few microliters of material containing radioactive precursor is stereotaxically introduced into a specific brain nucleus, and the appearance of radioactivity is determined at the next point of synaptic connection in a pathway. For example, radioactive protein gradually appears in the caudate nucleus after introduction of precursor into the substantia nigra, as the result of transport along an anatomically documented pathway. It is therefore possible to study the rate of axoplasmic transport along known internuncial systems in the brain. This raises the possibility in these known pathways of studying the effects of functional changes on the transport of substances along them.

The studies of axoplasmic transport have thus far produced several major findings. The first is that there are two obvious rates of axoplasmic transport, "fast" and "slow" (McEwen and Grafstein, 1968; Ochs, 1972), although there may be several others with intermediate rates (Karlsson and Sjöstrand, 1971a). The rate of fast transport varies with species and nerve and may vary between peripheral and central nervous system, but it tends to be several hundred millimeters per day, whereas the slow transport rate tends to be in the range of one to several millimeters per day (Ochs, 1972). The two processes are therefore separated by two orders of magnitude.

The composition of material transported by these two systems differs markedly. The proteins in the fast component are primarily associated with particles, although there are some soluble components, whereas more of the proteins transported in the slow component are soluble (McEwen and Grafstein, 1968). Glycoproteins are a prominent component of the rapidly transported material (Forman, McEwen, and Grafstein, 1971; Karlsson and Sjöstrand, 1971b; Zatz and Barondes, 1971). Microtubular protein represents a large percentage of the total soluble protein transported to nerve endings by the slow component (Feit et al., 1971).

The mechanism of axoplasmic transport remains obscure. It is known that protein synthesis is not required, at least for slow axoplasmic transport. Transport of previously labeled material will continue normally even after protein synthesis is inhibited by more than 95% (Barondes, 1968). Neither is the cell body required for this process, since transport occurs normally in an isolated axon following ligation near the cell soma or following transfer of the axon to an *in vitro* medium (Ochs, 1972). There is thus no motive force present in the neuronal soma that is required for the propulsion of substances to the nerve terminal. Energy is required for transport, and various inhibitors of oxidative phosphorylation block the transport process (Ochs, 1972). Colchicine and vinblastine block both fast and slow axoplasmic transport, either after local application along a nerve or administration to the region of cell bodies (Ochs, 1972). The last observation gave rise to a great deal of speculation about the role of microtubules in the propulsion of axoplasm, but the interpretation of these observations is unclear. In at least one well-documented situation, that of the crayfish central nervous system (Fernandez, Burton, and Samson, 1971), the application of colchicine completely stopped both slow and fast axoplasmic transport, but had no effect on the morphology of microtubules in glutaraldehyde-fixed preparations. However, this does not rule out the possible participation of microtubules in transport. Indeed most workers in the area of axoplasmic transport believe that the tubules or a contractile protein associated with neurons may be the motive force for axoplasmic transport (see Shelanski, *this volume*).

C. Regulation of Nerve Ending Function by Axoplasmic Transport

Given the known high rates of fast axoplasmic transport and the fact that interneurons in the central nervous system often have short axons, changes in the biosynthesis of proteins in nerve cell bodies could rapidly influence their nerve terminals. For example, given a rate of rapid transport of 240 mm/day, material could be transferred from the cell soma to the terminal within 1 hr in a neuron whose axon is 10 mm in length, in 6 min for a 1-mm axon, and in 36 sec for one 100 μ in length. In this view, the commonly held notion that the nerve cell body is functionally quite distant from the nerve terminal is incorrect. Rather, many of the interneurons in the nervous system are readily accessible to regulation by a change in the level of specific proteins that occurs in their cell bodies. Indeed, within 15 min after injection of radioactive leucine, isolated nerve endings are extensively labeled (Droz and Barondes, 1969), probably by transport of proteins from their cell bodies. It should also be pointed out that control would most likely result from a change in composition rather than a change in the rate of transport, since the latter would increase the arrival of all proteins at nerve terminals, whereas the consequence of the former would be highly selective.

D. Local Protein Synthesis at the Nerve Terminal

As is indicated above, this subject has received a great deal of attention, because it would provide a mechanism for regulating a specific nerve terminal. Studies of local protein synthesis in nerve terminals have mostly been done *in vitro,* using the synaptosomal fractions described elsewhere in this volume by Drs. Whittaker and Morgan. The incorporation of radioactive amino acid into protein by these fractions can be demonstrated under a variety of conditions. It also seems fairly clear that the mitochondria contained within the nerve ending, like mitochondria in general, can synthesize a restricted group of proteins. These are proteins required for mitochondrial function, but alterations in their synthesis could conceivably regulate nerve ending function. However, major attention has been directed to the possibility of nonmitochondrial protein synthesis, since this is considered more likely to play a regulatory role.

The major difficulty in interpreting studies of protein synthesis by nerve ending fractions is their contamination not only with mitochondria, but also with various kinds of membranes and a small but significant number of ribosome-containing vesicles presumably derived from endoplasmic reticulum. Indeed much of the *in vitro* protein synthesis found with synaptosomal fractions has been shown to be attributable to contaminants by electron microscope radioautography of the fraction after incubation with radioactive precursor. For example, Gambetti, Autilio-Gambetti, Gonatas, and Shafer (1972) found that almost half of the radioactivity remaining in the synaptosomal fraction after extensive washing was present in ribosome-containing vesicles, approximately 20% was associated with mitochondria, and the remainder was associated with nerve ending membranes. However, it is exceedingly difficult to conclusively demonstrate that this residual portion represents true protein synthesis rather than the absorption of amino acid or an interconversion of tritium into some other membrane product, particularly since only a tiny fraction of the radioactive precursor added to the incubation mixture was found to be incorporated into insoluble products after extensive washing.

Another attempt to contend with the problem of contamination has been made by contrasting the radioactive products synthesized by the nerve ending fraction with those made by microsomes or mitochondria, which are the major contaminants with known protein synthesizing capacity. Using this strategy, Ramirez, Levitan, and Mushynski (1972) have found that a fraction containing nerve ending membranes incorporates radioactive amino acid into only three distinct classes of protein products as determined by polyacrylamide gel electrophoresis, in contrast with the products incorporated by a mitochondrial fraction. This incorporation is totally inhibited by choloramphenicol, which inhibits mitochondrial but not microsomal protein synthesis. Using a similar strategy, unique proportions of radioactive products were found in the nerve ending fraction by Gilbert (1972) but incorporation in this system was inhibited by cycloheximide, which inhibits microsomal protein synthesis, and not by chloramphenicol. Whereas both reports are consistent with selective synthesis of certain products by the nerve ending fraction, the discrepancy between them indicates the need for further work to resolve this question. A similar strategy has been employed to study the incorporation of radioactive glucosamine into protein by nerve ending fractions (Dutton, Haywood, and Barondes, 1973). Although the evidence indicates that incorporation of glucosamine can be attributed to nerve ending particles rather than contaminants, much of the incorporated glucosamine is found associated with the mitochondria obtained by lysis of the nerve ending fraction.

VI. SUMMARY

Because of its regulatory functions, protein metabolism is of great importance in the nervous system. Mechanisms of regulation of amounts and functions of proteins are briefly reviewed and the techniques of evaluating protein metabolism in the nervous system are summarized. Regulation of nerve ending function by alterations in the composition of proteins transported in the axoplasm is considered and it is emphasized that in brain a change in the synthesis of proteins in the nerve cell body could influence the nerve ending in a matter of seconds. The status of current work on the possibility of nonmitochondrial protein synthesis at nerve endings is considered briefly.

REFERENCES

Banker, G., and Cotman, C. W. (1971): Characteristics of different amino acids as protein precursors in mouse brain: Advantages of certain carboxyl-labeled amino acids. *Archives of Biochemistry and Biophysics,* 142:565.

Barondes, S. H. (1968): Further studies of the transport of proteins to nerve endings. *Journal of Neurochemistry,* 15:343–350.

Barondes, S. H. (1969): Axoplasmic transport. In: *Handbook of Neurochemistry, Vol. II,* edited by A. Lajtha, pp. 435–446. Plenum Press, New York.

Barondes, S. H. (1970): Cerebral protein synthesis inhibitors block long-term memory. *International Review of Neurobiology,* 12:177–205.

Borisy, G., and Taylor, E. W. (1967): The mechanism of action of colchicine, binding of colchicine-^{3}H to cellular protein. *Journal of Cell Biology,* 34:525–533.

Droz, B. (1969): Protein metabolism in nerve cells. *International Review of Cytology,* 25:363–390.

Droz, B., and Barondes, S. H. (1969): Nerve endings: Rapid appearance of labeled protein shown by electron microscope radioautography. *Science,* 165:1131.

Dutton, G. R., Haywood, P., and Barondes, S. H. (1973): ^{14}C glucosamine incorporation into specific products in the nerve ending fraction *in vivo* and *in vitro. Brain Research, in press.*

Feit, H., Dutton, G. R., Barondes, S. H., and Shelanski, M. L. (1971): Microtubule protein: Identification in and transport to nerve endings. *Journal of Cell Biology,* 51:138–147.

Fernandez, H. L., Burton, P. R., and Samson, F. E. (1971): Axoplasmic transport in the crayfish nerve cord: The role of fibrillar constituents of neurons. *Journal of Cell Biology,* 51:176.

Fibiger, H. C., Pudritz, R. C., McGeer, P. L., and McGeer, E. G. (1972): Axonal transport in nigro-striatal and nigro-thalamic neurons: Effects of medial forebrain bundle lesions and 6-hydroxydopamine. *Journal of Neurochemistry,* 19:1697.

Forman, D. S., McEwen, B. S., and Grafstein, B. (1971): Rapid transport of radioactivity in goldfish optic nerve following injections of labeled glucosamine. *Brain Research,* 28:119–130.

Gambetti, P., Autilio-Gambetti, L. A., Gonatas, N. K., and Shafer, B. (1972): Protein synthesis in synaptosomal fractions: Ultrastructural radioautographic study. *Journal of Cell Biology,* 52:526.

Gilbert, J. M. (1972): Evidence for protein synthesis in synaptosomal membranes. *Journal of Biological Chemistry,* 247:6451.

Karlsson, J. O., and Sjöstrand, J. (1971a): Synthesis, migration and turnover of protein in retinal ganglion cells. *Journal of Neurochemistry,* 18:749.

Karlsson, J. O., and Sjöstrand, J. (1971b): Rapid intracellular transport of fucosi-containing glycoproteins in retinal ganglion cells. *Journal of Neurochemistry,* 18:2209.

Levitan, I. B., and Webb, T. E. (1970): Hydrocortisone-mediated changes in the concentration of tyrosine transaminase in rat liver: An immunochemical study. *Journal of Molecular Biology,* 48:339.

McEwen, B. S., and Grafstein, B. (1968): Fast and slow components in axonal transport of protein. *Journal of Cell Biology,* 38:494.

Montanaro, N., Novello, F., and Stirpe, F. (1971): Effect of alpha amanitin on ribonucleic acid polymerase II of rat brain nuclei and on retention of avoidance conditioning. *Biochemical Journal,* 125:1087.

Ochs, S. (1972): Fast transport of materials in mammalian nerve fibers. *Science,* 176:252.

Ramirez, G., Levitan, I. B., and Mushynski, W. E. (1972): Highly purified synaptosomal membranes from rat brain; incorporation of amino acid into membrane proteins *in vitro. Journal of Biological Chemistry,* 247:5382.

Schimke, R. J., and Doyle, D. (1970): Control of enzyme level in animal tissues. *Annual Review of Biochemistry,* 39:777.

Tomkins, G. M., Gelehrten, T., Granner, D., Martin, D., Samuels, H., and Thompson, E. (1969): Control of specific gene expression in higher organisms. *Science,* 166:1474.

Walsh, D. A., Krebs, E. G., Reimann, E. M., Brostrom, M. A., Crobin, J. D., Hickenbottom, J. P., Soderling, T. R., and Perkins, J. P. (1970): The receptor protein for cyclic AMP in the control of glycogenolysis. In: *Advances in Biochemical Psychopharmacology,* Vol. 3, edited by P. Greengard and E. Costa, pp. 265–285. Raven Press, New York.

Watson, J. D. (1970): *The Molecular Biology of the Gene.* Benjamin Press, New York.

Weiner, N. (1970): Regulation of norepinephrine biosynthesis. *Annual Review of Pharmacology,* 10:273.

Zatz, M., and Barondes, S. H. (1971): Rapid transport of fucosyl glycoproteins to nerve endings in mouse brain. *Journal of Neurochemistry,* 18:1125.

Proteins of the Nervous System
Raven Press, New York © 1973

Microtubules

Michael L. Shelanski*

I. INTRODUCTION

During the past decade, neurochemistry has followed the general trend in biochemistry toward subcellular correlation and moved from the analysis of the composition and activities of the total brain and its larger anatomical subdivisions to studies which are based on separation into cell types, portions of cells, and organelles. This change in emphasis is due in no small part to the refined techniques of electron microscopy and to the combination of microscopic and biochemical techniques for the separation of neurons, glia, synaptosomes, mitochondria, myelin, and other specialized fractions of nervous tissue. The application of cell culture techniques has also been of considerable importance in defining our chemical studies. Synaptosomal and cell culture approaches are both discussed in depth elsewhere in this volume by Dr. Herschman.

Although investigations of this sort have led to many interesting findings, we will confine our discussion to the microtubule, whose existence was unknown prior to the application of electron microscopy to the nervous system. Electron microscopic studies of the brain have shown that neurons are rich in long, unbranched, 240 Å diameter tubular structures (Fig. 1). These structures are identical in appearance to the microtubules of the mitotic spindle and the sperm flagellum. Microtubules are also found in the Schwann cells and mesaxon and in immature astrocytes (Peters, Palay, and Webster, 1970; Raine and Wisniewski, 1970), although rarely in mature astrocytes. While these structures are clearly not unique to brain tissue, their abundance in brain has led many neurobiologists to postulate important structural and functional roles for them.

The subunit protein of microtubules — tubulin — was originally described as a colchicine-binding protein. The initial isolation was performed from flagellar and ciliary microtubules (Shelanski and Taylor, 1967, 1968; Renaud, Rowe, and Gibbons, 1968; Stephens, 1968*a,b*), but it was apparent from comparative studies on colchicine-binding activity that brain and

---

* Present address: Department of Neurology and Neuropathology, Harvard Medical School, Boston, Mass. 02115.

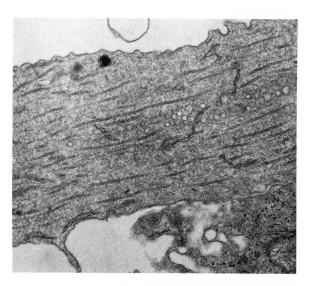

FIG. 1. Microtubules in a neurite of a neuroblastoma-glioblastoma hybrid. (Courtesy of Dr. M. Daniels.)

axoplasm were extraordinarily rich in this material (Borisy and Taylor, 1967*a,b;* Weisenberg, Borisy, and Taylor, 1968). More recent studies have shown tubulin to represent 15 to 40% of the soluble protein of brain extracts, depending on the species and age of the brain (Dutton and Barondes, 1969; Feit, Dutton, Barondes, and Shelanski, 1971; Bamburg, Shooter, and Wilson, 1973). Neuroblastoma cells in clonal culture are also very rich in tubulin (Olmsted, Witman, Carlson, and Rosenbaum, 1971). The abundance of tubulin, combined with the larger number of formed microtubules in the nervous system and the demonstration of relatively rapid turnover of the subunits (Feit, 1971), has reinforced the idea that tubulin and microtubules play an important role in nerve function.

The plant alkaloids colchicine and vinblastine bind to tubulin and cause an arrest of mitosis at metaphase. This is accompanied by a loss of spindle birefringence due to depolymerization of the spindle microtubules (Inoue, 1964). Colchicine produces a reversible depolymerization of microtubules in a variety of cell types (Porter, 1966), and similar effects are seen with other antimitotic alkaloids. Microtubules are also reversibly depolymerized by low temperatures (Tilney and Porter, 1967) and high hydrostatic pressures (Tilney, Hiramoto, and Marsland, 1966). Heavy water (D_2O) has the effect of stabilizing microtubules. Neural microtubules are similarly affected by colchicine and vinblastine (Wisniewski, Shelanski, and Terry, 1968). The homology between spindle tubules and neurotubules was initially demonstrated by Gonatas and Robbins (1964) and appears to hold on a biochemical as well as a structural basis.

II. PHARMACOLOGICAL OBSERVATIONS

Colchicine and vinblastine have been used extensively to study the role of microtubules in neuronal function. These experiments are subject to limitations; without very stringent controls, it is hard to be certain that the effects are exclusively on microtubules and that the microtubules are depolymerized or otherwise affected at all.

A number of workers have investigated the action of colchicine on axoplasmic flow (Karlsson and Sjöstrand, 1969; Kreutzberg, 1969; Fernandez, Burton, and Samson, 1971). The results indicate that both slow and fast flow can be abolished by colchicine or by vinblastine at reasonably low concentrations. Treatment with these agents is often accompanied by a tremendous proliferation of 100 Å diameter filaments and, in the case of the vinca alkaloids, by the formation of large paracrystalline structures in the cell body (Wisniewski et al., 1968; Bensch and Malawista, 1969), and it is possible that some of the effect on flow may be a mechanical damming action. In another case, the crayfish axon, flow is disrupted without complete disruption of the microtubules (Fernandez et al., 1971). These experiments have strongly implicated the microtubules in axoplasmic flow, but no evidence exists for the manner in which they function. They could be part of the motile apparatus or simply a means of keeping flow in an orderly pattern.

Colchicine also inhibits, reversibly, the outgrowth of axons from neuroblasts (Seeds, Gilman, Amano, and Nirenberg, 1970; Daniels, 1972, 1973) and neuroblastoma cells. This outgrowth can occur to an extent in the absence of protein synthesis and suggests that a considerable pool of microtubule subunits and other axon precursors must exist prior to neurite extension. This is almost identical to the behavior seen in the regenerating flagellum (Rosenbaum and Carlson, 1969).

Higher concentrations of colchicine and vinblastine have been reported to inhibit neurotransmitter release (Thoa, Wooten, Axelrod, and Kopin, 1972) and the release of hormones from a variety of endocrine cells (Lacy, Howell, Young, and Fick, 1968; Williams and Wolff, 1970). This inhibition has been proposed to be due to microtubule mediation of the release function. However, the doses of alkaloid used are often far above the minimum necessary for microtubule depolymerization and the question of side effects has not been satisfactorily answered. In the past few years the development of studies on muscle proteins in nonmuscle cells has progressed rapidly. A number of groups (Adelman and Taylor, 1969*a,b;* Weihing and Korn, 1969) have purified actin- and myosin-like proteins from slime molds, amoeba, and other cell types. Berl and Puszkin (1970) have worked on actin- and myosin-like proteins from brain and other workers have reported finding actin in neurons (Fine and Bray, 1971) and neuroblastoma cells. Recently, Berl and his co-workers have shown an exceptionally high concentration of actin- and myosin-like proteins in synaptosomes and have postulated a key role for these molecules in transmitter release (Berl, Puszkin, and Nicklas, 1973). Actin filaments are 50 to 60 Å in diameter, and thin filaments of this type are seen only rarely in neurons, except at the tip of the outgrowing axon (Tennyson, 1970; Yamada, Spooner, and Wessels, 1971). They are thinner than the 90 to 100 Å diameter neurofilaments and can bind heavy meromyosin in characteristic "arrowhead" complexes (Ishakawa, Bischoff, and Holtzer, 1969).

Colchicine has also been reported to destroy the clumping of concanavalin A binding sites on the surfaces of transformed cells (Ukena and Berlin, 1972).

The drugs colchicine and vinblastine bind to different sites on the tubulin molecule (Wilson, 1970), yet seem to affect the functions discussed here in similar ways. Whether any of these effects is due to a primary role of microtubules or whether they are secondary or tertiary effects is still to be ascertained.

Agents such as the nerve growth factor and cyclic AMP, which promote neuronal differentiation (Hsie and Puck, 1971), also promote the assembly of microtubules. Recent experiments indicate that dibutyryl cyclic AMP treatment might also decrease the susceptibility of microtubules to depolymerization at low temperature (Kirkland and Burton, 1972). Insulin promotes microtubular assembly in fat cells (Soifer, Brown, and Hechter, 1971) and in embryonic lens epithelia (Piatagorsky, Rothschild, and Wollberg, 1973); in the latter case this occurs in spite of a general depression of synthetic activity in the cell. Although it is likely that these agents affect microtubule assembly only indirectly, perhaps through mediation by calcium, it is interesting that considerable sequence homology has been reported between nerve growth factor and pro-insulin (Frazier, Angeletti, and Bradshaw, 1972).

This discussion of agents affecting microtubules is far from complete, but it does serve to illustrate the variety of neuronal functions which might be related to microtubules.

III. CHEMISTRY OF TUBULIN

A. Physical Chemical Features

Tubulin, the microtubular subunit, is a protein which has a molecular weight of 110,000 daltons and a sedimentation velocity of 6 Svedbergs (Shelanski and Taylor, 1967; Renaud et al., 1968; Weisenberg et al., 1968). On denaturation in 6 M guanidine-HCl or 8 M urea, the molecular weight falls to 55,000, suggesting that the native 6S species is a dimer composed of monomers of approximately equal molecular weights. On certain disc gel electrophoresis systems, the monomers are seen to run as separate closely spaced bands. Analysis of these bands reveals that the two subunits of the dimer are nonidentical on the basis of amino acid composition (Bryan and Wilson, 1971) and of peptide maps (Feit, Slusarek, and Shelanski, 1971; Fine, 1971). Thus far the subunits have not been resolved under less drastic conditions than sodium dodecyl sulfate or urea treatment.

Tubulin is an acidic protein with an isoelectric point in the range of 5.2 to 5.4. It appears that as many as four distinct tubulin subunit polypeptides of similar size may exist in brain, with perhaps five in cilia and flagella (Olmsted et al., 1971). The chemical relationship between the various chains visualized on isoelectric focusing has not been worked out.

Tubulin has no associated lipids. A number of workers (Falxa and Gill, 1969; Goodman, Rasmussen, DiBella, and Guthrow, 1970; Feit et al., 1971; Margolis, Margolis, and Shelanski, 1972) have reported small amounts of sugars in tubulin preparations. However, recent results by Eipper (1972) suggest that these sugars may be contaminants in the purification, and her tubulin preparations show only the faintest traces of sugars.

B. Nucleotide Binding

Microtubules from the cilia of *Tetrahymena* were demonstrated by Stephens, Renaud, and Gibbons (1967) to have 2 moles of guanine nucleotide bound per mole of tubulin dimer (120,000 g). A mixture of GTP and GDP was found, with some smaller amounts of GMP. Weisenberg et al. (1968) found that tubulin purified from brain had one molecule of guanine nucleotide, either GTP or GDP, tightly bound per 6S dimer and that this dimer was capable of binding another molecule of GTP in exchange with GTP in the incubation medium. This binding was fairly selective, with far lower levels of binding seen when either GDP or ATP was used. The tightly bound nucleotide does not exchange with GTP in the incubation medium even though the exchangeable site does so readily. However, neither nucleotide is covalently bound and both are released on acid precipitation of the protein. It is tempting to think of these sites as being allocated one to each monomer of the dimer. However, there is no evidence to support such an allocation at present, since all methods used to date to separate the monomers cause a total loss of nucleotide binding activity.

There is no competition between colchicine binding and nucleotide binding. In fact, GTP, GDP, and GMPPCP all stabilize colchicine binding and tubulin secondary structure against thermal denaturation (Ventilla, Cantor, and Shelanski, 1972).

C. Colchicine Binding

The hallmark of the cytoplasmic tubulin molecule has been its ability to bind the antimitotic alkaloid colchicine. Colchicine is bound directly to the 6S dimer but apparently not to nonspecific aggregates of tubulin (Shelanski and Taylor, 1968). There have been no clear reports of colchicine binding to the tubulin monomer, but there have been repeated suggestions of a smaller colchicine binding species. Borisy (1966) occasionally saw colchicine binding activity at 2.5S in brain extracts, and Robbins and Shelanski (1969) saw a rapidly migrating colchicine-binding peak on disc gel electrophoresis which had a sedimentation velocity in the 2.5S range when eluted from gels. Recently, Hammond and Bryan (1972) found that covalent linkage of a colchicine derivative to tubulin preparations resulted in the binding of the analogue to a low molecular weight entity. Whether this binding is to the monomer, to a colchicine binding peptide split from the dimer, or to an unrelated protein has not yet been determined.

Colchicine binds to a site on tubulin which is independent of the binding sites for GTP and the vinca alkaloids, but which appears to be identical with the site at which podophyllotoxin, another antimitotic alkaloid, acts (Wilson, 1970). The colchicine binding activity is labile under conditions traditionally used for tubulin purification, but can be stabilized indefinitely by the addition of sucrose to a final concentration of about 1 M (Frigon and Lee, 1972).

D. Tubulin Interactions with Vinblastine

Vinblastine, like colchicine, induces the depolymerization of cytoplasmic microtubules. However, it also causes the formation of large paracrystalline structures in the cytoplasm of treated cells (Bensch and Malawista, 1969). Vinblastine binds to tubulin (Owellen, Owens, and Donigian, 1972; Ventilla, 1972) and induces an ordered aggregation in solutions of purified tubulin (Weisenberg and Timasheff, 1970). The tubulin is precipitated in the presence of adequate concentrations of vinblastine and magnesium (Marantz, Ventilla, and Shelanski, 1969), and this precipitation can be used to purify tubulin from high-speed supernatants of brain homogenates (Olmsted, Carlson, Klebe, Ruddle, and Rosenbaum, 1970). The precipitates have a highly ordered paracrystalline structure closely resembling the structures seen in cells treated with vinblastine (Bensch, Marantz, Wisniewski, and Shelanski, 1969; Marantz and Shelanski, 1970). The paracrystals of tubulin may be dissolved by removal of vinblastine and magnesium, resulting in a species having a sedimentation velocity of 28–30S. It has not been possible to recover the native 6S form from tubulin purified in this manner.

Although vinblastine-induced assembly is a far cry from assembly into normal-appearing microtubules, it is useful for biochemical studies of the assembly process. Vinblastine-induced assembly proceeds only slightly in the absence of GTP even if GDP is substituted. Addition of GTP results in the rapid formation of characteristic paracrystals (Ventilla, Cantor, and Shelanski, *in preparation*). Assembly does not occur if β-methylene GTP (GMPPCP), a GTP analogue in which the γ-phosphate is not accessible for hydrolysis, is substituted for GTP (Ventilla, 1972). However, if prior to addition of vinblastine the protein is incubated at 37°C with GTP and the free GTP is subsequently removed, assembly will take place without GTP or in the presence of GMPPCP. This suggested that GTP must interact with the protein in a specific manner prior to assembly. A possible mechanism is one in which tubulin can bind a molecule of GTP at the *exchangeable* nucleotide binding site and hydrolyze the γ-phosphate of this GTP, utilizing it to convert a GDP at a *nonexchangeable* site to a GTP (Berry and Shelanski, 1972). This "transphosphorylated" protein would then be in an "active" form and able to assemble when vinblastine was added.

E. Assembly of Microtubules

After tubulin was purified, it became clear that it could not be reassembled into microtubules under any of the isolation conditions. Stephens (1968*b*) succeeded in reassembling detergent-dissociated outer doublet microtubules from sea urchin sperm flagella under conditions which required KCl and GTP. Tubules reassembled in this manner were unaffected by colchicine or low temperatures either during or after formation and had a considerable amount of detergent bound to them. It was difficult

to ascertain whether the problem in reassembly was due to some unap-
preciated factor or to some vital element being lost during tubulin purification. Weisenberg returned to supernatants of brain homogenates and
attempted reassembly of microtubules under a variety of buffer, salt,
temperature, and nucleotide conditions. He found microtubule assembly
only in cases in which the buffer had some ability to chelate calcium. He
then developed conditions for reassembly in which EGTA is used to chelate
free calcium (Weisenberg, 1972). Reassembly requires magnesium and
GTP as well as warm temperatures. Tubules reassembled under these conditions depolymerize when cooled to 4°C and are blocked in their assembly
by colchicine. Calcium causes a rapid loss of formed microtubules in such
suspensions. Under the same conditions, microtubules can be reassembled
from partially purified tubulin preparations (Weisenberg, 1972). However,
the ability to reassemble is lost if a two-step ammonium sulfate fractionation
precedes ion-exchange chromatography, as is the case in the usual method
of purification of tubulin from brain (Weisenberg et al., 1968). This may be
due to the loss of the nucleation factor described by Borisy and Olmsted
(1972). These workers discovered that microtubules could be reassembled
under low-calcium conditions similar to those described previously as long
as the supernatant was centrifuged at a force somewhat below $200,000 \times g$
for 1 hr. At higher forces, tubulin remained present but reassembly did not
occur. These workers attribute this phenomenon to the loss of ring-like
structures which could presumably serve as nucleating centers for microtubule assembly.

In the reassembly systems described, the tubules appear to be in active
exchange with free subunits in solution. Removal of free subunits will
shift the equilibrium away from tubules. Colchicine seems to function to
depolymerize tubules by blocking the participation of subunits in this
equilibrium and thus shifting it in favor of the subunits. The role of GTP
and "transphosphorylation" in assembly is not established, but either GTP
or ATP is necessary for assembly.

Tubulin, like actin, can be made to polymerize in the absence of added
nucleotide if agents such as sucrose are added to the solution. The assembly
of tubulin is favored by both sucrose (1 M) and glycerol (4 M), and will
proceed in the absence of added ATP or GTP, although in controls without
those agents no tubules are seen. The rate of assembly in 4 M glycerol
without GTP is, however, only one-tenth of the rate in glycerol with GTP
(Shelanski, Gaskin, and Cantor, 1973). Tubules assembled in glycerol are
not depolymerized by colchicine or low temperature. However, they cannot
initially be assembled at low temperature or in the presence of colchicine
and regain their usual lability when glycerol is removed. There is little or

no exchange between intact tubules in glycerol and free subunits. The reassembly of microtubules in glycerol can be used as an efficient purification method to obtain highly purified tubulin from brain homogenates. An active ATPase is co-purified with the tubulin in this purification and can be separated on sucrose gradients or by column chromatography.

These observations on microtubule assembly *in vitro* give some insights into the control of microtubule assembly *in vivo*. The ability of calcium to block tubule assembly suggests that the cell might use local control of the levels of calcium to regulate this process. GTP might also play a role in regulation of the rate of assembly. Since intracellular calcium levels are very low, calcium would be able to exert a rather exquisite control over tubule assembly. It is possible that the effects of agents such as cyclic AMP, insulin, and nerve growth factor on microtubule assembly might be mediated by calcium.

The fact that tubules can be assembled without added GTP demonstrated that GTP is not directly a part of the link between subunits in the tubule and that hydrolysis of the γ-phosphate is not an obligatory energy source for assembly.

IV. POSSIBLE ROLE OF THE MICROTUBULE IN THE NEURON

Earlier in this chapter we briefly reviewed experiments which implicated microtubules in neurite extension and preservation, in axoplasmic flow, in endocrine secretion, cell-surface site distribution, and ciliary and flagellar movement. The last of these is well studied, and flagellar and ciliary movement is almost certainly based on the interactions between the axonemal microtubules and the ATPase dynein (Gibbons, 1966) which is present as the small "arms" on the A-tubule of the outer doublet microtubules. Basically, the available information on microtubules can be viewed in two ways. In the first of these, the tubules are seen as skeletal structures which because of their ability to readily form and dissolve provide an ideal metastable cytoskeleton which can function in the formation of structures such as the reticulopods in foraminifera. In the nervous system, this view would have the axon begin to develop by the action of other cellular elements — perhaps actin and myosin acting on the membrane — and then after an initial outpouching the tubules would assemble and act to maintain the asymmetry of the structure. In this scheme, the ablation of axoplasmic flow by antimitotic agents would be explained away as a loss of order in flow due to loss of microtubule-bound or constrained compartments in which flow would normally take place efficiently. Certain problems exist with this most simple of approaches to microtubule function. It would seem that ordering and cytoskeletal functions in the neuron would be better served by more stable structures than the microtubules, perhaps by the neurofilaments, and that it would be very inefficient to devote so large a fraction of the cell's protein to these functions and to turn this protein over with a half-life as short as 4 days. These arguments do not disprove a purely cytoskeletal role for the microtubules, but they do go a long way toward explaining the author's unhappiness with such schemes.

The second approach is to think of the microtubule as a key component in a motility-transport system in the cell. Electron microscopic studies of microtubules in the nervous system have shown apparent cross-linking of tubules to synaptic vesicles (Jalfors and Smith, 1969) and to mitochondria (Raine, Ghetti, and Shelanski, 1971). In each of these cases the structures in question appear to be linked to the microtubules by short "arms." Similar arms are seen in spindle microtubules (McIntosh, Hepler, and Van Wie, 1969), and a detailed sliding tubule mechanism has been proposed which might account for the movements of mitosis. The force in such a model would quite possibly be generated by movements of the arms on the tubules. Similar movements of the arms might function in the transport of axoplasmic constituents. It is tempting to postulate that these arms are made of dynein-like protein, in analogy with the side arms on the ciliary and flagellar microtubules. The only firm identification of dynein from a cytoplasmic form has been from marine eggs by Weisenberg and Taylor (1968), and in this case the problem is complicated by the fact that the embryos of these forms are richly ciliated and dynein might be present as a ciliary precursor. A high molecular weight ATPase with ion activations similar to dynein is present in brain and neuroblastoma (Shelanski and Adelstein, *unpublished observations*), but its association with microtubules has not been firmly established.

It is also possible that force generation by the microtubule does not need a second component. A reordering of subunits to create a shorter form (Tilney, 1967) or the addition and subtraction of subunits along the length of the tubule could provide a method of shortening and possible force generation. It is clear that considerable further explanation of the chemistry and interactions of microtubules is needed before these questions can be finally resolved.

The manner in which microtubules might order the grouping of concanavalin A binding sites in membranes or how they might function in neurotransmission is made tantalizing by the observation of Feit and Barondes (1970) that there is a considerable quantity of particulate colchicine-binding activity in brain which may be associated with the synaptosomal membrane. This is rather unique to brain (Feit and Barondes, 1970; Williams and Wolff, 1970); however, it is possible that similar but less stable associations exist in other tissues as well. The exact role these presumptive membrane-associated subunits would play and whether they would act alone or in concert with other elements is in the realm of pure speculation.

Numerous models have been proposed for the action of fibrous proteins in axoplasmic transport and other neuronal functions, and many of these rely on some interplay between microtubules and actin-myosin systems (Rasmussen, 1970). There is no evidence for any direct molecular interactions between these proteins, but a possible link would be the differing effects of calcium on microtubules and on actin-myosin systems. Since few microtubules are seen in the nerve endings, one wonders why organelles which are so richly present in the axon seem to terminate at the origin of the synaptic expansion. At the same time, actin and myosin are said to be richly represented in this area (Berl et al., 1973). It is possible that vesicles and other constituents of axoplasm are transported down the axon in a manner which is mediated by the microtubule. When the ending is reached, the calcium concentration is higher and the tubules depolymerize, freeing the associated substances which in turn are exported from the cell by a calcium-facilitated system—actin and myosin. Such a system would be very economical from the standpoint of control and could possibly be electrically mediated, perhaps by an inward calcium current at the synapse. Extremely precise control of release could be accomplished in this manner.

V. CONCLUSION

I have tried in this review to cover the high points of microtubule chemistry and physiology. Much detailed information has been omitted and can be found in reviews on specialized aspects of the microtubule literature (i.e., Porter, 1966; McGee-Russell and Allen, 1971; Shelanski and Feit, 1972; Stephens, 1972). In the decade and a half since the description of microtubules, interest and work in these ubiquitous structures has grown rapidly. The challenge at this point is to unravel the secrets of their function or functions.

ACKNOWLEDGMENTS

The author is grateful to Drs. Robert Berry, Howard Feit, Matthew Daniels, and Marta Ventilla for many of the data presented here.

REFERENCES

Adelman, M. R., and Taylor, E. W. (1969*a*): Isolation of an actomyosin-like protein complex from slime mold plasmodium and the separation of the complex into actin- and myosin-like fractions. *Biochemistry*, 8:4964.

Adelman, M. R., and Taylor, E. W. (1969*b*): Further purification and characterization of slime mold myosin and slime mold actin. *Biochemistry*, 8:4976.

Bamburg, J. R., Shooter, E. M., and Wilson, L. (1973): Developmental changes in microtubule protein of chick brain. *Biochemistry (in press)*.

Bensch, K. G., and Malawista, S. (1969): Microtubular crystals in mammalian cells. *Journal of Cell Biology*, 40:95–107.

Bensch, K. G., Marantz, R., Wisniewski, H., and Shelanski, M. (1969): Induction *in vitro* of microtubular crystals by vinca alkaloids. *Science*, 165:495–496.

Berl, S., and Puszkin, S. (1970): Mg^{2+}-CA^{2+}-activated adenosine triphosphatase system isolated from mammalian brain. *Biochemistry*, 9:2057–2067.

Berl, S., Puszkin, S., and Nicklas, W. J. (1973): Actomyosin-like protein in brain. *Science*, 179:441.

Berry, R. W., and Shelanski, M. L. (1972): Interactions of tubulin with vinblastine and guanosine triphosphate. *Journal of Molecular Biology*, 71:71–80.

Borisy, G. G. (1966): Ph.D. thesis, Department of Biophysics, University of Chicago.

Borisy, G. G., and Olmsted, L. B. (1972): Nucleated assembly of microtubules in porcine brain extracts. *Science*, 177:1196–1197.

Borisy, G. G., and Taylor, E. W. (1967*a*): The mechanism of action of colchicine: Binding of colchicine-^{3}H to cellular protein. *Journal of Cell Biology*, 34:525–533.

Borisy, G. G., and Taylor, E. W. (1967*b*): The mechanism of action of colchicine: Colchicine binding to sea urchin eggs and the mitotic apparatus. *Journal of Cell Biology*, 34:535–548.

Bryan, J., and Wilson, L. (1971): Are cytoplasmic microtubules heteropolymers? *Proceedings of the National Academy of Sciences*, 68:1762–1766.

Daniels, M. P. (1972): Colchicine inhibition of nerve fiber formation *in vitro*. *Journal of Cell Biology*, 53:164–176.

Daniels, M. P. (1973): Fine structural changes in neurons and nerve fibers associated with colchicine inhibition of nerve fiber formation *in vitro*. *Journal of Cell Biology (in press)*.

Dutton, G., and Barondes, S. H. (1969): Glycoprotein metabolism in developing brain. *Science*, 166:1637–1638.

Eipper, B. (1972): Rat brain microtubule protein: Purification and determination of covalently bound phosphate and carbohydrate. *Proceedings of the National Academy of Sciences*, 69:2283–2287.

Falxa, M. L., and Gill, T. J. (1969): Preparation and properties of an alkylated brain protein related to the structural subunit of microtubules. *Archives of Biochemistry and Biophysics*, 135:194.

Feit, H. (1971): Metabolism of microtubule proteins in mouse brain. Ph.D. thesis. Department of Molecular Biology, Albert Einstein College of Medicine, Yeshiva University, New York.

Feit, H., and Barondes, S. H. (1970): Colchicine-binding activity in particulate fractions of mouse brain. *Journal of Neurochemistry*, 17:1355.

Feit, H., Dutton, G., Barondes, S. H., and Shelanski, M. L. (1971): Microtubule protein: Identification in and transport to nerve endings. *Journal of Cell Biology*, 51:138.

Feit, H., Slusarek, L., and Shelanski, M. L. (1971): Heterogeneity of tubulin subunits. *Proceedings of the National Academy of Sciences*, 68:2028–2031.

Fernandez, H. L., Burton, P. R., and Samson, F. E. (1971): Axoplasmic transport in the crayfish nerve cord. The role of fibrillar constituents of neurons. *Journal of Cell Biology*, 51:176.

Fine, R. (1971): Heterogeneity of tubulin. *Nature*, 233:283–284.

Fine, R. E., and Bray, D. (1971): Actin in growing nerve cells. *Nature*, 234:115–118.

Frazier, W. A., Angeletti, R. H., and Bradshaw, R. A. (1972): Nerve growth factor and insulin. *Science*, 176:482.

Frigon, R. P., and Lee, J. C. (1972): The stabilization of calf brain microtubule protein by sucrose. *Archives of Biochemistry and Biophysics*, 153:587–589.

Gibbons, I. R. (1966): Studies on the adenosine triphosphotase activity of 14S and 30S dynein from glia of tetrahymena. *Journal of Biological Chemistry*, 241:5590–5596.

Gonates, N. K., and Robbins, E. (1964): Homology between spindle tubules and neurotubules. *Protoplasma*, 59:25.

Goodman, D. B. P., Rasmussen, H., DiBella, F., and Guthrow, C. E., Jr. (1970): Cyclic adenosine 3',5' monophosphate-stimulated phosphorylation of isolated neurotubule subunits. *Proceedings of the National Academy of Sciences,* 67:652.

Hammond, S., and Bryan, J. (1972): Microtubule affinity labels. *Journal of Cell Biology,* 55:205a.

Hsie, A., and Puck, T. (1971): Morphological transformation of Chinese hamster cells by dibutyryl adenosine cyclic 3',5'-monophosphate and testosterone. *Proceedings of the National Academy of Sciences,* 68:358.

Inoue, S. (1964): In: *Primitive Motile Systems in Cell Biology,* edited by R. J. Allen and N. Kamiya, pp. 549–598. Academic Press, New York.

Ishakawa, H., Bischoff, R., and Holtzer, H. (1969): Formation of arrowhead complexes with heavy meromyosin in a variety of cell types. *Journal of Cell Biology,* 43:312.

Jalfors, U., and Smith, D. S. (1969): Association between synaptic vesicles and neurotubules. *Nature,* 224:710.

Karlsson, J.-O., and Sjöstrand, J. (1969): The effect of colchicine on the axonal transport of protein in the optic nerve and tract of the rabbit. *Brain Research,* 13:617–619.

Kirkland, W. L., and Burton, P. (1972): Cyclic adenosine monophosphate-mediated stabilization of mouse neuroblastoma cell neurite microtubules exposed to low temperature. *Nature,* 240:205.

Kreutzberg, G. W. (1969): Neuronal dynamics and axonal flow. IV. Blockage of intra-axonal enzyme transport by colchicine. *Proceedings of the National Academy of Sciences,* 62:722–728.

Lacy, P. E., Howell, S. L., Young, D. A., and Fick, C. J. (1968): New hypothesis of insulin secretion. *Nature,* 209:1177.

McGee-Russell, S. M., and Allen, R. D. (1971): Reversible stabilization of labile microtubules in the reticulopodial network of *Allogromia.* In: *Advances in Cell and Molecular Biology,* Vol. 1, pp. 153–184. Academic Press, New York.

McIntosh, J. R., Helper, P. K., and Van Wie, D. G. (1969): *Nature,* 224:659.

Marantz, R., and Shelanski, M. L. (1970): Structure of microtubular crystals induced by vinblastine *in vitro. Journal of Cell Biology,* 44:234–238.

Marantz, R., Ventilla, M., and Shelanski, M. L. (1969): Vinblastine-induced precipitation of microtubule protein. *Science,* 165:498.

Margolis, R. K., Margolis, R. U., and Shelanski, M. L. (1972): The carbohydrate composition of brain microtubule protein. *Biochemical and Biophysical Research Communications,* 47:432.

Olmsted, J. B., Carlson, K., Klebe, R., Ruddle, F., and Rosenbaum, J. (1970): Isolation of microtubule protein from cultured mouse neuroblastoma cells. *Proceedings of the National Academy of Sciences,* 65:129.

Olmsted, J. B., Witman, G. B., Carlson, K., and Rosenbaum, J. (1971): Comparison of microtubule proteins of neuroblastoma cells, brain, and *Chlamydamonas* flagella. *Proceedings of the National Academy of Sciences,* 68:2273.

Owellen, R. J., Owens, A. H., Jr., and Donigian, D. W. (1972): The binding of vincristine, vinblastine and colchicine to tubulin. *Biochemical and Biophysical Research Communications,* 47:685–691.

Peters, A., Palay, S., and Webster, H. deF. (1970): *Fine Structure of the Nervous System: The Cells and Their Processes.* Hoeber Medical Division of Harper and Row, New York.

Piatigorsky, J., Rothschild, S. S., and Wollberg, M. (1973): Stimulation by insulin of cell elongation and microtubule assembly in cultured embryonic chick lens epithelia. *Proceedings of the National Academy of Sciences (in press).*

Porter, K. R. (1966): In: *Ciba Foundation Symposium on Principles of Biomolecular Organization,* G. E. W. Wolstrenholme and M. O'Connor, editors, pp. 308–356. Little, Brown, Boston.

Raine, C. S., Ghetti, B., and Shelanski, M. L. (1971): On the association between mitochondria and microtubules within axons. *Brain Research,* 34:389–393.

Raine, C. S., and Wisniewski, H. (1970): On the occurrence of microtubules within mature astrocytes. *Anatomical Record,* 167:303.

Rasmussen, H. (1970): Cell communication, calcium ion and cyclic adenosine monophosphate. *Science,* 170:404.

Renaud, F. L., Rowe, A. J., and Gibbons, I. R. (1968): Some properties of the protein forming the outer fibers of glia. *Journal of Cell Biology,* 36:79.

Robbins, E., and Shelanski, M. L. (1969): Synthesis of a colchicine-binding protein during the HeLa cell life cycle. *Journal of Cell Biology,* 43:371–373.

Rosenbaum, J. L., and Carlson, K. (1969): Cilia regeneration in *Tetrahymena* and its inhibition by colchicine. *Journal of Cell Biology,* 40:415–425.

Seeds, N. W., Gilman, A. G., Amano, T., and Nirenberg, M. W. (1970): Regulation of axon formation by clonal lines of a neural tumor. *Proceedings of the National Academy of Sciences,* 66:160–167.

Shelanski, M. L., and Feit, H. (1972): Filaments and tubules in the nervous system. In: *Structure and Function of Nervous Tissue,* Vol. 6, edited by G. Bourne, pp. 47–80. Academic Press, New York.

Shelanski, M. L., Gaskin, F., and Cantor, C. R. (1973): Assembly of microtubules in the absence of added nucleotide. *Proceedings of the National Academy of Sciences,* 70:765.

Shelanski, M. L., and Taylor, E. W. (1967): Isolation of a protein subunit from microtubules. *Journal of Cell Biology,* 34:549.

Shelanski, M. L., and Taylor, E. W. (1968): Properties of the protein subunit of central pair and outer doublet microtubules of sea urchin flagella. *Journal of Cell Biology,* 38:304.

Soifer, D., Brown, T., and Hechter, O. (1971): Insulin and microtubules in rat adipocytes. *Science,* 172:269.

Stephens, R. E. (1968*a*): On the structural protein of flagellar outer fibres. *Journal of Molecular Biology,* 32:277.

Stephens, R. E. (1968*b*): Reassociation of microtubule protein. *Journal of Molecular Biology,* 33:517.

Stephens, R. E. (1972). In: *Biological Macromolecules,* Vol. 5., edited by S. Timasheff and G. Fasman, pp. 355–390. Marcel Dekker, New York.

Stephens, R. E., Renaud, F. L., and Gibbons, I. R. (1967): Guanine nucleotide associated with the protein of the outer fibres of glia and flagella. *Science,* 156:1606–1608.

Tennyson, V. M. (1970): The fine structure of the axon growth cone of the dorsal root neuroblast of the rabbit embryo. *Journal of Cell Biology,* 44:62.

Thoa, N. B., Wooten, G. F., Axelrod, J., and Kopin, I. J. (1972): Inhibition of release of dopamine-β-hydroxylase and norepinephrine from sympathetic nerves of colchicine, vinblastine or cytochalasin-B. *Proceedings of the National Academy of Sciences,* 69:520–522.

Tilney, L. G. (1967): *Journal of Cell Biology,* 34:327–343.

Tilney, L. G., Hiramoto, Y., and Marsland, D. (1966): Studies on the microtubules in Heliozoa. III. A pressure analysis of the role of these structures in the formation and maintenance of the axopodia of *Actinosphaerium nucleofilum* (Barrett). *Journal of Cell Biology,* 29:77–95.

Tilney, L. G., and Porter, K. R. (1967): Studies on the microtubules in Heliozoa. II. The effect of low temperature on these structures in the formation and maintenance of axopodia. *Journal of Cell Biology,* 34:327–341.

Ukena, T. E., and Berlin, R. D. (1972): Effect of colchicine and vinblastine on the topographical separation of membrane functions. *Journal of Experimental Medicine and Biology.*

Ventilla, M. (1972): Studies of microtubular proteins. Ph.D. thesis, Department of Chemistry, Columbia University, New York.

Ventilla, M., Cantor, C. R., and Shelanski, M. L. (1972): A circular dichroism study of microtubule protein. *Biochemistry,* 11:1554–1561.

Weihing, R., and Korn, E. D. (1969): Ameba actin: The presence of 3-methylhistidine. *Biochemical and Biophysical Research Communications,* 35:906.

Weisenberg, R. C. (1972): Microtubule formation in vitro in solutions containing low calcium concentrations. *Science,* 177:1104–1105.

Weisenberg, R. C., Borisy, G. G., and Taylor, E. W. (1968): The colchicine-binding protein of mammalian brain and its relation to microtubules. *Biochemistry,* 7:4466.

Weisenberg, R. C., and Taylor, E. W. (1968): Studies on ATPase activity of sea urchin eggs and isolated mitotic apparatus. *Experimental Cell Research*, 53:372.

Weisenberg, R. C., and Timasheff, S. N. (1970): Aggregation of microtubule subunit protein. Effects of divalent cations, colchicine and vinblastine. *Biochemistry*, 9:4110.

Williams, J. A., and Wolff, J. (1970): Possible role of microtubules in thyroid secretion. *Proceedings of the National Academy of Sciences*, 67:1901.

Wilson, L. (1970): Properties of colchicine binding protein from chick embryo brain. Interactions with vinca alkaloids and podophyllotoxin. *Biochemistry*, 9:4999.

Wisniewski, H., Shelanski, M. L., and Terry, R. D. (1968): Effects of mitotic spindle inhibitors on neurotubules and neurofilaments in anterior horn cells. *Journal of Cell Biology*, 38:224.

Yamada, K. M., Spooner, B. S., and Wessels, N. K. (1971): Ultrastructure and function of growth cones and axons of cultured nerve cells. *Journal of Cell Biology*, 49:614.

Proteins of the Nervous System
Raven Press, New York © 1973

Studies of Axoplasmic Transport*

Diana Johnson Schneider

I. AXOPLASMIC TRANSPORT AS A NEUROANATOMICAL METHOD

Early work on axoplasmic flow, much of which is reviewed in this volume, showed that a steady stream of newly synthesized protein flows from neuronal somata to their axon terminals. Several authors (see Taylor and Weiss, 1965; Lasek, Joseph, and Whitlock, 1968) suggested and demonstrated that a neuroanatomical method for tracing long pathways could be based on axoplasmic flow, since the distribution of newly synthesized proteins from neurons at the locus of the isotope injection might easily be traced in serial autoradiographs following the administration of a radioactively labeled amino acid.

Until quite recently, most anatomical methods for tracing pathways in the central nervous system involved placing localized lesions within the brain or spinal cord and visualizing the resulting axonal degeneration with one of a number of silver staining procedures which selectively impregnate degenerating material (Nauta and Gygax, 1954; Fink and Heimer, 1967). Alternatively, degenerating axons and terminals could be recognized in the electron microscope (Gray and Guillery, 1966). Although studies using the degeneration methods have vastly increased our knowledge of neuronal connections in the brain, they have two serious limitations. Axons passing through the injured region, whose cells of origin lie elsewhere in the brain, are invariably interrupted by the lesion and, of course, undergo degeneration. In many cases, a series of overlapping lesions could establish the true source of a particular pathway, but very often the complexity of the region in question is such as to preclude this approach; the source of origin of many of the brain's pathways has therefore remained obscure. A second practical difficulty with the degeneration methods is that axonal degeneration sometimes occurs proximal to the site of a lesion, and it may be difficult to establish the polarity of the pathways under investigation if recurrent collaterals are involved. There are a number of additional drawbacks to the degeneration methods, including the capriciousness of the stains themselves,

---

* As in the author's other chapter, this chapter presents in summary form recent research material presented at the conference on *Proteins of the Nervous System*.

the wide variation in the time required for different pathways to degenerate, and the difficulty in making even approximate estimates of the numbers of axons or terminals contributed by a pathway.

Cowan, Gottlieb, Hendrickson, Price, and Woolsey (1972) have recently shown that the axoplasmic transport of radioactively labeled proteins can serve as the basis of a neuroanatomical method for tracing connections in the central nervous system which obviates most of the complications inherent in the degeneration methods. Basically, the method consists of injecting a concentrated solution of a tritiated amino acid (^{3}H-leucine or ^{3}H-proline are particularly suitable for this purpose) into a small region of the brain or spinal cord and allowing the animal to survive until the newly synthesized proteins have been transported to the axon terminals of the labeled cells. The distribution of radioactive proteins is then traced in serial autoradiographs of the brain or cord. Since the neuronal soma is the major, if not the exclusive, site of protein synthesis, the terminals of fibers passing through the labeled area will not be labeled. The polarity of the pathway can be established unequivocally because the transport of newly synthesized protein is normally unidirectional. Finally, axoplasmic flow is a physiological process that proceeds at a definable rate, and therefore the amount of protein reaching the terminal field of a particular class of cells probably bears a simple relationship to the number of terminals in the field, although admittedly this assumption at present lacks direct proof. Since what one observes are varying densities of silver grains in the exposed autoradiographs, certain quantitative aspects of the pathway can be investigated.

Restricted areas of the brain have been labeled by injecting small volumes of concentrated tritiated amino acid ($\sim$ 0.1 μl of 10 μC/μl ^{3}H-leucine or ^{3}H-proline) with a Hamilton microsyringe (Fig. 1). Careful microscopic examination of these specimens showed that areas of gray matter quite close to the intensely labeled regions had only background levels of radioactivity. Injections made through micropipettes have labeled far smaller populations of neurons than the ones shown in Fig. 1.

In order to show that fibers of passage do not incorporate and transport label, injections were made into several fiber pathways, including the corpus callosum, lateral olfactory tract, optic nerve, and ventral hippocampal commissure. Under these circumstances the bundles of fibers become heavily labeled, presumably due to the uptake of the label and subsequent protein synthesis by the glial cells in the vicinity of the injection. However, there was no evidence of label in the distal parts of the fiber system (e.g., after midline injections of the corpus callosum, its lateral parts and the cortical fields in which they terminate were unlabeled). These experiments indicate either that there is no protein synthesis in these axons or that, if

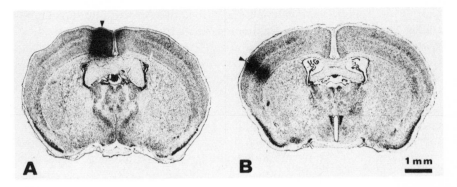

FIG. 1. Injections into two areas of the mouse cortex. Each injection consisted of 5 μC of ^{3}H-leucine in 0.5 μl of saline, and the animals survived for 24 hr after the injection. Auto-radiographs were exposed for 2 weeks. A: An injection into medial SI motor cortex. B: Injection into SI face area. Note the limited spread of the label. (From Cowan et al., 1972.)

the axons do synthesize protein, the products are not transported in de-tectable amounts. One can therefore conclude that whatever labeled termi-nals are identified belong only to neurons whose somata have been labeled by the injected material.

In view of recent reports of retrograde axoplasmic flow (Kristensson and Olson, 1971; LaVail and LaVail, 1972) and of protein synthesis in axon terminals (Cotman and Taylor, 1971), it has been important to prove that protein is not synthesized in significant amounts in axon terminals and then retrogradely transported to the cell body, which would complicate the inter-pretation of experiments based on axoplasmic flow. This was demonstrated in the chick visual system, where the retina receives a strong centrifugal projection from the isthmo-optic nucleus (ION) of the midbrain (Cowan and Powell, 1963). Subsequent to the injection of ^{3}H-leucine into the vitreous of the eye, there was heavy labeling of the retina and considerable transport of protein to the optic tectum, the main terminus of the optic nerve. However, the cell bodies in the ION were not labeled, although their terminals in the retina (Dowling and Cowan, 1966) must have been exposed to a high concentration of isotope. These and other similar experi-ments have shown that there is no detectable retrograde transport of whatever proteins may be synthesized in axon terminals. Of course, these results do not contradict the evidence for retrograde axonal transport, which may involve proteins originally synthesized in the cell soma or other macro-molecules taken up by axon terminals.

It has been important to identify the subcellular location of both the rapid and slowly transported materials. Electron microscopic autoradiographic studies showed that a large fraction of the rapidly transported proteins are distributed to axon terminals (Fig. 2). When the eye of a monkey was injected with ³H-leucine and the animal was allowed to survive only long enough for the rapidly transported materials to reach the lateral geniculate nucleus, approximately 50% of the grains were located over optic nerve fiber terminals, and only 25% were over the myelinated preterminal segments of the axons. The remaining grains were located over neuronal somata, dendrites, glia, and blood vessels. In experiments with longer survival times, in which the slowly transported protein has reached the

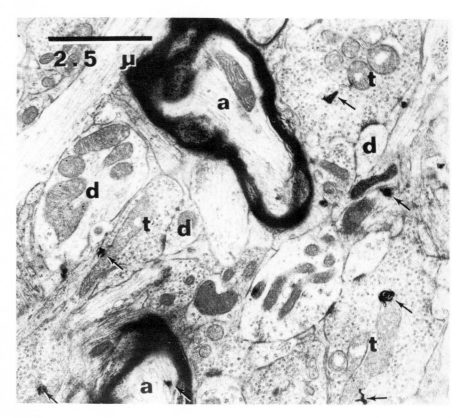

FIG. 2. An electron microscopic autoradiograph from lamina 6 of the lateral geniculate body of a monkey. ³H-Leucine (100 μC) was injected into the contralateral eye and the animal allowed to survive for 3 days. Note that most of the silver grains are over terminals (t), but that one is over a myelinated axon (a). Dendrites are labeled (d). (From Cowan et al., 1972.)

geniculate, the relative number of grains over terminals and preterminals was almost exactly reversed (Hendrickson, 1972). These experiments, in conjunction with those described below, show that the location of labeled materials transported in the rapid component can be used to define the location of the terminal field of the labeled pathway.

Perhaps the most critical test of the autoradiographic method was to show that pathways traced with it corresponded in detail with earlier descriptions based on degeneration methods. This has been shown for several pathways, among which the commissural projection of the hippocampus is one of the most instructive examples. Degeneration studies had shown that fibers projecting through the ventral hippocampal commissure to the contralateral hippocampus terminate only on the basal dendrites and the inner four-fifths of the apical dendritic tree, whereas the cell somata and the outer one-fifth of the apical dendrites do not receive such contralateral projections. When the cells of origin of the commissural pathway were labeled, the pattern of grains in the terminal fields corresponded exactly to the pattern of degeneration seen in earlier experiments (D. I. Gottlieb and W. M. Cowan, *in preparation;* Fig. 3). Although the details of the quantitative uses of the autoradiographic method are beyond the scope of this review, it is worth mentioning that the relative heights of the peaks in graphs such as the one shown in Fig. 3 give reliable estimates of the relative intensity of pathways, and that similar quantitative analyses have been made for other pathways in the CNS.

Earlier work on axoplasmic flow demonstrated the continuous flow of protein from the somata of peripherally located neurons, such as retinal ganglion cells and dorsal root ganglion cells, along their axons to their axon terminals. This recent work shows that this process is shared by central neurons and that small areas of the brain may be labeled by appropriately placed injections of radioactive precursors. Only neurons whose somata are directly exposed to the label can incorporate it for subsequent transport; axons passing through the labeled zone will not synthesize protein and their terminals will not be labeled. This finding may be of importance for biochemical as well as anatomical studies of axoplasmic flow. Since the discovery of axoplasmic flow, the question of the nature of the transported protein has been of paramount importance and this question is still under active investigation. These anatomical studies suggest that axoplasmic flow from central as well as peripheral neurons may now be studied biochemically.

The possibility of using radioautography following axoplasmic transport as a neuroanatomical mapping method has also been examined by Neale, Neale, and Agranoff (1972), using the goldfish visual system. Following the

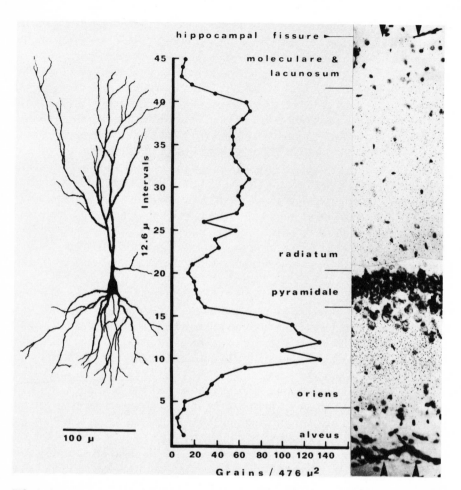

FIG. 3. An experiment illustrating the use of the autoradiographic method for localizing terminal fields. An injection of ^{3}H-leucine was made into the source of origin of the commissural fibers to the hippocampus in the rat. The animal was allowed to survive long enough for only rapidly transported material to reach the opposite hippocampus. The right-hand panel shows an autoradiograph of part of the terminal field in the contralateral hippocampus. The graph shows the grain density as a function of depth in the central portion of the autoradiograph marked by the arrowheads. Note that the grain density is low over the alveus, the st. pyramidale, and the st. moleculare and lacunosum, but high in the st. oriens and the st. radiatum. This corresponds well to the pattern of degeneration seen after interrupting the commissural pathway. The drawing on the left illustrates the appearance of a typical pyramidal cell as seen in Golgi preparations and is included to show the basal and apical dendrites on which the commissural fibers terminate. (From Cowan et al., 1972.)

injection of ³H-proline into the vitreous, labeled protein was observed predominantly in the contralateral optic tectum (Fig. 4). The highest concentrations of grains were found in a discrete area medial to the marginal fiber layer, in the external plexiform layer containing retinal axons and

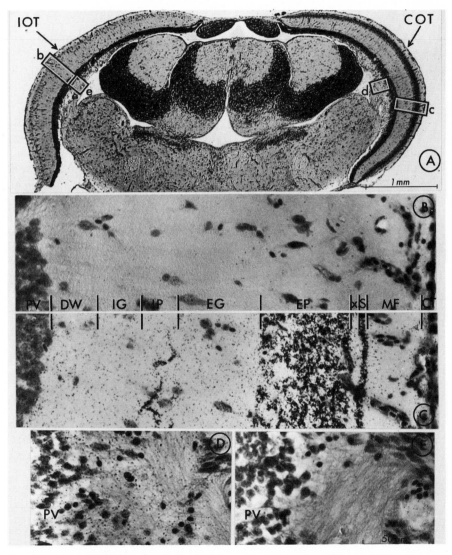

FIG. 4. Light microscopic radioautography in the visual system of the goldfish following the injection of ³H-proline into the vitreous. *B−E* are higher magnifications of regions *b−e* in A. (From Neale et al., 1972.)

nerve endings, in the internal plexiform layer, and in the periventricular layer, areas which appear to correspond to retinal synaptic regions detected by axonal degeneration (Roth, 1969).

II. AXOPLASMIC FLOW IN THE VISUAL SYSTEM

Karlsson and Sjöstrand (1971a,b; 1972a,b) have examined the axoplasmic flow process in the retinal ganglion cells of the rabbit, which project to the lateral geniculate and superior colliculus. The rabbit visual system is particularly well suited to such studies because more than 95% of the fibers from the retina terminate on the contralateral side.

Four flow rates were observed in this system: 150, 40, 6 to 12, and 2 mm/day. The relative amounts of material arriving with the rapid phase varied depending on the source of label, but larger amounts arrived in the superior colliculus. The rapid phase contained large amounts of membranous components, whereas most of the soluble proteins were in the slow phase. The turnover rate of material in the slow phase was approximately 10 days, when calculated either on the basis of total protein or a single protein, such as vinblastine-precipitable material.

The amount of protein transported to the terminals of the retinal ganglion cells was calculated, based on the assumptions that: (1) the retinal ganglion cells take all their leucine from the vitreous body; (2) the injected ^{3}H-leucine is evenly distributed in the vitreous; (3) incorporation is essentially complete within 1 hr; (4) leucine represents 7.7% of the amino acid residues of the transported proteins, and the average residue weight is 115; and (5) the total number of axons is approximately 260,000. It was then calculated that: (1) each retinal ganglion cell produces 60×10^{-12} g protein for transport each day; (2) this represents 15% of the total protein content each day; and (3) the total protein transported is 8×10^{-6} g/day to the superior colliculus and 8×10^{-6} g/day to the lateral geniculate.

Levels of radioactivity in the optic nerve and optic tract remained high at a time when maximal incorporation was observed at the nerve terminals. The pattern of radioactive decay in the fibers indicated two components, one representing material moving through the axon, the second that of material remaining *in situ*. An appreciable amount of material thus appeared to remain in the axon.

When ^{3}H-fucose was used to label glycoproteins, the labeled material was transported in the fast phase (Figs. 5 and 6), and the labeled material was more stable than that labeled with ^{3}H-leucine. It was evident that a considerable amount of the label was localized to the peripheral parts of the axoplasm and to the axolemma. Again, a significant amount of material

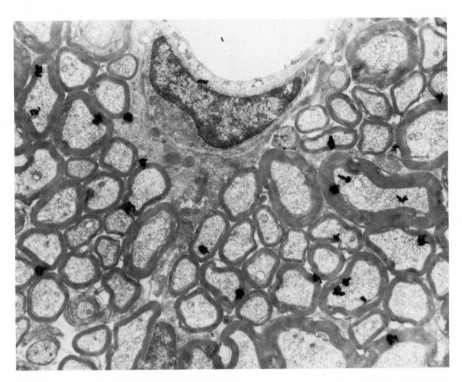

FIG. 5. Electron microscopic autoradiograph of the optic tract 48 hr after injection of ³H-fucose. The autoradiographic silver grains are mainly distributed over the myelin sheath and peripheral parts of the axoplasm. × 7,000. (L. E. Eriksson, H.-A. Hansson, J.-O. Karlsson, and J. Sjöstrand, *in preparation*.)

remained in the optic tract. A comparison of the amounts of material transported to the axon terminals following the injection of different label sources is shown in Table 1 for the rabbit, rat, and chick. In comparison to perikaryal macromolecular synthesis, the proteins of rapid axonal transport in all species studied were characterized by a high fucose content.

Similar results have been obtained in the goldfish visual system by Forman, Grafstein, and McEwen (1972). After the injection of ³H-fucose, glycoproteins were transported to the tectum within 24 hr in the fast phase; no labeled material was transported in the slow component of axoplasmic flow. There is no evidence for incorporation of fucose at the nerve ending following transport; rather, the fucose is incorporated into protein in the cell soma prior to transport.

A similar system has been used to study the role of proteins in synaptic

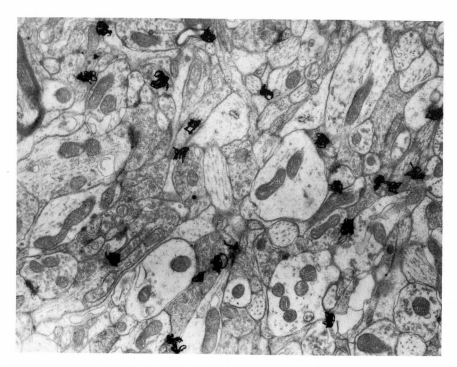

FIG. 6. Electron microscopic autoradiograph of the superior colliculus 48 hr after injection of ³H-fucose. Autoradiographic silver grains are mainly related to the synaptic terminals, filled with vesicles, of retinal ganglion cells. × 15,200. (From Eriksson et al., *in preparation*.)

functions (Cuénod and Schonbach, 1971; Schonbach and Cuénod, 1971; Schonbach, Schonbach, and Cuénod, 1971, 1973; Boesch, Marko, and Cuénod, 1972; Perisic and Cuénod, 1972). Marko and Cuénod (1972) have recently examined the contribution of the fast and slow components of axoplasmic flow to the assembly of proteins in different portions of the synaptic apparatus.

Proteins and glycoproteins were labeled by intraocular injection of ³H- and ¹⁴C-proline and ³H-fucose, respectively. Synaptic subfractions were isolated from the contralateral optic lobe (Whittaker, Michaelson, and Kirkland, 1964) at 1 and 14 days, at which times the fast and slow flows, respectively, have reached the nerve endings in this region.

A threefold increase in specific activity of the fast-flowing material relative to the homogenate was found in two fractions (F and G), which were shown by electron microscopy to contain synaptic ghosts; the activity

TABLE 1. Comparison between retinal incorporation and axonal transport to the terminals in the lateral geniculate body and the superior colliculus of adult rabbits, adult rats, and chick embryos

Animal	Precursor	Macromolecule	Axonal transport phase	Transport ratio[a]	Reference
Adult rabbit	leucine	protein	rapid (I) rapid (II) slow (IV)	1.4 2.0 7.8	Karlsson and Sjöstrand, 1971a " "
	fucose	glycoprotein	rapid (I + II)	4.7	Karlsson and Sjöstrand, 1971b
	uridine	RNA	slow (IV)	0.03 (LGB[b] only)	Jarlstedt and Karlsson, 1973
Adult rat	leucine	protein	rapid	1.4	Sjöstrand and Hansson, 1971
	fucose	glycoprotein	rapid	8.9	Sjöstrand and Hansson, 1971
Chick embryo (18 days)	leucine	protein	rapid	1.7	Marchisio and Sjöstrand, 1972
	fucose	glycoprotein	rapid	5.4	Marchisio and Sjöstrand, 1972

[a] Maximal amount of protein-bound radioactivity transported to the terminal region in percent of maximal amount incorporated into retinal proteins.

[b] LGB = lateral geniculate body.

of the slow-flowing material was not enriched in any of the fractions (Fig. 7). The relative activity of the soluble fractions from nerve endings (O) was below 1 in both cases, and the synaptic vesicle fraction (D) showed a specific activity virtually identical to that of the homogenate. That this activity is representative of the vesicles themselves rather than of impurities was indicated by an increased relative specific activity when Ficoll gradients were used rather than sucrose (Morgan, Wolfe, Mandel, and Gombos, 1971), since these gradients were found to yield purer vesicles.

The total activity in the tectum was higher at 14 days than at 1 day in all fractions, with most of this activity in fractions which predominantly contain mitochondria (Fig. 8). The distribution of radioactivity 1 day after intraocular injection of ^{3}H-fucose was similar to that seen with ^{14}C-proline (Table 2). However, the amount of transported activity was substantially greater with fucose, representing 16% of retinal precipitable activity as compared with 3% for proline.

Di Giamberardino has examined the transport of glycoproteins in the ciliary ganglion of the chicken, which receives fibers from the nucleus of Edinger-Westphal (Di Giamberardino, Bennett, Koenig, and Droz, 1972; Di Giamberardino and Bennett, 1972; Bennett and Koenig, 1972). In agreement with the observations of other workers, he has found that fucosyl glycoproteins migrate with the fast phase of the axonal flow. Moreover, he

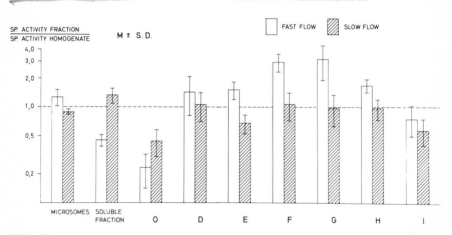

FIG. 7. Distribution of the specific activity of proteins in various tectal fractions referred to the specific activity of the proteins in the homogenate. ^{3}H- or ^{14}C-Proline was injected intraocularly 14 days (slow flow) and 1 day (fast flow) before sacrifice. Columns O and D to I refer to the fractions after osmotic shock of crude mitochondria (Whittaker et al., 1964). Values are from eight experiments for fast flow and from six experiments for slow flow. Note the enrichment in activity at 1 day for fractions F and G. (From P. Marko and M. Cuénod, *in preparation*.)

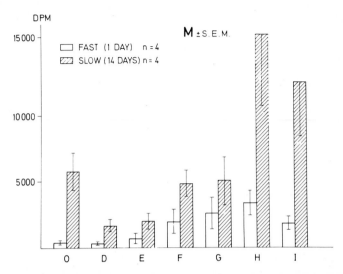

FIG. 8. Total radioactivity present in proteins of crude mitochondrial subfractions after osmotic shock. Labeled proline (50 μC) was injected intraocularly 1 day (fast flow) and 14 days (slow flow) before sacrifice. (From P. Marko and M. Cuénod, *in preparation*.)

TABLE 2. *Specific activity of tectal proteins 1 day after intraocular injection of 50 μC* ³H-fucose and 25 μC ¹⁴C-proline

Fraction	³H	³H / ³H-Hom	¹⁴C	¹⁴C / ¹⁴C-Hom	³H / ¹⁴C
Homogenate	4,250	1.00	490	1.00	8.7
Crude nuclei	4,960	1.17	695	1.42	7.2
Microsomal	5,960	1.40	620	1.27	9.6
Soluble	865	0.20	225	0.46	3.8
O	770	0.18	225	0.46	3.4
D	3,385	0.79	430	0.88	7.8
E	11,825	2.77	955	1.95	12.4
F	14,040	3.29	1,135	2.31	12.4
G	15,180	3.57	1,265	2.58	12.0
H	4,175	0.98	455	0.93	9.2
I	2,280	0.54	290	0.59	7.9

suggested that a small fraction of the transported glycoproteins could move with the slow phase, since the broad peak of label recorded in axons and in nerve endings persists after the arrival of the first slowly transported proteins. Subcellular fractionation of the whole ciliary ganglion indicated that these glycoproteins accumulate in fractions rich in mitochondria and membranes. It is not yet possible to rule out the possibility of a reutilization of labeled fucose. Dutton, Haywood, and Barondes (1973) have examined the incorporation of label into glycoproteins of mouse brain subcellular fractions following the intracranial administration of glucosamine. Marked differences in the labeling kinetics during the first 4 hr of incorporation were previously found for leucine, fucose, and glucosamine (Zatz and Barondes, 1971). When calculated as the ratio of nerve ending to total soluble protein, a slow increase was observed with leucine. For fucose, a sharp increase from a low to a high ratio was observed after 2 hr. An early high ratio with no lag was maintained during this period with glucosamine. It was thus suggested that, although fucosyl glycoproteins of the nerve ending fraction are synthesized in the nerve cell bodies and transported by rapid axoplasmic flow and that leucine-containing protein appears at the nerve terminal predominantly by slow axoplasmic flow, a substantial proportion of the glucosamine in the soluble macromolecules of the nerve ending fraction is incorporated locally by the nerve endings themselves. Hence, glycoproteins from the various subcellular fractions (Whittaker et al., 1964) were studied after 1 hr *in vivo* incorporation of ^{14}C-glucosamine, at a time before fucose-labeled glycoproteins appear at the nerve endings via fast axoplasmic flow.

Glycopeptides prepared from this material and separated by size using gel filtration showed that there was a predominant ^{14}C-glucosamine-containing glycopeptide associated with the nerve ending fraction with an apparent molecular weight of 1,250. This constituted a larger percentage of the labeled glycopeptides associated with the nerve ending fraction as compared to the other subcellular fractions. Also, its relative synthesis was greater in mice pretreated for 2 hr with acetoxycycloheximide to deplete the brain of protein sugar acceptors. After 4 hr of *in vivo* labeling, other, larger glycopeptides constituted a greater percentage of the total labeled glycopeptides derived from the nerve ending fraction, suggesting transport of glucosamine-containing glycoproteins to the nerve ending fraction during this time.

After *in vitro* labeling of the nerve ending fraction with ^{14}C-glucosamine, a single class of labeled glycopeptides was found with the same apparent molecular weight as the predominant labeled glycopeptide in the nerve ending fraction after 1 hour *in vivo* labeling. Furthermore, similarly labeled microsomal and mitochondrial fractions were less active in incorporating glucosamine than the nerve ending fraction. The results indicate that ^{14}C-glucosamine is incorporated into specific products by the nerve ending fraction, which is relatively insensitive to protein synthesis inhibition, and that this glycosylation cannot be attributed to contamination with membranes derived from the Golgi apparatus, endoplasmic reticulum, or free mitochondria. Recent results suggest that a substantial portion of the product found after *in vitro* labeling is associated with the mitochondria-rich components of the lysed nerve ending fraction. The mitochondria contained within the nerve ending may, therefore, be the major site of this glycosylation.

REFERENCES

Bennett, G. C., and Koenig, H. L. (1972): Transport axonaux de glycoprotéines aux terminaisons nerveuses du ganglion ciliaire de poulet aprés injection intraventriculaire cérébrale de fucose-³H. *Journale de Microscopie*, 14:18–19a.

Boesch J., Marko, P., and Cuénod, M. (1972): Effects of colchicine on axonal transport of proteins in the pigeon visual pathway. *Neurobiology*, 2:123–132.

Cotman, C. W., and Taylor, D. A. (1971): Autoradiographic analysis of protein synthesis in synaptosomal fractions. *Brain Research*, 29:366–372.

Cowan, W. M., Gottlieb, D. I., Hendrickson, A. E., Price, J. L., and Woolsey, T. A. (1972): The autoradiographic demonstration of axonal connections in the central nervous system. *Brain Research*, 37:21–51.

Cowan, W. M., and Powell, T. P. S. (1963): Centrifugal fibers in the avian visual system. *Proceedings of the Royal Society, Series B*, 158:232–252.

Cuénod, M., and Schonbach, J. (1971): Synaptic proteins and axonal flow in the pigeon visual pathway. *Journal of Neurochemistry*, 18:809–816.

Di Giamberardino, L., and Bennett, G. C. (1972): Cinétique de renouvellement des protéines dans les terminaisons nerveuses du ganglion ciliaire de poulet: Comparaison des données de la radioautographie et du fractionnement cellulaire. *Journal de Microscopie*, 14:39–40a.

Di Giamberardino, L., Bennett, G. C., Koenig, H. C., and Droz, B. (1972): Differential renewal of proteins and glycoproteins in chicken ciliary ganglion. *Federation of European Biological Societies 8th Meeting, Abstract*, p. 157.

Dowling, J. E., and Cowan, W. M. (1966): An electron microscope study of normal and degenerating centrifugal fiber terminals in the pigeon retina. *Zeitschrift für Zellforschung*, 71:14–28.

Dutton, G. R., Haywood, P., and Barondes, S. H. (1973): *Brain Research (in press)*.

Fink, R. P., and Heimer, L. (1967): Two methods for selective silver impregnation of degenerating axons and their synaptic endings in the central nervous system. *Brain Research*, 4:369–374.

Forman, D. S., Grafstein, B., and McEwen, B. S. (1972): Rapid axonal transport of [³H]-fucosyl glycoproteins in the goldfish optic tectum. *Brain Research*, 48:327–342.

Gray, E. G., and Guillery, R. W. (1966): Synaptic morphology in the normal and degenerating nervous system. *International Review of Cytology*, 19:111–182.

Hendrickson, A. E. (1972): Electron microscopic distribution of axoplasmic transport. *Journal of Comparative Neurology*, 144:381–398.

Jarlstedt, J., and Karlsson, J.-O. (1973): Evidence for axonal transport of RNA in mammalian neurons. *Experimental Brain Research (in press)*.

Karlsson, J.-O., and Sjöstrand, J. (1971a): Synthesis, migration and turnover of protein in retinal ganglion cells. *Journal of Neurochemistry*, 18:749–767.

Karlsson, J.-O., and Sjöstrand, J. (1971b): Rapid intracellular transport of fucose-containing glycoproteins in retinal ganglion cells. *Journal of Neurochemistry*, 18:2209–2216.

Karlsson, J.-O., and Sjöstrand, J. (1972a): Axonal transport of proteins in retinal ganglion cells. Amino acid incorporation into rapidly transported proteins and distribution of radioactivity to the lateral geniculate body and the superior colliculus, *Brain Research,* 37:279–285.

Karlsson, J.-O., and Sjöstrand, J. (1972*b*): Axonal transport of proteins in retinal ganglion cells. Characterization of the transport to the superior colliculus. *Brain Research,* 47:185–194.

Kristensson, K., and Olson, Y. (1971): Retrograde axonal transport of protein. *Brain Research,* 29:363–365.

Lasek, R., Joseph, B. S., and Whitlock, D. G. (1968): Evaluation of a radioautographic neuroanatomical tracing method. *Brain Research,* 8:319–336.

LaVail, J. H., and LaVail, M. M. (1972): Retrograde axonal transport in the central nervous system. *Science,* 176:1416–1417.

Marko, P., and Cuénod, M. (1972): Origin of proteins in synaptic organelles. *Experientia,* 28:729.

Marko, P., Susz, J.-P., and Cuénod, M. (1971): Synaptosomal proteins and axoplasmic flow; Fractionation by SDS polyacrylamide gel electrophoresis. *Federation of European Biological Societies Letters,* 17:261–264.

Morgan, I. G., Wolfe, L. S., Mandel, P., and Gombos, G. (1971): Isolation of plasma membranes from rat brain. *Biochimica et Biophysica Acta,* 241:737–751.

Nauta, W. J. H., and Gygax, P. A. (1954): Silver impregnation of degenerating axons in the central nervous system: A modified technic. *Stain Technology,* 29:91–93.

Neale, J. H., Neale, E. E., and Agranoff, B. W. (1972): Radioautography of the optic tectum of the goldfish after introcular injection of ³H-proline. *Science,* 176:407–410.

Perisic, M., and Cuénod, M. (1972): Synaptic transmission depressed by colchicine blockade of axoplasmic flow. *Science,* 175:1140–1142.

Roth, R. L. (1969): Optic tract projections in representatives of two fresh-water teleost families. *Anatomical Research,* 163:253.

Schonbach, J., and Cuénod, M. (1971): Axoplasmic migration of protein: A light microscopic autoradiographic study in the avian retinotectal pathway. *Experimental Brain Research,* 12:275–282.

Schonbach, J., Schonbach, C., and Cuénod, M. (1973): Distribution of transported proteins in the slow phase of axoplasmic flow. An electron microscopical autoradiographic study. *Journal of Comparative Neurology (in press).*

Schonbach, J., Schonbach, C., and Cuénod, M. (1971): Rapid phase of axoplasmic flow and synaptic proteins: An electron microscopical autoradiographic study. *Journal of Comparative Neurology,* 141:485–498.

Sjöstrand, J., and Hansson, H.-A. (1971): Effect of colchicine on the transport of axonal protein in the retinal ganglion cells of the rat. *Experimental Eye Research,* 12:261–269.

Taylor, A. C., and Weiss, P. (1965): Demonstration of axonal flow by the movement of tritium-labeled protein in mature optic nerve fibers. *Proceedings of the National Academy of Sciences,* 54:1521–1527.

Whittaker, V. P., Michaelson, I. A., and Kirkland, R. J. A. (1964): The separation of synaptic vesicles from nerve-ending particles ("synaptosomes"). *Biochemical Journal,* 90:293–305.

Zatz, M., and Barondes, S. H. (1971): Particulate and solubilized fucosyl transferases from mouse brain. *Journal of Neurochemistry,* 18:1125.

Index